AF736992

Pediatric Electromyography

Hugh J. McMillan • Peter B. Kang
Editors

Pediatric Electromyography

Concepts and Clinical Applications

Springer

Editors
Hugh J. McMillan
Division of Neurology
Children's Hospital of Eastern Ontario
University of Ottawa
Ottawa, ON
Canada

Peter B. Kang
Division of Pediatric Neurology
Shands Children's Hospital
University of Florida College of Medicine
Gainesville, FL
USA

ISBN 978-3-319-61360-4 ISBN 978-3-319-61361-1 (eBook)
DOI 10.1007/978-3-319-61361-1

Library of Congress Control Number: 2017953446

© Springer International Publishing AG 2017
This work is subject to copyright. All rights are reserved by the Publisher, whether the whole or part of the material is concerned, specifically the rights of translation, reprinting, reuse of illustrations, recitation, broadcasting, reproduction on microfilms or in any other physical way, and transmission or information storage and retrieval, electronic adaptation, computer software, or by similar or dissimilar methodology now known or hereafter developed.
The use of general descriptive names, registered names, trademarks, service marks, etc. in this publication does not imply, even in the absence of a specific statement, that such names are exempt from the relevant protective laws and regulations and therefore free for general use.
The publisher, the authors and the editors are safe to assume that the advice and information in this book are believed to be true and accurate at the date of publication. Neither the publisher nor the authors or the editors give a warranty, express or implied, with respect to the material contained herein or for any errors or omissions that may have been made. The publisher remains neutral with regard to jurisdictional claims in published maps and institutional affiliations.

Printed on acid-free paper

This Springer imprint is published by Springer Nature
The registered company is Springer International Publishing AG
The registered company address is: Gewerbestrasse 11, 6330 Cham, Switzerland

To my family, for their unwavering patience, tolerance, and flexibility.

—Hugh J. McMillan

To my wife Christina and our children Marian, Audrey, Louisa, and Marcus, who were very patient for many evenings as I disappeared into our home office to work on this book, and to my parents, Kwang Soo Kang and Moon Kil Kang, whose wise and enduring guidance set me on the path that eventually led me to this project.

—Peter B. Kang

Foreword

The late H. Royden Jones, Jr. (1936–2013) was a giant in the field of pediatric electromyography. A highly skilled and caring physician, he trained countless pediatric and adult neurologists and neurophysiologists throughout his long career at the Lahey Clinic and Boston Children's Hospital. His former residents and fellows now work across North America and around the world. He and two coauthors wrote what is generally recognized to be the first comprehensive textbook of pediatric electromyography which was published in 1996. We both had the privilege of training with Royden and benefited enormously from his mentorship as well as his boundless energy, kindness, and knowledge.

Hugh McMillan thanks Pierre Jacob, M.D., for introducing him to the world of neurophysiology and to Daniel Keene, M.D., for his mentorship. He is grateful to the outstanding teachers and mentors during his fellowship training: Basil T. Darras, M.D.; H. Royden Jones, Jr., M.D.; Peter B. Kang, M.D.; James A. Russell, D.O.; and Jayashri Srinivasan, M.B.B.S.

Peter Kang had the great fortune to be trained and inspired by many talented neuromuscular neurologists over the years. These include John T. Sladky, M.D., his first child neurology mentor in medical school; Mark J. Brown, M.D., and Shawn J. Bird, M.D., who taught him the basics of electromyography during residency; Gihan Tennekoon, M.D., and Richard S. Finkel, M.D., who taught him much about neuromuscular disease in childhood during residency; and Seward B. Rutkove, M.D., Elizabeth Raynor, M.D., H. Royden Jones, Jr., M.D., and Basil T. Darras, M.D., who trained him during his fellowship in clinical neurophysiology and electromyography. Basil Darras also served as a wonderful mentor during his junior faculty years at Boston Children's Hospital and Harvard Medical School. He benefited greatly from sage advice imparted over the years by Arthur K. Asbury, M.D., Robert C. Griggs, M.D., and Edward M. Kaye, M.D.; and the support of his faculty department chairs Joseph J. Volpe, M.D., Scott L. Pomeroy, M.D., Ph.D., and Scott A. Rivkees, M.D. He owes these mentors a great debt for all of their encouragement and support for many years.

We are very grateful to the talented colleagues who contributed valuable chapters to this book, many of whom we met at the biennial Paediatric EMG Congress organized for two decades by Matthew Pitt and Royden Jones.

We both thank the talented staff at Springer for this wonderful opportunity to share the very special skills of performing electromyography on the youngest and most vulnerable of our patients, especially Joanna Bolesworth, who first approached us about this project, Rajesh Sekar for supervising production of the book, and André Tournois, who provided valuable support throughout the project.

The goal of pediatric electromyography is to perform a valuable diagnostic study in as gentle a manner as possible when prompt diagnosis is crucial. We hope that this book will help encourage the lifelong acquisition of the skills needed to perform these studies properly and facilitate timely neuromuscular diagnoses for many years to come.

Ottawa, ON, Canada — Hugh J. McMillan
Gainesville, FL, USA — Peter B. Kang

Contents

Contributors

Megan Crone, M.D., F.R.C.P.C. Alberta Children's Hospital, University of Calgary, Calgary, AB, Canada

Basil T. Darras, M.D. Division of Clinical Neurology, Neuromuscular Center, Boston Children's Hospital, Harvard Medical School, Boston, MA, USA

Jahannaz Dastigir, D.O. Atlantic Health System, Goryeb Children's Hospital, Morristown, NJ, USA

Jim Dowling, M.D., Ph.D. Hospital for Sick Children, University of Toronto, Toronto, ON, Canada

Karin Edebol Eeg-Olofsson, M.D., Ph.D. University of Uppsala, Uppsala, Sweden

Department of Clinical Neurophysiology, University Hospital Uppsala, Uppsala, Sweden

Alier J. Franco, Ph.D. Children's Hospital of Philadelphia, Nashville, TN, USA

Cyril Gitiaux, M.D., Ph.D. Department of Neurophysiology, Reference Center for Neuromuscular Diseases, Paris Descartes University, Necker Enfants Malades Hospital, Paris, France

Hernan D. Gonorazky, M.D. Hospital for Sick Children, University of Toronto, Toronto, ON, Canada

Gregory G. Heuer, M.D., Ph.D. University of Pennsylvania, Philadelphia, PA, USA

Children's Hospital of Philadelphia, Philadelphia, PA, USA

Joe F. Jabre, M.D. David Geffen School of Medicine at UCLA, Los Angeles, CA, USA

Peter B. Kang, M.D., F.A.A.N., F.A.A.P. Division of Pediatric Neurology, Shands Children's Hospital, University of Florida College of Medicine, Gainesville, FL, USA

Ioannis Karakis, MD, PhD, MSc, FAAN, FAANEM, FAES Department of Neurology, Emory University School of Medicine, Atlanta, GA, USA

Nancy L. Kuntz, M.D. Northwestern Feinberg School of Medicine, Ann & Robert H Lurie Children's Hospital of Chicago, Chicago, IL, USA

Wendy K.M. Liew, M.B.Ch.B., M.R.C.P.C.H., F.A.M.S SBCC Baby and Child Clinic, Neurology Centre, Singapore, Singapore

John C. McHugh, MB, BCh, BaO, M.D., M.R.C.P.I. Department of Clinical Neurophysiology, Our Lady's Children's Hospital, Crumlin and AMNCH; Academic Unit of Neurology, Trinity College, Dublin, Ireland

Hugh J. McMillan, MD, MSc, FRCPC, FAAN Division of Neurology, Children's Hospital of Eastern Ontario, University of Ottawa, Ottawa, ON, Canada

Matthew C. Pitt, M.D., F.R.C.P. Clinical Neurophysiology, Great Ormond Street Hospital for Children, NHS Foundation Trust, London, UK

Susana Quijano-Roy, M.D., Ph.D. Unité de Maladies Neuromusculaires, Service de Neurologie, Réeducation et Réanimation Pédiatriques, AP-HP, Hôpital R. Poincaré, Hôpitaux Universitaires Paris-Ile-de-France-Ouest, (U1179- INSERM-UVSQ), Université de Versailles, Garches, France

Francis Renault, M.D., A.I.H.P., A.C.C.A. Neurophysiology Unit, Armand-Trousseau University Hospital, Paris, France

Bhaskar Roy, M.B.B.S., M.M.S.T. Beth Israel Deaconess Medical Center, Harvard Medical School, Boston, MA, USA

Seward B. Rutkove, M.D. Beth Israel Deaconess Medical Center, Harvard Medical School, Boston, MA, USA

Monique M. Ryan, M.Med. B.S., F.R.A.C.P. Murdoch Childrens Research Institute, The Royal Children's Hospital, University of Melbourne, Melbourne, Australia

John T. Sladky, M.D. Professor of Pediatrics and Neurology, University of Florida College of Medicine, Shands Children's Hospital, Gainesville, FL, USA

Jiri Vajsar, M.D., M.Sc., F.R.C.P.C. Hospital for Sick Children, University of Toronto, Toronto, ON, Canada

Kerry A. Vaughan, M.D. Hospital of the University of Pennsylvania and University of Pennsylvania Healthcare System, Philadelphia, PA, USA

Part I
Basic Concepts

Chapter 1
Historical Perspective of Electrodiagnosis

John T. Sladky

In constructing a historical context in which to view the discipline of electrodiagnostic medicine, it is difficult to determine a logical starting point. It is an elementary argument to assert that the biological underpinnings of the discipline date easily back to Galvani and Volta in the eighteenth century. Although these scientific pioneers played seminal roles in characterizing the role of electricity in the function of muscle and nervous tissue, some would credit even earlier observers with reporting the phenomenology that Galvani characterized as "the energy of life". Ultimately, it is the translational process of applying fundamental biological principles to the investigation of human disease, which has permitted the evolution of our discipline. Admitting a large measure of arbitrariness reinforced by a limited historical perspective of the scientific zeitgeist of successive eras of neurobiologists, I have cobbled together a decidedly imperfect, but well intentioned, snapshot of the conceptual ontogeny of electrodiagnostic medicine and its adaptation to pediatrics. I should apologize to bioengineers who will note that I have given short shrift to the technical aspects of the development of clinical electrophysiology. The evolution of our discipline has not been predominantly hypothesis driven but rather has been a captive of technology and has grown at a logarithmic pace as new methodologies have been adapted to investigate human neuromuscular physiology. Let me add one further disclaimer; I have not attempted to acknowledge the role of individual contributions to the body of knowledge but rather the evolution of our ongoing integration of basic scientific information into the understanding of the biological substrate of neuromuscular disease.

Notions regarding the role of what came to be understood as electrical properties in the animation and maintenance of vitality among humans and surrounding fauna date back at least to the Greeks and Romans. Practitioners at the time utilized electrical stimulation for the treatment of a range of perceived ailments. The logistics of

---

J.T. Sladky, M.D.
Professor of Pediatrics and Neurology, University of Florida College of Medicine,
Shands Children's Hospital, Gainesville, FL, USA
e-mail: jsladky@ufl.edu

© Springer International Publishing AG 2017

H.J. McMillan, P.B. Kang (eds.), *Pediatric Electromyography*,
DOI 10.1007/978-3-319-61361-1_1

this procedure required the application of torpedo fish to a patient's skin. The torpedo fish is an electric ray with electroplax organs located on each side of the head. These electric generators accorded the animal an efficient means to ward off predators and to subdue prey. The patient was persuaded to step on the animal as might occur while wading in the ocean. It was assumed that the resultant painful electrical shock experienced by the patient would imbue vigor to the recipient or provide salutary effects for a variety of common afflictions. These practices likely provided a historical context that underpinned widely held notions that conceived of electricity as the "animus" or "life force" that initiated and maintained muscle activity.

By the beginning of the eighteenth century, three well-established schools of thought dominated the hypothetical discussion of what provided the mechanistic nexus between intent and the execution of motor action. The traditionalist position, advocated by Descartes, averred that an "ephemeral force" traveled along the peripheral nerve and animated the muscle. The more pragmatic Thomas Willis felt that a vital fluid passed through hollow tubes represented by the peripheral nerves and the fluid activated the contractile mechanism in the muscle. A somewhat less tenable position was championed by Isaac Newton who conceived of a vibratory signal transmitted along the nerve which was informed by the frequency and amplitude of the oscillatory activity. Within this theoretical/philosophical milieu resided the advocates of electricity as a more plausible mechanism of signal transduction in nerve and muscle.

The ability to generate, store and direct static electricity using electrostatic generators and the Leyden jar, a technology developed by the mid-eighteenth century, instigated a wave of experimentation and perhaps an even larger swell of therapists providing treatments with tactile and visually impressive effects for common and uncommon ailments, unfortunately with little or no tangible benefit, at least for the patient. Dr. Aloisio Luigi Galvani was one of those scientists working in the final quarter of the eighteenth century drawn to the new field of inquiry based on electrical stimulation. I have read multiple iterations of the anecdotal description of the seminal experiment, none quite alike. The essential element seems to be that while Galvani and an assistant were dissecting a nerve/muscle preparation in a frog, an errant spark from a nearby electrostatic generator reached the operator resulting in an electrical spark transduced via forceps to the exposed tissue within the operating field resulting in a muscular contraction in the frog's distal leg. Despite the scintillating visual and auditory overlay that the discharge of static electricity brought to the laboratory, Galvani needed a more controlled stimulus for his experimental models. He devised an alternative method using linked pairs of dissimilar metallic electrodes to produce a direct current source for stimulation of nerves and muscles in a more regulated fashion. Galvani worked in relative silence for over a decade before finally publishing his work in 1791 [1]. In this treatise, he asserted his conclusions that electrical energy or "animal electric fluid" was demonstrably the signal transduction medium in neuromuscular transmission and muscle activity.

Acknowledging the above, it seems reasonable to assert that the modern era of clinical electrophysiology began in mid-nineteenth century Paris with Dr. Guillaume-Benjamin-Armand Duchenne du Boulogne (1806–1875). By the

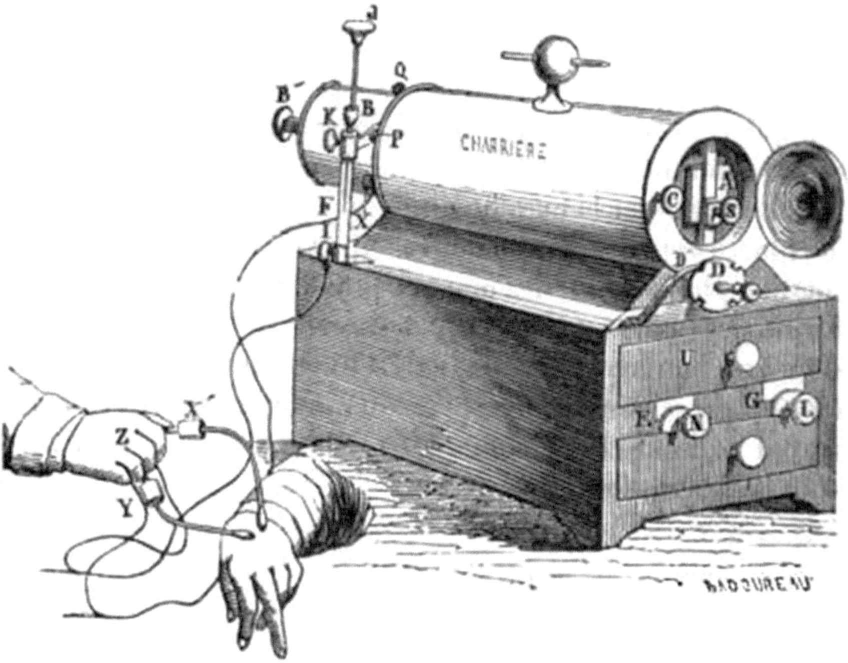

Fig. 1.1 Duchenne's handmade direct current electrostimulation device. Non-invasive surface electrodes could be placed for precise stimulation of small muscles of the hand and face

turn of the nineteenth century, many practitioners in Europe and North America endorsed electrotherapy for a host of neuropsychiatric and other conditions. Duchenne conceived of using electrical stimulation of muscle and nerve for diagnostic purposes [2]. He devised a portable direct current source along with a series of specialized surface electrodes, which permitted non-invasive stimulation of nerve and muscle and obviated the complication of wound infection that frequently ensued after placement of subcutaneous electrodes, which was the custom at that time (Fig. 1.1). He understood that stimulation of the nerve triggered contraction of a constellation of functionally related muscles and developed electrodes for the isolation and stimulation of individual muscles to investigate their specific role in volitional movements. Early in his career he became interested in the muscles of facial animation and in utilizing "localized faradization" (focused electrostimulation of individual muscles or muscle groups) to distinguish upper from lower motor neuron facial paralysis (Fig. 1.2). Duchenne designed and built his stimulating device to permit individual or trains of repetitive electrical stimuli to be selectively delivered to individual or constellations of muscles. His aim at the bedside was to be able to elicit a convincing supramaximal stimulus and to grade the resultant contractile response using visual and tactile measures, which could be incorporated into serial testing protocols. He applied lessons gleaned from these studies to the evaluation of appendicular muscles affected by nerve or spinal cord injury.

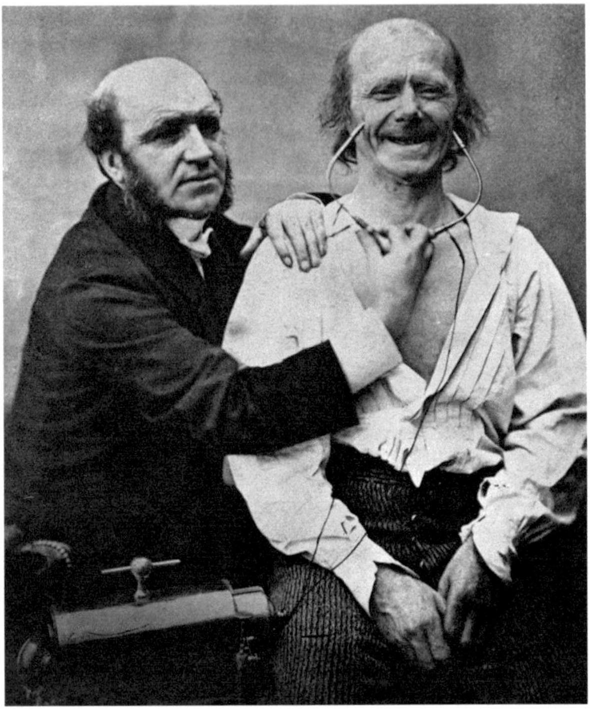

Fig. 1.2 "Faradization" of facial muscles. Duchenne used this device to distinguish upper from lower motor neuron palsies. He also used the techniques he developed to investigate the relationship between facial expression and emotion. He observed an association between involvement of the extraocular muscles along with the lower facial muscles when the smile was born out of happiness as opposed to social convenience. The term "Duchenne smile" has joined the formal lexicon of academic physiognomy to denote the sincerity of the facial expression

Poliomyelitis was endemic among the children of mid-nineteenth century Paris, especially in crowded urban environments where public hygiene was limited. Although the communicable nature of the disease was gaining recognition, a mechanistic understanding of the cause of paralysis was lacking. It was commonly held that the paralysis in this disease was "essential" in nature, an obfuscational proposition that declared that the pathogenic process existed in a realm beyond the ken of contemporary medical science and hence, was indescribable and unknowable. Duchenne, thought to be somewhat of a contrarian among his colleagues, noted homologies in his observations of electrical muscle and nerve stimulation in patients with facial palsy, poliomyelitis and spinal cord injuries. He used electrostimulation of muscles and nerves to examine patients with spinal cord diseases, including those presumed to be poliomyelitis, to characterize patterns of affected muscles as excitable or not. He demonstrated that those atrophic muscle groups, which were unresponsive to direct electrical stimulation, generally did not recover while contiguous muscles, which exhibited a tangible response to supramaximal electrical stimulation, would exhibit the capacity to regain function. He was able to discern that this testing could be performed early in the disease and might provide important prognostic insights. Given the high incidence of poliomyelitis in urban centers of the period and the fact that most of the acutely affected were children since a majority of adults were rendered immune by prior infection, children constituted a large segment of Duchenne's patients. He focused on this experience in his writings and in didactic sessions with his fellow neurologists in Paris. Imagine Duchenne explicating the fine points of the electrodiagnostic evaluation of a child with acute paralysis before Charcot and his contemporaries at the Hôpital Universitaire Pitié-Salpêtrière during the 1860s. Duchenne correctly inferred that the site of the primary lesion in poliomyelitis must be the anterior horn cells in the spinal cord. At the time, autopsy studies in individuals with poliomyelitis had been performed on patients with longstanding paralysis who died from unrelated causes. Visual inspection of post mortem pathological specimens of the spinal cord failed to demonstrate evidence of definite abnormality. Microscopic anatomy of the spinal cord, however, had not been studied in this disease. Duchenne argued that the key to understanding the pathogenesis lay in a more scrupulous examination of the spinal cord in these patients. Over the ensuing decade, Duchenne's hypothesis was confirmed by several observers, including his younger colleague Dr. Jean-Martin Charcot in a paper published in 1870. Duchenne came to be highly regarded for his clinical and pathophysiological acumen and was referred to by Charcot as "mon maître en neurologie" or my mentor in neurology.

Duchenne first illustrated the superficial phenomenology of brachial plexus palsy in 1862 in association with a photograph of a 6 year old boy exhibiting the sequellae of a brachial plexus injury sustained at birth. Even before that publication, he had recognized a stereotypical constellation of features which he termed "obstetric palsy of the brachial plexus". It required another decade to collect and publish his anatomical observations on three patients with that injury in 1872. Duchenne surmised that the injury was related to traction of the head against the after coming shoulder with concomitant injury to the plexus in the course of delivery of an infant with shoulder dystocia. It is fitting that the baton was metaphorically passed in this fashion as Dr. Wilhelm Heinrich Erb (1840–1921) published his findings on the physiological and anatomical substrates for this malady in 1874 [3]. Erb was familiar with Duchenne and his opinions regarding the disease along with his studies of anatomy and clinical electrophysiology. He freely acknowledged his colleague's precedence in describing the nature of the injury. Erb's singular contribution was the amalgamation of electrophysiology and neuroanatomy with the use of electrodiagnostic methods to localize the site of the anatomic lesion to the upper trunk of the brachial plexus. He employed a needle electrode inserted at the medial border of the supraclavicular fossa beneath the insertion of the sternocleidomastoid to stimulate the brachial plexus near the confluence of cervical nerve roots five and six at the origin of the upper trunk. Tetanic stimulation at that site in normal subjects elicited a constellation of simultaneous muscle contractions resulting in the assumption of what was described as a "fencer's posture" with abduction of the shoulder, flexion of the biceps and supination of the forearm. The agonist muscles activated by electrical stimulation of the brachial plexus near "Erb's point" predicted the pattern of weakness resulting from an injury to the upper trunk of the brachial plexus at that site. Anatomic studies confirmed Erb's notion of the localization of the injury with evidence of consequent chronic denervation in muscles downstream from the injury.

There are many interesting analogies and distinctions within the personal and professional lives of Duchenne and Erb that deserve more attention than can be provided here. Both came from working class families. Duchenne was never warmly embraced by the medical establishment in Paris. He was never inducted into the

Academy of Sciences in his native France. He was, however, internationally known and later in his career was elected to membership in prestigious academic societies in multiple countries outside of France. He also established close relationships with several of the seminal figures in clinical neurology working in Paris, probably the epicenter of clinical neuroscience at the time. Duchenne was highly regarded in that circle and was referred to by Charcot as "my mentor in neurology". Erb, by contrast, migrated from his rural beginnings in the Bavarian countryside to Heidelberg, one of the most prestigious academic institutions in Europe, for his education where he studied under Dr. Jakob Henle and Dr. Nikolaus Friedreich. He remained on the faculty at the University for the balance of his career with the exception of a 3 year hiatus when he accepted the position and served as Chair of Internal Medicine at the University of Leipzig from 1880–1883. He returned to Heidelberg to accept an appointment as Chair of Internal Medicine after Friedreich's death. Like Duchenne, Erb viewed neurology as an independent field of inquiry within the discipline of medicine and played a seminal role of establishing the field of clinical neurology as a unique academic and clinical niche in the biological sciences.

The evolution of clinical electrodiagnosis at the outset of the twentieth century would be held in abeyance while technical progress continued in research laboratories focusing on signal processing and characterization in nerve and muscle. Though the cathode ray tube, the basis for the development of the oscilloscope, was invented just before 1900, the triggered sweep oscilloscope would not become widely available for clinical applications until after the Second World War.

Like so many arenas in pediatrics new translational approaches are usually hand me downs from our adult colleagues who have developed these experimental techniques among populations competent to provide informed consent until their safety and reliability has been confirmed. Such was the case with clinical electrodiagnosis which by the mid-1950s had been embraced at multiple centers as a potential means to refine and focus the evaluation of patients with neuromuscular disease.

In Rochester, Minnesota, Dr. Edward H. Lambert, a neurophysiologist, and Dr. Peter J. Dyck, who specialized in peripheral nerve histopathology, collaborated on a landmark study of individuals and kinships with dominantly inherited neuropathy conforming to a diagnosis of Charcot-Marie Tooth disease (CMT). The patients included in this study were phenotypically similar and were all members of kinships with what appeared to be dominantly inherited peripheral neuropathies. In 1957, Thomas and Gilliatt reported the observation of profound slowing of motor nerve conduction velocity in an individual with a phenotype consistent with CMT [4]. It was discovered that clinically similar patients with this disease were heterogeneous based on sensory and motor nerve conduction studies and could be segregated into two groups based on the motor conduction velocity of the ulnar and median nerves in the forearm. They divided the patients into those with conduction velocities above and below 35 m/s and correlated those groups with histopathology from sural nerve biopsies. This work codified the clinical, electrodiagnostic and histopathological characteristics of these patients and provided the biological substrate for the initial classifications of demyelinating or axonal CMT. They showed that these clinical traits bred true within the kinships and hence could infer that there were probably independent autosomal dominant genes involved in producing the distinctive electrophysiological and histopathological phenotypes associated with the demyelinating and axonal forms of the disease. Later the nosology would evolve into hereditary motor and sensory neuropathy types I and II (HMSN I and HMSN II), though many still use the traditional terminology CMT1 and CMT2. After that came the deluge.

It was understood that CMT was dominantly inherited but the disease seemed entirely capricious in terms of its age of onset and pace of progression in affected individuals. Families wanted to know whether their toddler was affected and as much information as could be garnered regarding what the future might hold for that child. In order to begin to attempt to answer some of these questions it was necessary to understand more about the developmental biology of the peripheral nervous system in children, more specifically, the ontogeny of motor conduction velocity as a function of age. To that end, Lambert set out to characterize age specific normative values for ulnar motor nerve conduction in a cohort including 6 premature infants, 42 term newborns and 98 children less than 15 years of age [5]. He and his colleagues showed that saltatory conduction in the ulnar motor nerve changes significantly with age and that what may be normal nerve conduction velocity in a toddler would be classified as consistent with demyelinating CMT if it were documented in an adult. The fact of the evolution of nerve conduction velocity with age was not a revelation, however, without a precise understanding of the normative values for electrophysiological measurements at different ages in children, the technology held limited value in the evaluation and management of children with neuromuscular disease.

At nearly the same time, Dr. Fritz Buchtal in Copenhagen and Dr. Ingrid Gamstorp, a child neurologist in Uppsula, Sweden were grappling with similar issues in the context of newborn infants of different conceptional ages in the neonatal nursery and later in childhood. Buchtal set out to systematically study cohorts of infants born at different gestational ages to develop accurate normative data for nerve conduction measurements in infants. Not surprisingly, he was able to demonstrate that nerve conduction velocities in infants were dependent on the age since conception and could be used to quite accurately predict the conceptional age of a newborn or an older infant independent of the age of the child from birth. Gamstorp evaluated motor conduction in median, ulnar and peroneal nerves in normal individuals ranging in age from newborn to adult [6]. Nerve conduction velocities, like EEG patterns, were stereotypical in their tempo of growth toward an apogee in the mid-first decade and ultimately a regression in later adulthood.

By the 1970s clinical electrophysiology had been widely validated as a useful tool for the study of neuromuscular disease in children. While these techniques were becoming widely employed in adult populations, their application in younger individuals remained largely confined to tertiary pediatric centers. There were, perhaps, two handfuls of neurologists who were vocal advocates for the incorporation of electrodiagnostic techniques into the evaluation of pediatric neuromuscular disease. Only a few stood on the front lines and developed centers dedicated to expanding our understanding of the neurobiology of clinical electrophysiology codifying that knowledge in the medical literature and passing down lessons learned in the clinical laboratory to residents and fellows. One of the most prominent among them was Dr. H. Royden Jones, Jr. (1936–2013). After training in neurology and electrophysiology at the Mayo Clinic where he came under the influence of Lambert, he moved to the Boston area and joined the Lahey Clinic staff in 1972. In 1978, he became Director of the EMG laboratory at Boston Children's Hospital where, over the next 35 years, he molded the thinking and practice of the next generation of pediatric clinical neurophysiologists. Among many accomplishments, he, along with Dr. Charles F. Bolton and Dr. C. Michel Harper, Jr., wrote and published what was for years the only widely known textbook of pediatric EMG [7]. It is heartening to see that this expertise has been passed on from experimental physiologists and adult neurologists to a growing cohort of child neurologists who are applying classic principles to make these useful diagnostic techniques available to a broader group of infants, children, and adolescents around the world.

References

1. Galvani L. De Viribus Electricitatis in motu Musculari Commentarius. Lelio della Volpe: Bologna; 1791.
2. Duchenne GB. De l'Electrisation Localisee et de son Application a la Physiologie, a la Pathologie et a la Therapeutique. Paris: Bailliere; 1855. p. 926.
3. Watt AJ, Niederbichler AD, Yang LJ, Chung KC. Wilhelm Heinrich Erb, M.D. (1840 to 1921): a historical perspective on Erb's palsy. Plast Reconstr Surg. 2007;119(7):2161–6.
4. Gilliatt RW, Thomas PK. Extreme slowing of nerve conduction in peroneal muscular atrophy. Ann Phys Med. 1957;4(3):104–6.
5. Thomas JE, Lambert EH. Ulnar nerve conduction velocity and H-reflex in infants and children. J Appl Physiol. 1960;15:1–9.
6. Gamstorp I. Normal conduction velocity of ulnar, median and peroneal nerves in infancy, childhood and adolescence. Acta Paediatr Suppl. 1963;52(Suppl 146):68–76.
7. Jones HR Jr, Bolton CF, Harper CM Jr. Pediatric clinical electromyography. Philadelphia: Lippincott-Raven; 1996. p. 487.

Chapter 2
Anatomy and Physiology of Peripheral Nerves

Hugh J. McMillan

Neurophysiologists must demonstrate knowledge of the gross anatomy and location of peripheral nerves and muscles in order to carry out nerve conduction studies and electromyography (see Chaps. 4, 5, 6, 7, 9 and 10). However, they must also be aware of the microanatomy of nerves and as well as basic physiology in order to understand factors that can influence optimal timing of tests and/or how artifacts can influence NCS/EMG test results.

Gross Anatomy

The peripheral nervous system includes the motor and sensory neurons, peripheral nerves, neuromuscular junctions and muscles.

Motor neurons, also known as anterior horn cells, are located in the ventral gray matter of the spinal cord. Their axonal projections or motor nerves extend from the spinal cord as ventral roots eventually innervating skeletal muscle. Each group of muscles innervated by any given level of the spinal cord is referred to as belonging to the same myotome. Sensory neurons, also known as dorsal root ganglia, lie outside of the spinal cord. Their projections extend in two directions; proximally towards the dorsal root of the spinal cord and distally towards an area of the body from which they carry sensory stimuli. The distinct region of skin innervated by each sensory level of the spinal cord is known as a dermatome. Nerve roots and their related diseases are covered in Chap. 17.

Although the most proximal segments of the motor (ventral) and sensory (dorsal) roots travel separately, the efferent motor fibers and afferent sensory fibers travel

H.J. McMillan, MD, MSc, FRCPC, FAAN
Division of Neurology, Children's Hospital of Eastern Ontario, University of Ottawa, Ottawa, ON, Canada
e-mail: hmcmillan@cheo.on.ca

© Springer International Publishing AG 2017

H.J. McMillan, P.B. Kang (eds.), *Pediatric Electromyography*,
DOI 10.1007/978-3-319-61361-1_2

together as mixed nerves just distal to the dorsal root ganglia. There are a total of 31 spinal nerves at five different spinal levels; 8 cervical, 12 thoracic, 5 lumbar, 5 sacral and 1 coccygeal nerve roots. In addition, 10 of the 12 cranial nerves (CN III to XII) are considered part of the peripheral nervous system and will be covered in Chap. 15.

Classification of Peripheral Nerves

Peripheral nerves are typically mixed meaning that they carry both sensory and motor fibers. However there are several examples of pure sensory nerves (e.g., lateral femoral cutaneous nerve) or pure motor nerves (e.g., posterior interosseous nerve) that branch off directly from a plexus or a larger nerve. Nerves contain various types of fibers including: (1) large myelinated, (2) small myelinated and; (3) small unmyelinated axons (Table 2.1).

Large myelinated fibers are preferentially tested by nerve conduction studies since their larger diameter (12–20 μm) axons allow these fibers to conduct the fastest of all motor fibers (70–120 m/s). Myelination of these axons further increases conduction velocity by enabling saltatory conduction which will be discussed in detail below. Myelin is produced by supportive Schwann cells that wrap or layer each axon in a fatty, protective spiral coat with numerous layers. Layering of myelin is seen quite nicely on electron microcopy (ultrastructure) of peripheral nerves (Fig. 2.1). The total thickness of myelin in a mature nerve is approximately 2/3 the diameter of the axon. Large myelinated fibers include: (1)

Table 2.1 Peripheral nerve fiber types

Fibre type	Diameter (μm)	Conduction Velocity (m/s)	Myelination	Function
Afferent fibers				
IA	12–20	70–120	Large myelinated	From muscle spindles
IB	12–20	70–120	Large myelinated	From Golgi tendon organs
II	6–12	30–70	Small myelinated	From Meissner's and Pacinian corpuscles & endings in skin & connective tissue
III	2–6	4–30	Small myelinated	From skin; pressure afferents
IV	<2	<2	Small unmyelinated	From skin; pain (pin-prick), temperature afferents
Efferent fibers				
Alpha	12–20	70–120	Large myelinated	To skeletal muscles
Gamma	3–8	15–40	Small myelinated	To intrafusal fibers of muscle spindles
B	1–3	5–15	Small myelinated	To pre-gangliononic autonomic efferents
C	<1	<2	Small unmyelinated	To post-ganglionic autonomic efferents

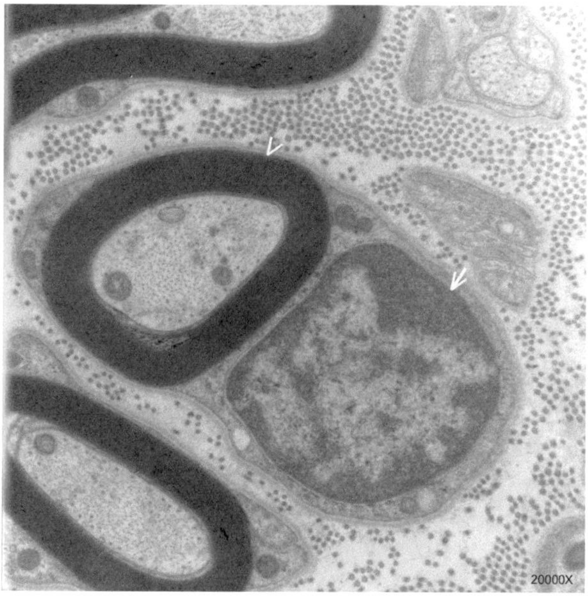

Fig. 2.1 Ultrastructural image of a normal, large myelinated peripheral nerve (*arrow head*). The axon is seen in cross-section and has been wrapped in layers or spirals of protective myelin by the adjacent Schwann cell (*arrow*). *Photo credit: Dr. Jean Michaud, Department of Pathology, Children's Hospital of Eastern Ontario*

afferent fibers from muscle spindles and Golgi tendon organs which relay important information about joint position and stretch which is critical for our reflexes as well as; (2) motor efferent fibers travelling from the motor neurons to skeletal muscles. Peripheral nerve myelination progresses significantly during the first few years of life as is reflected in the normal neonatal ulnar nerve motor conduction velocities of 20–35 m/s which increase to adult normal values (>50 m/s) by 3–5 years of age [1].

Small myelinated fibers are approximately half the diameter of large fibers and not surprisingly conduct more slowly than their larger counterparts. Examples of small myelinated afferent fibers include axons extending from Meissner and Pacinian corpuscles. These are touch receptors located near the surface of the skin. When the corpuscle is deformed by pressure, the nerve endings are stimulated. They are well adapted to feeling rough surfaces and detecting vibration such that they respond to transient touch rather than sustained pressure. Small myelinated efferent fibers also supply the intrafusal fibers of muscle spindles as well as preganglionic autonomic efferents.

Small unmyelinated fibers are the smallest axons (<2 mm) and due to their extremely slow conduction velocity (<2 m/s) cannot be tested by conventional nerve conduction studies. Neurophysiologists must be aware of the limitations of testing such that when a small fiber neuropathy is suspected on clinical grounds, ancillary testing is considered as appropriate (see Chap. 19). Examples of small unmyelinated afferent fibers include sensory fibers carrying information regarding pain (pin-prick) and temperature sense. Small unmyelinated efferent fibers innervate post-ganglionic autonomic organs.

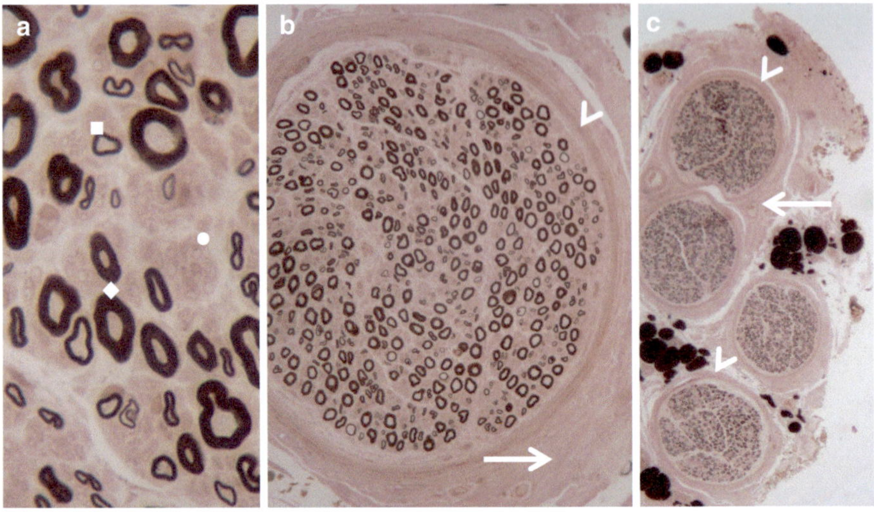

Fig. 2.2 Normal peripheral nerve sections stained with p-phenylenediamine at (**a**) high power shows large myelinated axons (*diamond*), small myelinated axons (*square*) and unmyelinated axons (*circle*) all surrounded by endoneurium; (**b**) medium power shows a fascicle containing many axons surrounded by perineurium (*arrow head*) which in turn is surrounded by epineurium (*arrow*); (**c**) low power demonstrates how the epineurium (*arrow*) binds together multiple fascicles and also contains arterioles. *Photo credit: Dr. Gerard Jansen, Department of Pathology, The Ottawa Hospital Civic Campus*

Nerve Microanatomy

Each peripheral nerve fiber or axon is surrounded by multiple levels of connective tissue. Endoneurium surrounds individual axons. Individual axons are clustered into fascicles that are surrounded by a layer of connective tissue called perineurium. This in turn is surrounded by a thicker layer of epineurium that binds together multiple perineurial-bound fascicles as well as arterioles (Fig. 2.2).

Physiology

Signal transmission along peripheral nerves is based upon the presence of a stable electrochemical charge across the cell membrane of an axon, with a mechanism for rapid and reversible changes of that charge in response to stimuli.

The difference in electrochemical charge at baseline is referred to as a resting membrane potential. Ion pumps, typically requiring energy provided by adenosine triphosphate (ATP), are responsible for transporting ions such as Na^+, K^+, Cl^- and Ca^{2+} into or out of the cell to establish electrical and chemical concentration gradients. Typically, resting membrane potentials of most glial cells is approximately −75 mV (i.e., the cytoplasm is negative compared to the extracellular matrix). Phospholipid bilayers are hydrophobic, thereby preventing charged particles from easily moving through membranes. Despite this, functional ion pumps are required to prevent ions

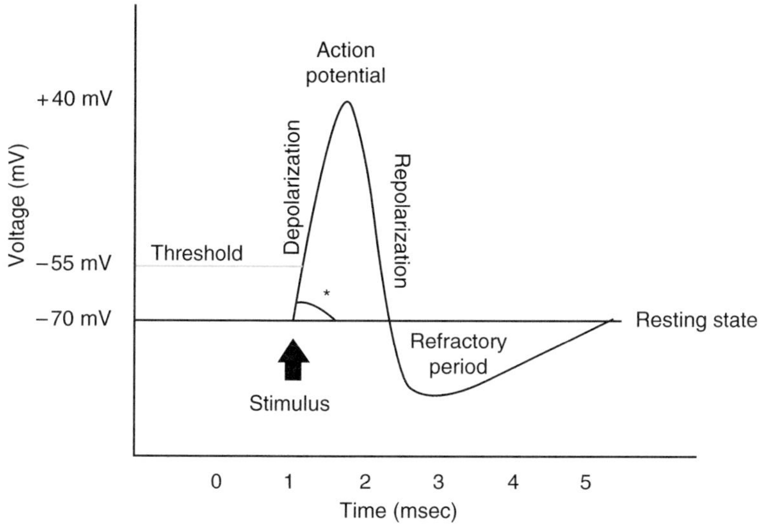

Fig. 2.3 Action potential and the associated changes in membrane voltage. The initial horizontal line represents the resting membrane potential (−70 mV). A stimulus (*arrow*) triggers local sodium channels to open which increase the membrane potential. If insufficient sodium (Na^+) channels open the membrane potential does not exceed threshold and a failed potential ensues (*asterix*) where the resting membrane potential is re-established If sufficient Na^+ channels open and the threshold is surpassed, an all-or-none action potential is generated. The depolarization phase is characterized by Na^+ channels opening and the influx of Na^+ ions increasing the membrane potential from −70 mV to +40 mV. This change triggers Na^+ channels to close and K^+ channels to open. The repolarization phase is characterized by an efflux of K^+ and a return of the membrane potential to −90 mV. Since this surpasses the resting potential this is known as the refractory period. The Na^+K^+-ATPase pump re-establishes the concentration of ions and the resting membrane potential

from eventually diffusing across their electrochemical concentration gradients which would result in the loss of the resting membrane potential.

Ion channels are proteins that span cell membranes and can allow the passage of specific ions through an otherwise impermeable lipid bilayer. Specific factors can trigger a conformational change in ion channel proteins, causing them to open and permit the rapid influx or efflux of ions. Ion channels can be stimulated to open by; (1) binding with a ligand (i.e., a neurotransmitter); (2) local changes in voltage (i.e., propagation of an action potential); (3) local stress or pressure (i.e., common trigger for sensory mechanoreceptors) as well as; (4) phosphorylation which more typically results in prolonged configuration changes that can modulate the resting membrane potential.

Nerve-to-nerve and nerve-to-muscle signal transmission occurs via an action potential where adjacent voltage-gated ion channels open in a stepwise manner. Action potentials have several key characteristics. First there is a threshold for the initiation of an action potential. In the case of mechanoreceptors in the skin, small amounts of pressure will cause some sodium channels to open, thereby raising the membrane potential. If the potential is raised beyond a threshold value then adjacent voltage-gated sodium channels will open, triggering an influx of sodium ions that represents the initiation of an action potential (Fig. 2.3). This action potential is self-propagating, spreading along the length of the axon as voltage gated channels open in succession much as dominos fall in a line. If the threshold is not reached then the ion pumps will work to reestablish the resting membrane potential, and an action potential is not generated. The influx of sodium channels reverses the membrane potential from about −70 mV to +40 mV. At this point the sodium channels close and the potassium channels open. The efflux of potassium lowers the membrane potential to approximately −90 mV which repolarizes the membrane. At this time the potassium channels close. The $Na^{+}K^{+}$-ATPase pump will work to reestablish the resting membrane potential, but the brief period of time that the membrane potential remains below −70 mV is known as the absolute and relative refractory periods, namely the time where it is impossible and then more difficult for a second action potential to be generated.

Saltatory Conduction

Schwann cells perform a similar function for peripheral nerves as that of oligodendrocytes within the central nervous system. Schwann cells provide an insulating coat of myelin to a single axonal segment of a peripheral nerve. Peripheral nerve myelin shows differences from its central counterpart, namely a greater proportion of myelin basic protein (MBP) as well as the presence of peripheral myelin protein 22 (PMP22) and myelin protein zero (MPZ or P_0) [2]. Overall, myelin functions to insulate the axon and increase the electrical resistance across the cell membrane. Each segment of myelin is interrupted by short, unmyelinated gaps known as the nodes of Ranvier. The high resistance along the myelinated segments prevents the electrical current from leaving the axon, allowing action potentials to 'jump' from one node of Ranvier to the next, thereby enabling the axon to to propagate action potentials at much higher conduction velocities (70–120 m/s) which are characteristic of large myelinated nerves. The jumping of conduction is referred to as saltatory conduction.

Effects of Demyelination

Segmental demyelination due to either local nerve compression or inflammation can disrupt specific segments of myelin along a peripheral nerve axon, while other segments will remain intact. Even though the axon itself retains its structural integrity, an action potential cannot propagate normally along a myelinated nerve if a segment of that nerve is demyelinated. The explanation for this is that the voltage gated ion channels are normally located only at each node of Ranvier, thus a demyelinated stretch of an axon has very different electrophysiologic properties than a naturally unmyelinated axon. The end result is typically failure of conduction along that stretch of the axon, giving rise to the phenomenon of conduction block.

Peripheral neuropathies will be covered in Chap. 18. Once the offending agent has been removed, peripheral nerve remyelination will occur. However the remyelinated segments are typically shorter, with a corresponding increase in the number of nodes of Ranvier along the remyelinated portion of the axon, which can give rise to permanent alterations in the axon's electrophysiology properties [3, 4].

Injury and Regrowth (Sequence of Events Post-injury)

Axonal injury is another important consideration for the neurophysiologist. When an axon is severed it is no longer possible for an action potential to be transmitted. The proximal segment, which remains in continuity with the anterior horn cell or dorsal root ganglia, will receive nourishment from the cell body and thus remain intact. However, the portion of the axon distal to the site of injury will undergo Wallerian degeneration whereby it degenerates in an anterograde manner. Abnormalities will become apparent on nerve conduction studies 3–10 days post-injury [5, 6].

Peripheral nerve injury has been classified by Seddon into three categories. Neuropraxia is the mildest and is associated with a focal demyelination without associated axonal loss. Full recovery typically occurs over days to weeks as the Schwann cells remyelinate the affected segments. Patients suffering from neuropraxia may suffer from weakness and/or paresthesia as well as pain at the site of injury. Nerve conduction studies are preserved except perhaps at stimulation sites that are proximal to the demyelinated segment(s), as the action potentials cross the site of injury. Nerves affected by neuropraxia may demonstrate conduction block (i.e., decreased compound motor action potential (CMAP) amplitudes across the site of injury) and/or focal slowing of conduction velocity across the affected area. Needle EMG may demonstrate decreased recruitment but no active denervation (i.e., positive sharp waves or fibrillation potentials) is seen since axonal continuity persists. Axontmesis is moderate in severity, and describes the partial or complete loss of axonal continuity; however, some surrounding perineurium and/or epineurium remains intact. This is important for potential recovery as sprouting will appear from the proximal axon tips within a week of the injury and slowly grow by about 1 mm per day (1 inch per month). If there is some continuity of neural elements and/or connective tissue, then the potential for reinnervation is greater. Neurotmesis is the most severe classification of nerve injury, where there is no continuity of neural or connective tissue. As such the potential for recovery is more guarded without an anatomical pathway for reinnervation to occur. Nerve transfers and/or grafting may be considered in such cases given the uncertain potential for spontaneous recovery. Aberrant or erroneous reinnervation can occur particularly following neurotmesis. Perhaps the most familiar example is a facial synkinesis that can occur after Bell palsy. This can be manifested as involuntarily contraction of the orbicularis oris (blinking) with contraction of other ipsilateral facial muscles [7].

Neuromuscular Transmission

The neuromuscular junction (NMJ) is the connection between a motor nerve and the muscle fiber that it innervates. It is not a physical connection but is represented by the apposition of the terminal bouton and the motor endplate on the muscle fiber. Signaling via neurotransmitters across this gap enables nerve action potentials to be translated into physical muscle contractions.

As the action potential reaches the end of the motor axon, the change in resting potential triggers the opening of voltage gated calcium channels. Calcium binds to synaptotagmin which triggers the release of packets or vesicles of acetylcholine from the terminal. Acetylcholine is released into the synaptic cleft, traveling from the terminal bouton to the motor endplate where it binds to nicotinic acetylcholine receptors (AChRs). AChRs are examples of ligand-gated ion channels. The binding of acetylcholine results in local depolarization and generation of an excitatory post-synaptic potential (EPSP). Unlike the action potential which is self-propagating, the EPSP demonstrates a decrement in both time (as the ion pumps work to restore the resting potential) and space (as the change in membrane potential becomes less as it travels farther from its site of initiation). Adjacent EPSPs are summative and if sufficient ligand-gated ion channels are stimulated the resulting EPSP will surpass the threshold, triggering a muscle action potential that ultimately leads to a physically palpable muscle contraction. Disorders of neuromuscular transmission will be discussed in Chap. 21.

Muscle Contraction

Muscle fibers generate contractile force that is initiated by motor nerves. The term motor unit is applied to a single motor neuron and all the muscle fibers that it innervates. Most muscles contain several hundred motor units.

Muscle contraction is initiated when a sufficient number of acetylcholine molecules bind to the acetylcholine receptors (i.e., ligand-gated channels) of a motor endplate, triggering a local depolarization of the muscle membrane. Muscle fibers have similar electrical properties to those of large unmyelinated axons. After the ligand-gated channels trigger the initial depolarization, a muscle action potential then propagates along the muscle membrane (also known as the sarcolemma) via voltage gated sodium channels. The action potential also triggers voltage gated calcium channels to open at terminal tubules (t-tubules) throughout the sarcolemma. Calcium is stored in the t-tubules, which are invaginations or intracellular extensions of the sarcolemma. The opening of calcium channels leads to an influx of calcium ions into the cytoplasm, activating the contraction of proteins within the sarcomere that generates the actual mechanical force of muscle contraction.

The sarcomere is the basic contractile unit of muscle. Several key filaments exist. Actin filaments are known as the "thin filaments". They are anchored at the dark

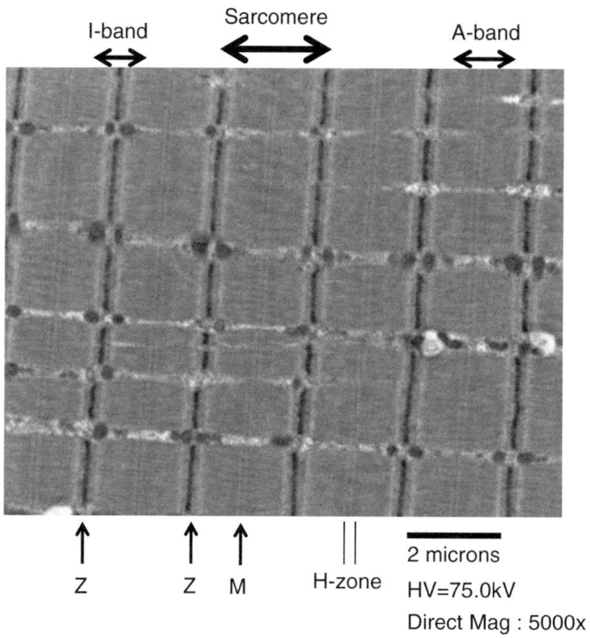

Fig. 2.4 Ultrastructural image (electron microscopy) of a normal skeletal muscle fiber that is contracted. These myofibers are comprised of alternating dark and light bands each representing the basic contractile unit of muscle known as the sarcomere. Individual sarcomeres are bordered by the dark, vertical Z-lines which act as anchors to which actin filaments attach. The lighter I-bands represent actin without overlying myosin. The darker A-band represents actin with overlying myosin. During muscle contraction, actin filaments are pulled over myosin causing shortening of the I-band as seen in this photo. *Photo credit: Dr. Jean Michaud, Department of Pathology, Children's Hospital of Eastern Ontario*

stripes within the muscle known as the Z-line (Fig. 2.4). One sarcomere is measured as the distance between two adjacent Z-lines. The actin filaments give rise to two 'bands' that are visible by electron microscopy. The I-band is the segment of actin that does not have overlying myosin filaments; it is located immediately next to the Z-band to which it is anchored. The A-band is the segment of actin that does have overlying myosin. Myosin filaments are known as the "thick filaments". The H-zone is the area containing myosin without overlying actin filaments. The M-line is a thin line in the center of the myosin molecule that is formed by cross-connecting elements of cytoskeleton.

Calcium binds to another protein called troponin which causes tropomyosin to slide over actin and muscle contraction to occur. Energy from adenosine triphosphate (ATP) is required to release the myosin head from actin allowing the muscle to relax. It is notable that ATP expenditure is directly related to relaxation of the sarcomere rather than its contraction. This is referred to as the sliding filament theory of muscle contraction.

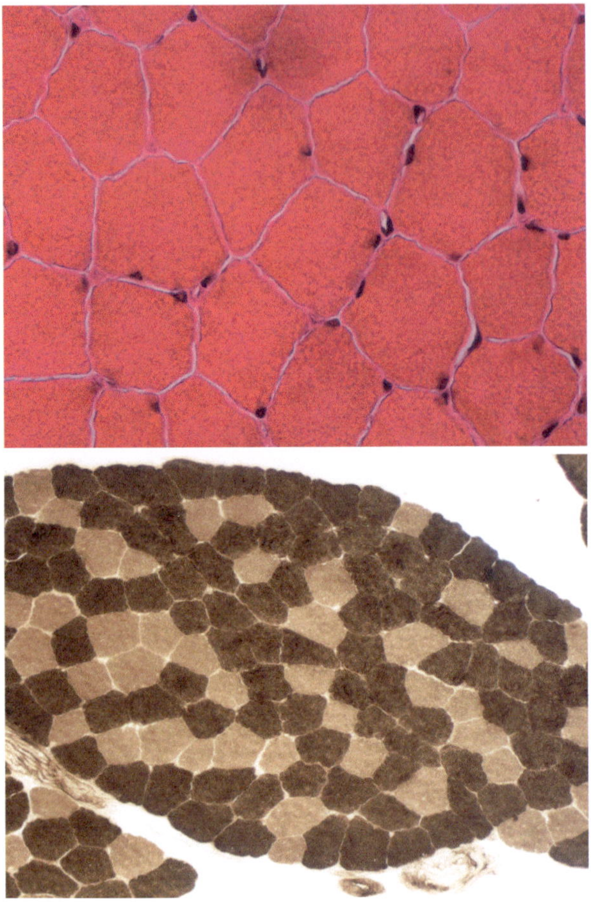

Fig. 2.5 Microscopic view of normal skeletal muscle seen in cross section, H&E (60× magnification) and ATPase 9.4 staining (20× magnification) showing Type 1 and Type 2 muscle fibers. *Photo credit: Dr. Jean Michaud, Department of Pathology, Children's Hospital of Eastern Ontario*

Disorders of the sarcomere can give rise to a variety of muscle diseases, most notably congenital myopathies which will be discussed in Chap. 22.

Classification of Skeletal Muscle Fibers

Skeletal muscle fiber types cannot be reliably distinguished on routine Hematoxylin and Eosin (H&E) staining, though sometimes type I fibers may appear darker due to a higher concentration of mitochondria. To distinguish among fiber types consistently, other stains are preferred.

Type 1 fibers are known as slow-twitch oxidative fibers. They demonstrate high oxidative and low glycolytic activity. These fibers are resistant to fatigue and subsequently used in longer-duration, lower-intensity exercise such as low-intensity jogging and maintenance of posture. The abundance of mitochondria in these fibers causes them to stain darkly on preparations for oxidative enzymes such as nicotinamide adenine dinucleotide tetrazolium reductase (NADH-TR), cytochrome oxidase and succinic dehydrogenase. They also stain darkly on ATPase preparations at pH 4.6 and lightly at pH 9.4. Type 1 fibers correspondingly have low glycogen content (Fig. 2.5).

Type 2 fibers can be divided into two subtypes: Type 2B, also known as fast-twitch glycolytic fibers, demonstrate high glycolytic and low oxidative activity. They are sensitive to fatigue and are recruited for short-duration, high-intensity exercises such as sprinting. The lower abundance of mitochondria in these muscles causes them to stain lightly with preparations for oxidative enzymes thereby differentiating them from Type 1 fibers. Type 2A fibers show an intermediate pattern. Although they are fast-twitch they are more fatigue resistant than Type 2B fibers, and are thus known as fast-twitch oxidative fibers. They show a mix of oxidative and glycolytic capacity thereby showing an intermediate pattern of staining for oxidative enzymes (most noticeable on ATPase preparations at pH 4.6).

Knowledge of fiber type variability can help distinguish among forms of congenital myopathies and metabolic muscle diseases. Of note, type 1 and type 2 muscle fibers show similar electrophysiological properties on routine needle EMG studies, and such examinations cannot distinguish between them.

References

1. Thomas JE, Lambert EH. Ulna nerve conduction velocity and H-reflex in infants and children. J Appl Physiol. 1960;15:1–9.
2. Shy ME, Garbern GY, Kamholz J. Hereditary motor and sensory neuropathies: a biological perspective. Lancet Neurol. 2002;1:110–8.
3. Smith KJ, Hall SM. Nerve conductions during peripheral demyelination and remyelination. J Neurol Sci. 1980;48:201–19.
4. Fullerton PM, Gilliatt RW, Lascelles RG, Morgan-Hughes JA. The relation between fibre diameter and internodal length in chronic neuropathy. J Physiol Lond. 1965;178:26.
5. Pilling JB. Nerve conduction during Wallerian degeneration in man. Muscle Nerve. 1978;1(1):81.
6. Chaudhry V, Cornblath DR. Wallerian degeneration in human nerves: serial electrophysiological studies. Muscle Nerve. 1992;15(6):687–93.
7. Kimura J, Rodnitzky RL, Okawara SH. Electrophysiological analysis of aberrant regeneration after facial nerve paralysis. Neurology. 1975;25:989–93.

Chapter 3
Approach to Electrodiagnostic Testing in Children

Peter B. Kang

Performing nerve conduction studies and electromyography in children shares the same fundamental principles with electrodiagnostic studies performed in adults. The nerves and muscles available for testing are mostly the same, electrode placement is similar, and data interpretation relies on the same basic physiology. However, there are nevertheless important differences that should be emphasized. Without sedation, younger children as well as those with developmental delay or cognitive impairment will often have difficulty tolerating the comprehensive nerve conduction studies involving as many as a dozen different motor and sensory nerves as well as extensive needle examination of multiple extremities that is more typical of adult studies. Older children and adolescents are more likely to tolerate the scale of testing that is familiar to adult neurophysiologists.

Do the limitations of the extent of testing that are typically present in a non-sedated study imply that pediatric electromyography is merely an abbreviated form of adult electromyography, or that all pediatric studies should be performed under sedation? The answer to both questions is no. The practical constraints happen to be compatible with the types of questions that are asked in different age groups. Infants and toddlers, in whom the technical challenges are most dramatic, often present for evaluation of generalized neuromuscular disorders rather than focal lesions such as mononeuropathies. This may include motor neuron disease and generalized myopathies. To address such questions requires not so much the examination of a set list of nerves and muscles but an accurate assessment of enough representative nerves and muscles in enough extremities to yield a conclusion with an acceptable level of diagnostic certainty. On the other hand, older children and adolescents are more likely to present with focal complaints that necessitate assessment for mononeuropathies. Exceptions do occur, an example being the evaluation of Erb's palsy in infants.

P.B. Kang, M.D., F.A.A.N., F.A.A.P.
Division of Pediatric Neurology, Shands Children's Hospital, University of Florida College of Medicine, Gainesville, FL, USA
e-mail: pbkang@ufl.edu

© Springer International Publishing AG 2017

H.J. McMillan, P.B. Kang (eds.), *Pediatric Electromyography*,
DOI 10.1007/978-3-319-61361-1_3

In a child, it is almost always possible to obtain an electrodiagnostic study without sedation that is complete enough to answer the specific question at hand. For such a study to be successfully performed, the neurophysiologist must be patient, adaptable, and experienced in working with children. The assistance of other personnel, such as neurophysiology fellows and technologists, can be invaluable, but care must be taken not to fill the room with too many staff, as the introduction of numerous new faces simultaneously in an unfamiliar environment may increase the risk of frightening the child. When available, a child life specialist who is experienced with guiding children through medical procedures can also help soothe and calm the child during the study. Parents should generally be permitted and encouraged to be present to support and comfort the child, unless the child is being examined under sedation or general anesthesia in a procedure room where family members are prohibited from staying.

Knowledge of technical considerations will also help minimize discomfort and maximize the tolerance of the child for the study. When performing nerve conduction studies, the desire to use the lowest current needed should be balanced against the desirability of delivering as few stimulations as possible. Sensory studies should generally be performed prior to motor studies since smaller stimulation intensity is required. Gradually increasing the stimulation intensity by 1–2 milliampere (mA) at a time will likely result in the delivery of more stimulations than needed. Conversely, a rapid increase in intensity has the potential to startle and alarm the child. A reasonable compromise is to raise the current by about 5 mA increments until a reproducible, maximal sensory nerve action potential (SNAP) amplitude is obtained. For sensory nerve conduction studies in particular, it should be remembered that currents above 20–30 mA are rarely needed to obtain a supramaximal sensory nerve action potential. Supramaximal motor responses sometimes require higher currents, but often not. Except when specifically indicated to help answer the specific electrophysiologic question, F responses are usually not helpful and are uncomfortable for children, and should be elicited selectively. H reflexes are often exceedingly painful for young children and should only be obtained in rare circumstances in this age group. For the needle examination, the smallest concentric bipolar electrode commercially available is 25 mm in length and 0.3 mm in diameter (30 gauge) with a 0.03 mm^2 recording area. This thin needle electrode should be used in almost all circumstances for children and adolescents, unless a specific muscle is too deep to be sampled accurately by this electrode.

An informal poll conducted in 2015 by the author among a group of ten expert pediatric neurophysiologists yielded the following information about practice habits around the world. Local analgesia was used always by two neurophysiologists and sometimes by six others. Conscious sedation was used always by one neurophysiologist and sometimes by four others. General anesthesia was used sometimes by two neurophysiologists. These results suggest that in experienced hands, electromyography may be performed successfully in the majority of children either without any anesthesia or with the use of local analgesia only. A prospective, large-scale survey of children and their parents after electromyography found that the level of pain reported was equivalent or less than that of venipuncture by the majority of families [1].

Local analgesia is favored by some neurophysiologists and may be a practical and helpful option for some children in certain settings. Topically applied creams are most commonly used, while infiltrative drugs are rarely used, especially as the latter may introduce artifact. A popular topical cream used for many procedures is the eutectic mixture of local anesthetics (more commonly known as EMLA), which consists of lidocaine 2.5% and prilocaine 2.5%. EMLA has been documented to reduce pain for venipuncture in infants [2] and children [3], vaccinations in infants [4] and children [5, 6], and other intramuscular injections in infants and children [7]. The disadvantage of using EMLA is the prolonged lag time before onset of analgesia, which may be as long as an hour, though some children will experience pain reduction earlier [8].

Another popular cream delivers amethocaine, now known as tetracaine, with the brand name Ametop, which is favored by some neurophysiologists due to a shorter time to onset of analgesia, typically 30 min [9, 10]. Several studies have suggested greater potency of amethocaine compared to EMLA in children [11–13], while another study indicated equivalent efficacy [14], and another suggested that EMLA was more efficacious than amethocaine [15]. However, amethocaine has been more expensive than EMLA, at least in some markets [9].

There are two challenges to the use of such topical creams in the setting of a pediatric electromyography laboratory. First, the cream must be applied in advance of the needle examination, ideally at least an hour ahead of time for EMLA and 30 min ahead of time for amethocaine/tetracaine. If the cream is applied before the nerve conduction studies are performed, that may provide sufficient or nearly sufficient time for onset of analgesia. The second challenge is that the neurophysiologist must guess which muscles are most likely to require needle examination. In some situations the choice of muscles is predictable, but not in others. It is worth noting that distraction techniques have been found to be as effective as EMLA cream for children receiving venipuncture in one study [16].

A subcutaneous analgesia option favored by some neurophysiologists is jet-injected lidocaine, marketed under the brand name J-Tip, which makes use of a carbon dioxide cartridge to propel the lidocaine into the subcutaneous tissue. The J-tip has been shown to reduce pain associated with venipuncture [17] and lumbar puncture [18] in children. One study suggests that the J-tip may be more efficacious than EMLA cream in reducing pain associated with intravenous catheter insertion in children [19]. Vapocoolant sprays have been adopted to reduce procedural pain in both adults and children [20], and one report indicates effective pain reduction in adults undergoing electromyography [21].

Conscious sedation or general anesthesia may be helpful in selected circumstances to facilitate the adequate assessment of a child for a particular question. Toddlers, as well as children with significant cognitive impairment, are most likely to require conscious sedation or general anesthesia overall. Infants will often tolerate enough examination to answer the question at hand, but for certain evaluations such as the assessment of Erb's palsy, conscious sedation or general anesthesia may augment the quality of the study. Older children and adolescents should only require conscious sedation or general anesthesia in rare cases if they are unusually anxious and the family refuses to even attempt a study in the regular electromyography laboratory. Whenever conscious sedation or general anesthesia is used, it should be kept in mind that though nerve conduction studies will be easier to obtain, needle examination will be limited to assessment of spontaneous activity only, unless an arrangement can be made with the anesthesiologist (with the prior knowledge and consent of the family) that the sedation or anesthesia be "lightened up" sufficiently to permit some withdrawal to pain and thus assessment of some motor units, usually in a limited number of muscles. Such titration is only practical for drugs with short half-lives, such as propofol.

A child who undergoes conscious sedation becomes drowsy and may fall asleep, but is generally able to maintain a natural airway. In contrast, a child who undergoes general anesthesia is completely unconscious and should be unarousable, and typically requires airway support. There are a variety of medications that have been used to induce conscious sedation or general anesthesia in children for the purposes of performing nerve conduction studies and needle electromyography. They include benzodiazepines (sedation and anxiolysis), nitrous oxide (dissociation and analgesia), propofol (may act as a sedative or general anesthetic agent depending on the dose), morphine (analgesia), and ketamine (sedation and analgesia). Nitrous oxide has been documented to reduce pain during venous cannulation in children [22, 23]. A technical point that should be kept in mind is that F responses may be suppressed by some of these drugs, especially nitrous oxide and propofol [24]. Sevoflurane has been used in the setting of pediatric electromyography, but it may not always be ideal, especially as it carries a malignant hyperthermia risk that some children undergoing these evaluations may be susceptible to. Sevoflurance also obscures F responses. Neuromuscular blockade should never be used, as a significant proportion of children being studied may have neuromuscular disorders that would react poorly to such medications. One common agent used for neuromuscular blockade, succinylcholine, also presents a risk of malignant hyperthermia.

In summary, the approach to maximizing the comfort of children undergoing electromyography while optimizing the quality of the data obtained varies across the globe. The vast majority of children, when approached properly by staff who are experienced in performing these studies in this age group, are able to tolerate an informative study with distraction techniques or local analgesia only.

References

1. Alshaikh NM, Martinez JP, Pitt MC. Perception of pain during electromyography in children: a prospective study. Muscle Nerve. 2016;54(3):422–6.
2. Biran V, Gourrier E, Cimerman P, Walter-Nicolet E, Mitanchez D, Carbajal R. Analgesic effects of EMLA cream and oral sucrose during venipuncture in preterm infants. Pediatrics. 2011;128(1):e63–70.
3. Tak JH, van Bon WH. Pain- and distress-reducing interventions for venepuncture in children. Child Care Health Dev. 2006;32(3):257–68.
4. Taddio A, Nulman I, Goldbach M, Ipp M, Koren G. Use of lidocaine-prilocaine cream for vaccination pain in infants. J Pediatr. 1994;124(4):643–8.

5. Abuelkheir M, Alsourani D, Al-Eyadhy A, Temsah MH, Meo SA, Alzamil F. EMLA(R) cream: a pain-relieving strategy for childhood vaccination. J Int Med Res. 2014;42(2):329–36.
6. Cassidy KL, Reid GJ, McGrath PJ, Smith DJ, Brown TL, Finley GA. A randomized double-blind, placebo-controlled trial of the EMLA patch for the reduction of pain associated with intramuscular injection in four to six-year-old children. Acta Paediatr. 2001;90(11):1329–36.
7. Carbajal R, Biran V, Lenclen R, Epaud R, Cimerman P, Thibault P, et al. EMLA cream and nitrous oxide to alleviate pain induced by palivizumab (Synagis) intramuscular injections in infants and young children. Pediatrics. 2008;121(6):e1591–8.
8. Lullmann B, Leonhardt J, Metzelder M, Hoy L, Gerr H, Linderkamp C, et al. Pain reduction in children during port-a-cath catheter puncture using local anaesthesia with EMLA. Eur J Pediatr. 2010;169(12):1465–9.
9. Herd DW, Newbury C, Brown PM. Cost benefit analysis of amethocaine (Ametop) compared with EMLA for intravenous cannulation in a children's emergency department. EMJ. 2010;27(6):456–60.
10. Bishai R, Taddio A, Bar-Oz B, Freedman MH, Koren G. Relative efficacy of amethocaine gel and lidocaine-prilocaine cream for Port-a-Cath puncture in children. Pediatrics. 1999;104(3):e31.
11. Arrowsmith J, Campbell C. A comparison of local anaesthetics for venepuncture. Arch Dis Child. 2000;82(4):309–10.
12. Romsing J, Henneberg SW, Walther-Larsen S, Kjeldsen C. Tetracaine gel vs EMLA cream for percutaneous anaesthesia in children. Br J Anaesth. 1999;82(4):637–8.
13. Lawson RA, Smart NG, Gudgeon AC, Morton NS. Evaluation of an amethocaine gel preparation for percutaneous analgesia before venous cannulation in children. Br J Anaesth. 1995;75(3):282–5.
14. Choy L, Collier J, Watson AR. Comparison of lignocaine-prilocaine cream and amethocaine gel for local analgesia before venepuncture in children. Acta Paediatr. 1999;88(9):961–4.
15. van Kan HJ, Egberts AC, Rijnvos WP, ter Pelkwijk NJ, Lenderink AW. Tetracaine versus lidocaine-prilocaine for preventing venipuncture-induced pain in children. Am J Health Syst Pharm. 1997;54(4):388–92.
16. Lal MK, McClelland J, Phillips J, Taub NA, Beattie RM. Comparison of EMLA cream versus placebo in children receiving distraction therapy for venepuncture. Acta Paediatr. 2001;90(2):154–9.
17. Lunoe MM, Drendel AL, Levas MN, Weisman SJ, Dasgupta M, Hoffmann RG, et al. A randomized clinical trial of jet-injected lidocaine to reduce venipuncture pain for young children. Ann Emerg Med. 2015;66(5):466–74.
18. Ferayorni A, Yniguez R, Bryson M, Bulloch B. Needle-free jet injection of lidocaine for local anesthesia during lumbar puncture: a randomized controlled trial. Pediatr Emerg Care. 2012;28(7):687–90.
19. Jimenez N, Bradford H, Seidel KD, Sousa M, Lynn AM. A comparison of a needle-free injection system for local anesthesia versus EMLA for intravenous catheter insertion in the pediatric patient. Anesth Analg. 2006;102(2):411–4.
20. Cohen Reis E, Holubkov R. Vapocoolant spray is equally effective as EMLA cream in reducing immunization pain in school-aged children. Pediatrics. 1997;100(6):E5.
21. Moon YE, Kim SH, Choi WH. Comparison of the effects of vapocoolant spray and topical anesthetic cream on pain during needle electromyography in the medial gastrocnemius. Arch Phys Med Rehabil. 2013;94(5):919–24.
22. Paut O, Calmejane C, Delorme J, Lacroix F, Camboulives J. EMLA versus nitrous oxide for venous cannulation in children. Anesth Analg. 2001;93(3):590–3.
23. Vetter TR. A comparison of EMLA cream versus nitrous oxide for pediatric venous cannulation. J Clin Anesth. 1995;7(6):486–90.
24. Dueck MH, Oberthuer A, Wedekind C, Paul M, Boerner U. Propofol impairs the central but not the peripheral part of the motor system. Anesth Analg. 2003;96(2):449–55.

Part II
Nerve Conduction Studies

Chapter 4
Sensory Studies

John C. McHugh

Introduction

Sensory nerve conduction studies in children are generally well tolerated and easy to perform. It is intended that this chapter be read in conjunction with Chap. 5 (motor nerve conduction studies) in order to gain an overall view of nerve conduction studies (NCS) in children.

Many authoritative texts already describe NCS techniques in great detail in adults, therefore this discussion will focus on the studies as they pertain to children [1, 2]. The overall technical details will of course be similar but important differences exist when performing and interpreting NCS in adults compared to children. For example, the relatively smaller distances being measured in children have the potential to have a greater proportional impact upon the calculations of latencies and conduction velocity. There is also an even greater need for empathy and kindness when performing neurophysiological testing upon the pediatric patient. Lastly there is a need for careful advanced planning since neurophysiological testing in children may need to be limited to the absolute minimum number of studies required to answer the clinical question. While the latter points may also be applicable for adult patients, it is particularly relevant for children who may show less tolerance of the test particularly when pathology is present and as such higher stimulation intensity may be required.

J.C. McHugh, MB, BCh, BaO, M.D., M.R.C.P.I.
Department of Clinical Neurophysiology, Our Lady's Children's Hospital,
Crumlin and AMNCH, Academic Unit of Neurology, Trinity College Dublin, Dublin, Ireland
e-mail: John.McHugh@olchc.ie

© Springer International Publishing AG 2017

H.J. McMillan, P.B. Kang (eds.), *Pediatric Electromyography*,
DOI 10.1007/978-3-319-61361-1_4

Strategic Planning

Despite the advances of molecular testing over the last decade, the overall use of EMG/NCS in children <18 years old continues to rise, although a recent review noted that the demand for EMG testing in younger children (<5 years old) may have diminished [3]. Most referrals stem from neurologists, both from specialists and non-specialists in neuromuscular medicine. The remaining referrals are received from orthopaedic surgeons, rheumatologists, pain specialists and other physician groups. The most common reasons for referral are evaluation of polyneuropathy or mononeuropathies followed by evaluations of symptoms affecting multiple limbs (e.g., weakness or pain).

The starting point for planning a set of NCS is to ensure that a specific clinical question is posed [4]. Clinical history and physical examination must guide the testing that is to be performed since neurophysiological testing is essentially an extension of the physical examination. Most neurophysiologists or neurologists will first attempt nerve conduction studies and electromyography (NCS/EMG) on an awake or non-sedated child. Most children will typically tolerate electrophysiological testing unless there is a comorbid diagnosis (e.g., autism, severe global developmental delay) that creates a barrier to physician-patient communication, or severe anxiety and/or pain may limit testing. The time spent obtaining a history and performing a clinical examination also affords the physician an opportunity to establish rapport with the child or adolescent and gain his/her trust. This may be particularly helpful where anxiety and/or apprehension are factors.

Laboratories may have guidelines and/or protocols that are intended for use in patients with specific clinical problems. However, the NCS/EMG in children must be tailored according to: (1) the question posed by the referring physician; (2) the individual child's clinical signs and symptoms and; (3) the likelihood that he/she will tolerate electrophysiological tests required to answer the clinical question. For these reasons it is important to plan the study in advance. One helpful way of determining how to prioritize the order in which nerves will be studied for a particular problem is to ask; "If this study must end prematurely what is the minimum number of nerves in descending order of importance that must be tested to answer the clinical question?" Posing such a question allows a pragmatic and rational study to take shape and is a useful mental exercise. Even if such scenarios are not frequently encountered it nevertheless maximizes the likelihood that valuable information can be obtained.

Sensory nerve conduction studies are the most rational starting point for almost all electrophysiological studies. Since most sensory nerves are located superficially they require low stimulation intensity compared to motor nerve studies. Much information is to be gained from intact lower extremity sensory nerve action potentials (SNAP) as normal amplitude, morphology and velocity are extremely helpful at excluding a length-dependent, large-fiber polyneuropathy. However, even for clinical problems involving sensory symptoms and/or areflexia it is typically necessary to pursue additional testing. Intact SNAPs and absent or reduced motor responses may lead to speculation about a neuronopathy (including motor neuron disease), myopathy, or certain disorders of the neuromuscular junction. In a patient presenting with weakness, the finding of reduced or absent SNAP assists in localizing the lesion distal to the dorsal root ganglion (i.e., within the distal nerve root or anterior primary ramus, plexus or peripheral nerve) [5]. Reduced SNAP amplitudes are not consistent with a primary disorder of motor neurons or a primary disorder of muscle or neuromuscular transmission. In this manner the NCS/EMG study will proceed iteratively and can adapt to the findings in a way that integrates knowledge and narrows down potential clinical differential diagnoses.

First Impressions—How to Approach the Child and Parents

It is advisable that some written information should be forwarded to parents in advance of NCS regarding the nature of the test. It is useful to describe the environment of the test and estimate roughly how long the test should take. Effort on these points ahead of meeting the patient can go a long way to achieving some calm at the time of the appointment. The neurophysiologist should introduce himself/herself to the child and to the parents, making particular effort to allow the child to feel comfortable in the environment.

Parents and children will want to know what the testing involves and what it will feel like. In covering these points, it is important to balance their need and right to information about the test with the potential for creating unmerited apprehension particularly in regard to the tolerability of the test. For nerve conduction studies, it is my practice to avoid using the words: electrode, stimulator and shock. Instead, I prefer to use the terms: sticker, battery and pulse, zap or tickle. When asked if the test is going to hurt it can be useful to liken the sensation one feels when they bang their funny bone or after one walks on a carpet and touches a door handle.

Consent

Written consent is not a requirement for non-sedated NCS in most if not all institutions and any effort to introduce more formal consent procedures for reasons of propriety only serves to increase parental anxiety in the author's view. After explaining the test and the reasons for carrying it out, there is value for the neurophysiologist to begin and work quickly to complete the test. This must be carried out with a calm demeanor so as to avoid the appearance of being rushed or worse still actually rushing the test.

Getting Started

Invite the child to sit with the parent during the test. Older children are usually comfortable sitting by themselves on the examination chair or table. For children under five, it is often helpful to ask them to sit on a parent's knee. For all children, it is advisable to ask them to remove their shoes which has the three-fold benefit of allowing accurate measurement of height before the test, exposing the feet for testing where needed, and minimizing consequences of being kicked during the study.

For babies, it is typically best to carry out studies in the arms of a parent or caregiver, though a cooperative infant may tolerate studies on an examination table. The use of swaddling during the test can minimize unwanted movement artefacts but also acts as a comfort measure and can even facilitate sleep in very young patients. The use of feeding during a test may also help to pacify a young baby, although in general it is the author's preference to avoid this unless it is necessary.

Establishing a rapport with the child and his/her parents is invaluable to the examination. One cannot be too prescriptive on this point. To some extent there is an individualized approach for everyone when it comes to dealing with children. This will be a reflection of the neurophysiologist's own personality, age and level of experience with children. Within the room, toys, teddy bears and stickers may provide helpful diversions and incentives for younger children. For the older ones, ready-made distraction is available by talking about the equipment itself. Most children over the age of six (and many below) will engage with the idea of playing a game using the EMG computer. It may be worth noting that most small handheld electronic devices including phones do not generate 60 Hz artifact or other appreciable electrical artifacts with standard filter settings.

Pre-test Measurements and Considerations

Height should be measured routinely in all cases before NCS. In contrast to adults, in whom SNAP amplitudes diminish to some small extent in the very tall, height is not directly important for understanding sensory NCS in children [6]. However, it is relevant to some parameters in motor NCS (Chap. 5) and therefore it should be registered before testing.

It is important to have a thermometer available for measurement of skin temperature. Temperature affects the velocity of conduction for large fiber sensory and motor nerves such that cooling of a limb diminishes conduction velocity and warming increases it [7]. The duration and area of the recorded potentials are also affected such that a broader potential of increased area is obtained at lower temperatures and this can be modeled in a linear fashion. Temperature also has an effect on the amplitude of compound nerve or muscle action potentials such that amplitudes tend to be larger during cooling although the relationship is non-linear. The optimal skin temperature for NCS is ≥32 °C at the wrist and ≥30 °C at the ankle. Warming of limbs should be undertaken when skin temperatures are below this level. In reality, many laboratories do not routinely engage in limb warming pre-test unless the peripheries are very cold and precise measurement of conduction velocity is essential, e.g. to distinguish a demyelinating from an axonal neuropathy based on strict velocity criteria. Whilst making this differentiation is usually straight forward in most cases, borderline conduction velocity slowing in the setting of cold peripheries and small SNAPs poses a problem and limb warming might need to be considered in such instances.

Although short term effects on conduction velocity can be observed after 2–3 minutes of limb immersion in warm water, more rigorous studies reveal that longer durations of immersion are required to achieve adequate warming of nerve [8]. For this and other reasons, a practical suggestion is to aim to avoid cold limbs by keeping room temperature warm and allowing the patient sufficient time to acclimatize to being indoors before carrying out the study. Furthermore, although subject to theoretical objections, the use of a correction factor can be considered (adding 4% of the measured sensory conduction velocity for every degree below the minimum expected value). For a more in-depth exploration of temperature and its implications for NCS please refer to Chap. 11 (Artifacts) and/or the excellent minimonograph of Denys [7].

Brief Overview of Physiology and Equipment

The basic operations of all EMG machines are similar. To perform nerve conduction studies, there is an electrical stimulator which comprises a cathode (negative pole) and an anode (positive pole). The flow of current between the two poles induces localized changes in the distribution of charge across the underlying nerve membrane such that the nodal portion of membranes beneath the cathode becomes relatively more positive intracellularly. This depolarization from resting membrane potential is what triggers the nerve action potential to occur at nodes of Ranvier adjacent to the cathode. The action potential will propagate itself in both an antidromic and orthodromic direction along the nerve. Antidromic sensory nerve conduction studies occur when an action potential travels in the opposite direction from the normal physiological afferent sensory response. Orthodromic nerve conduction studies occur when the action potential is propagated in the normal physiological direction. The latter is particularly useful for eliminating motor artifact in mixed nerves of the hand and/or feet. Surface electrodes are placed over the skin in an area corresponding to the normal physiological course of a specific sensory nerve. Many laboratories tend to rely primarily on either antidromic or orthodromic sensory studies for the most commonly studied nerves, but others use a standardized mix of the two approaches.

Stimulating electrodes vary in design. Bar electrodes are encased in molded plastic and have a fixed spacing between anode and cathode. In pediatric NCS, it is usually necessary to have at least two sizes available: studies in patients over 18–24 months can be achieved using conventional adult stimulators with spacing of 2–3 cm between anode and cathode; studies in newborns and infants ideally require smaller stimulators (1 cm spacing or less) [9]. Ring electrodes can be used for digital stimulation. Subcutaneous needle stimulation with surface anode (e.g., for lateral femoral cutaneous nerve of the thigh) can be helpful in some instances but is not used commonly in children and as such will not be discussed further here. A well-equipped laboratory that performs studies in children should have an array of different surface electrodes available for different circumstances.

A supramaximal stimulus is one which is sufficient to stimulate all of the large fiber axons within the nerve such that a compound nerve action potential is measured, meaning that its amplitude cannot be augmented by further increases in stimulus intensity. For sensory studies, short duration (usually 0.1 ms) square wave pulses are increased to achieve a maximal sensory nerve action potential (SNAP). In children, discomfort is reduced by having some appreciation of the range of stimulus intensities that is likely to produce a supramaximal SNAP for each nerve at a given site. In this way, the number of stimuli can be kept to a minimum. As a very simple guide, sensory stimulation (at 0.1 ms durations) should rarely be increased beyond 40–50 mA in a child, and never beyond 10–20 mA in the digits. For many sensory nerves, supramaximal SNAPs will be achieved at stimulus intensities of 10–20 mA but this, of course, varies according to: the specific nerve and site; the density and volume of intervening soft tissue; and the degree of myelination (which is influenced in turn by age and by the presence of nerve pathology).

SNAPs are recorded using active and inactive surface electrodes, otherwise referred to as G1 and G2 or (sometimes E1 and E2) where E is short for electrode and G refers to grid. These are placed in line on the skin overlying the nerve of interest. The recorded wave-form is usually triphasic comprising a positive, negative and then a second positive component. This is produced by the passage of the action potential through a tissue volume conductor, which can be modelled simply as a cylinder with positive-negative dipoles at its leading and trailing end [10]. The direction of the recorded potential difference is determined by what E1 (G1) sees relative to E2 (G2) at a given time and this will change with movement of the dipole towards and then away from the recording electrode pair. The shape and relative amplitudes of the three phase-components is determined by the orientation, inter-electrode spacing and distance of the surface electrodes relative to the action potential generator, i.e., the nerve. These factors are controlled for by the rules which govern electrode placement, which will be discussed below. Of note, a simpler biphasic potential (the norm for compound muscle action potentials in motor studies) can also be seen in some sensory studies, for example in antidromically recorded digital SNAPs; this occurs because of the peculiar effects of positive far field potentials (as opposed to local potentials) [10]. When these arise, they are seen equally by active and inactive electrodes and accordingly they do not register as a potential difference—therefore the first visible potential difference appears to arise directly under E1 (G1) and not in advance of it.

Shock artifacts are visible in every sensory recording in children. Indeed the absence of shock artifact should alert the neurophysiologist to some form of recording failure; the most common reason for this being disconnection of the recording leads to the amplifier after cleaning. The relatively short distances between stimulating and recording electrodes in children is a technical difficulty since spread of the shock artifact more readily contaminates the potential of interest and in some instances can obscure it entirely. Electrical isolation of the stimulator is a feature of most modern EMG machines which helps to reduce shock artifact, as does the use of shielded cables for stimulation. Other measures which can be adopted in the pediatric EMG laboratory include: avoiding excessively short distances between stimulus and recording sites; using alcohol-rubs to dry the skin before testing to reduce skin impedances; changing the surface electrode stickers; placement of the ground electrode between stimulating and recording electrodes. On rare occasions it may be necessary to further reduce skin impedance by gently abrading the skin before testing, however this is a technique used primarily in adults and is not generally recommended for children. Another tip which can be useful in situations of particular difficulty is to change the shape of the stimulus from a monopolar to biphasic square wave; this can also remove or alleviate shock contamination but should not be relied upon as an alternative to scrupulous skin preparation and electrode application.

Nerve Selection

The question of which nerve(s) to study is influenced primarily by the clinical question that is to be answered. However, some age-related factors must also be considered. For infants the sensory nerves that are routinely studied include: median, ulnar and medial plantar nerves. In children and adolescents the sensory nerves that are routinely studied include: median, ulnar, dorsal ulnar cutaneous, radial, superficial peroneal and sural nerves. Less commonly the lateral and medial antebrachial cutaneous nerves can be studied.

Electrode Placement for Sensory NCS

The positioning of stimulating and recording electrodes should be anatomically the same in children as for adult patients. The difference is that limb lengths vary considerably between child- and adulthood and therefore the distances between stimulating and recording electrodes in adults must be adjusted for the child. Therefore, in children it is more useful to position electrodes in relation to surface anatomical landmarks rather than at fixed linear distances.

The following section will deal with how to carry out sensory conduction studies in children for all of the commonly studied nerves. It should be noted that nerves can be stimulated in either direction—orthodromically or antidromically. There is no one correct method and in most instances ortho- or antidromic testing uses exactly the same electrode placements, simply swapping the stimulating and recording electrode pairs as required. The direction of recording does not affect nerve conduction velocity but the amplitude of sensory nerve action potentials (SNAPs) will vary depending on the approach used, and thus reference ranges may vary depending on which approach is adopted. In my own laboratory, a mixture of anti- and orthodromic testing is used: orthodromic testing is favored in the hands and in the feet, whereas antidromic testing is generally preferred at more proximal sites.

Illustrations of electrode placements are provided in Figs. 4.1, 4.2, 4.3, 4.4, 4.5, 4.6, 4.7, 4.8 and 4.9. Tables 4.1 and 4.2 provide descriptions of electrode placements for both antidromic and orthodromic approaches.

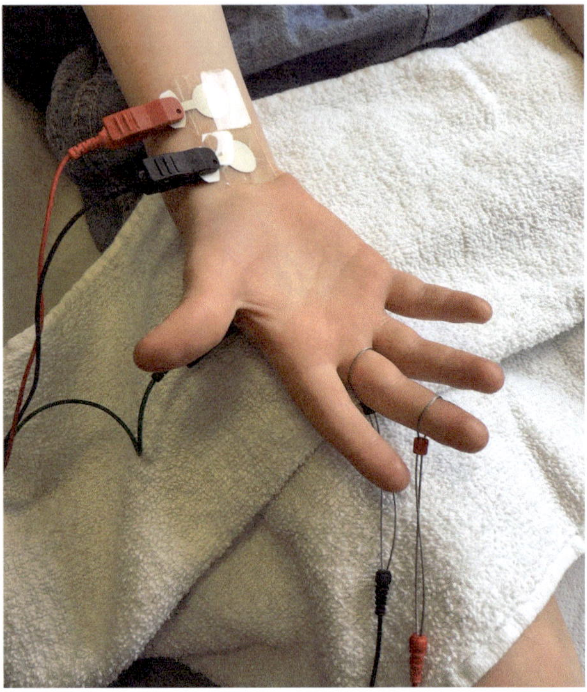

Fig. 4.1 Median digit III orthodromic study recording over the median nerve at the wrist and stimulating digit III

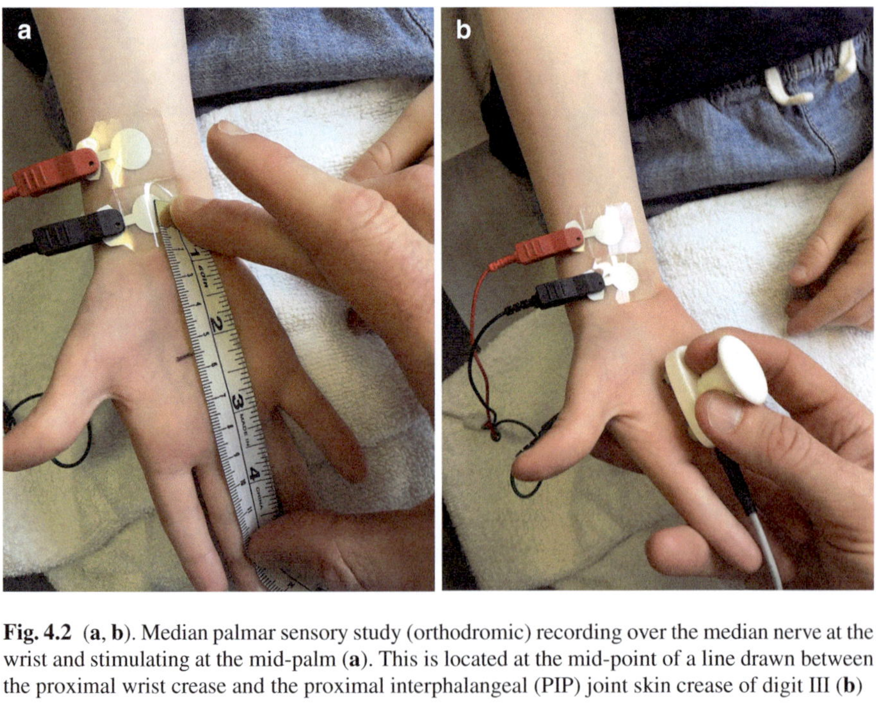

Fig. 4.2 (**a**, **b**). Median palmar sensory study (orthodromic) recording over the median nerve at the wrist and stimulating at the mid-palm (**a**). This is located at the mid-point of a line drawn between the proximal wrist crease and the proximal interphalangeal (PIP) joint skin crease of digit III (**b**)

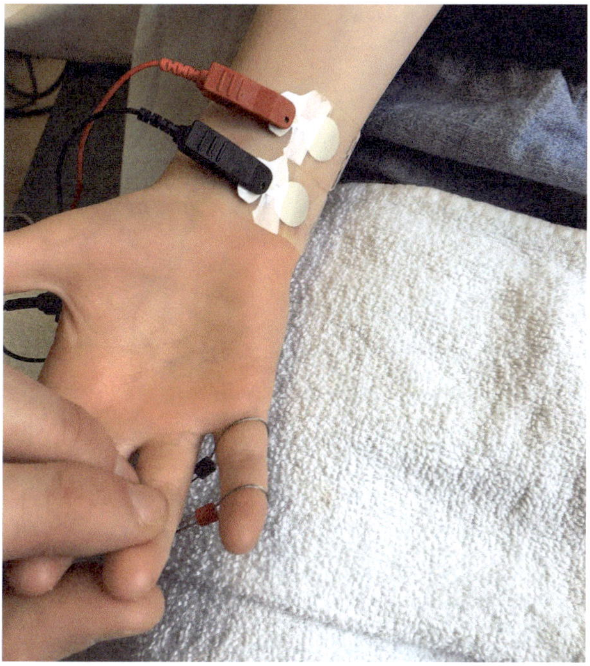

Fig. 4.3 Ulnar digit V orthodromic study recording over the ulnar nerve at the wrist and stimulating digit V with ring electrodes

Stimulation and Recording

In adults, it is customary and acceptable to average the recorded sensory signal over a train of 5–20 stimuli to optimize the recorded waveform and facilitate measurement and marking of specific latencies and amplitudes. Some neurophysiologists use the repetitive stimulation setting at frequencies of 1–2 Hz to collect a reasonable number of potentials rapidly, thus needing only 5–10 seconds to acquire a single averaged SNAP. The same approach can be adopted in pediatric patients although some experienced practitioners advocate the use of single shocks in order to minimize discomfort and maximize compliance with testing. My view is that single supramaximal shocks may be adequate, particularly where the response is normal but I prefer to use averaging and to deliver repetitive shocks that increase from the point where a child can feel nothing to the point where they appreciate a "tickle". I find that it is useful to maintain stimulation at this level for a few seconds to gain the child's confidence and disperse any lingering parental anxiety about the test. I then play a game with the child, encouraging them to inspect the baseline noise as it waves on the screen (I refer to it as "the sea"). I invite the child to tell me when they see a dolphin or other sea creature emerge from it. As I increase the stimulus to the point where the SNAP becomes visible, I whisper that it will be a bit "ouch" for just a second, then quickly increase to supramaximal and finish stimulation by marveling at how large the response is (at least in cases where the SNAP is recordable). It is important that

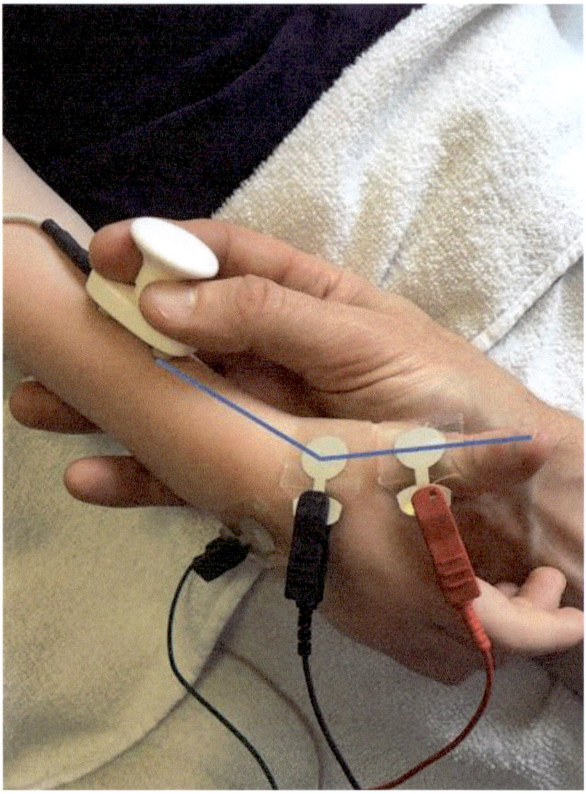

Fig. 4.4 Superficial radial antidromic study. The distance between cathode and G1 is approximately the same as the distance from G1 to the tip of the thumb

the first nerve study should succeed as it lays a platform of confidence which permits further testing to occur. If this approach is unsuccessful, especially in infants and younger children who may not fully comprehend such interactions, an alternative approach is to capture two similar individual SNAPs and display them separately on the report to convey to others that the SNAP is reproducible and not artifactual.

The sweep speeds, screen amplification and filter-settings can be changed easily on digital machines (belying the decades of development and technological sophistication that have culminated in modern EMG equipment). Amplification settings of 10 μV per screen division (10 μV/D) and sweep speed settings of 1 ms/D are a common default for sensory NCS. These can be changed or increased as necessary so as to optimize visualization and marking of the waveform on the screen. Default filter settings of 2 Hz–20 kHz are standard in NCS to reduce high frequency noise and low frequency artifacts [1].

Measurements in NCS are primarily concerned with only two things: size and speed. The size of the sensory nerve action potential (SNAP) provides an estimate of the number of healthy functioning sensory neurons within the nerve being tested. The sensory conduction velocity and associated latencies provide information that relates to the fastest conducting myelinated fibers within the nerve. NCSs are insensitive to

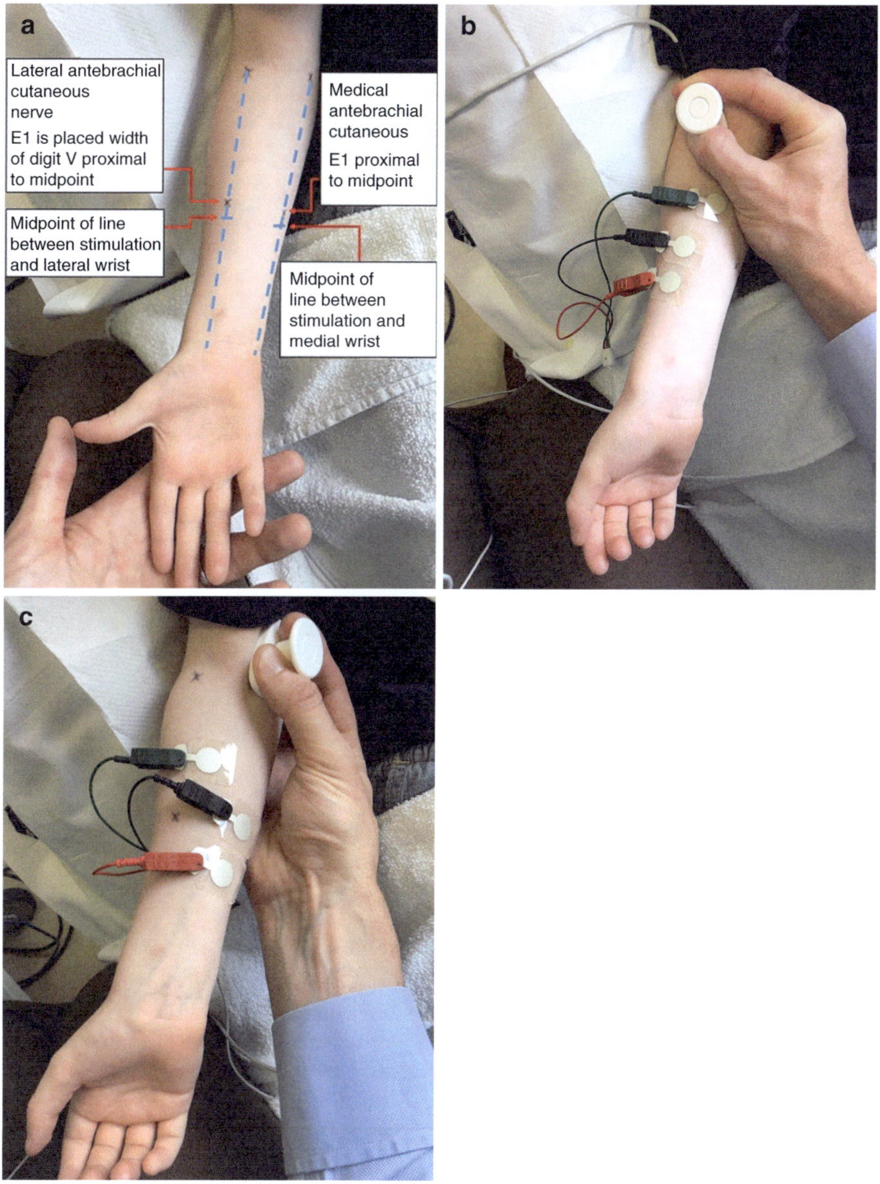

Fig. 4.5 (**a**–**c**). Limb measurements (**a**) for antidromic recording of lateral (**b**) and medial (**c**) antebrachial cutaneous nerves of the forearm

the functioning of small diameter and unmyelinated nerve fibers, the physiology of which must be interrogated by other means that will not be discussed here.

Size and speed in sensory NCS are described primarily in terms of amplitude (measured in microvolts; μV), and velocity (measured in meters per second; m/s). Other

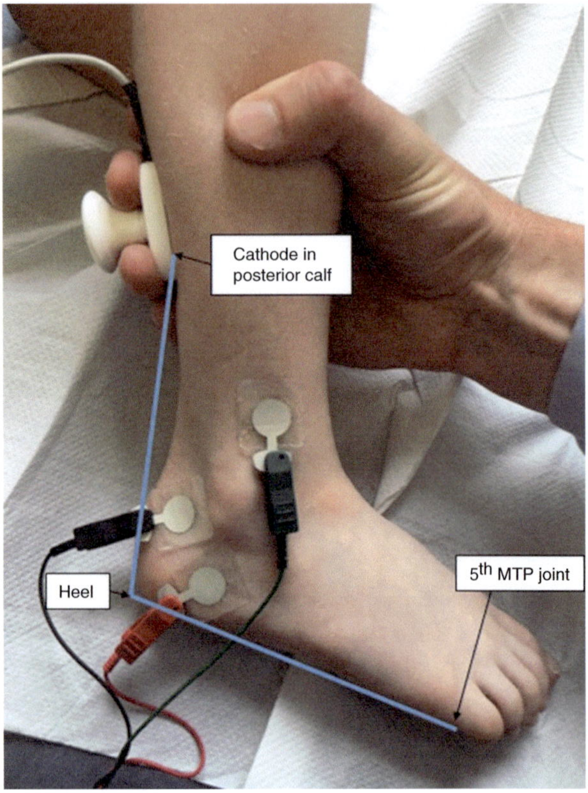

Fig. 4.6 Sural sensory antidromic study stimulating behind the calf, the same distance above the inferior heel as the 5th metatarsophalangeal (MTP) joint is anterior to it; recording is postero-lateral to the lateral malleolus

parameters include individual latency measurements, the shape of the waveform and its duration and area. These measurements are defined by placing markers of latency and amplitude on the compound potential; most modern EMG programs will do this automatically but the markers should be inspected routinely and edited if placed erroneously, especially in some antidromic sensory studies where an artifactual motor waveform sometimes appears. The computer analyzes the waveform and automatically defines latency of onset (for biphasic potentials), first and second positive and negative peaks as well as the zero-crossing line that follows the negative peak.

Calculations of velocity are derived from these measurements by dividing the distance between stimulating and recording electrodes by the time (in milliseconds) from stimulus to onset or peak. The specific latency chosen to calculate velocity varies between different laboratories. My preference is to mark onset latency (for biphasic potentials) or first positive peak latency for triphasic potentials; these correspond to the contributions of the fastest conducting fibers. An alternative practice is to choose the negative peak latency: this has the advantage of being more consistently identifiable but will underestimate the velocity of the very fastest axons contributing to the potential. Analysis of the duration and area of the negative component of the waveform provides a useful index of temporal dispersion, which will be increased in cases of demyelination.

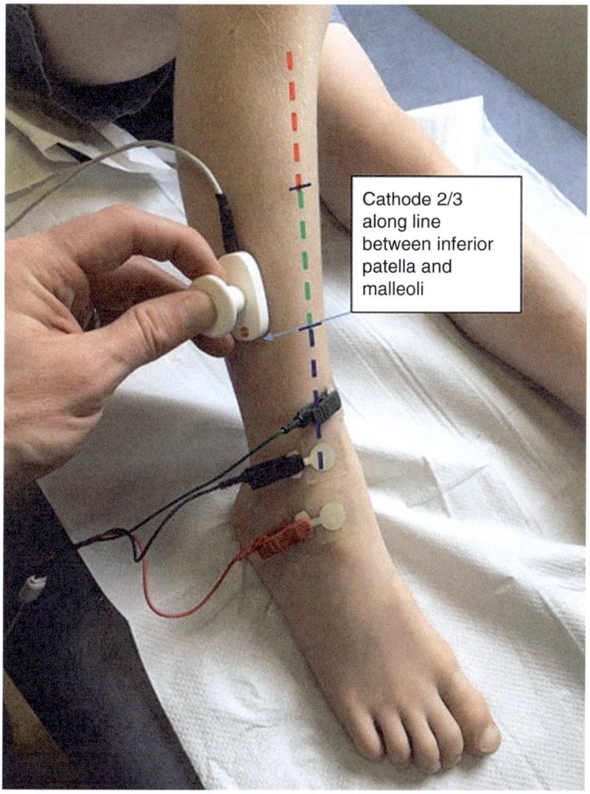

Fig. 4.7 Superficial peroneal sensory study stimulating over the lateral leg and recording at the ankle

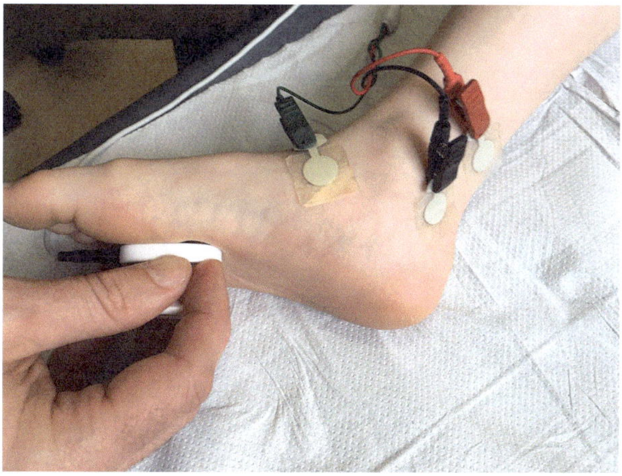

Fig. 4.8 Medial plantar orthodromic study stimulating at the medial arch (anode just proximal to the 1st MTP head) and recording behind the medial malleolus

Amplitude may be calculated in different ways: baseline to negative peak; from the midpoint of a "tilted" line connecting positive peaks to the negative peak; or from negative to positive peak.

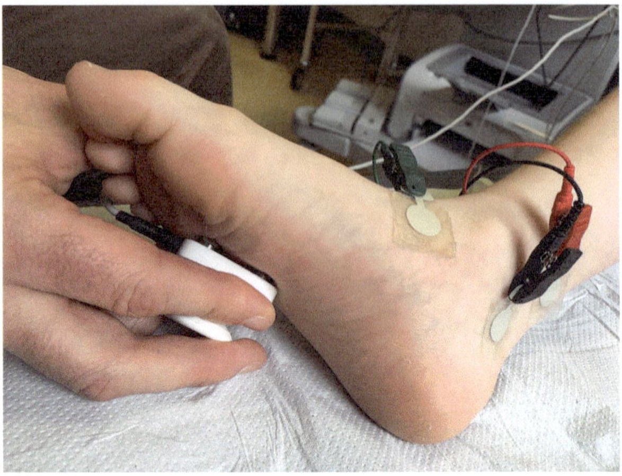

Fig. 4.9 Lateral plantar orthodromic sensory study stimulating over the lateral sole (between 4th and 5th metatarsal bones) and recording behind the medial malleolus

Table 4.1 Positioning of Electrodes for Upper Limb Sensory Nerve Conduction Studies

	Stimulation site	Recording site
Median nerve		
Antidromic	Stimulator placed at the wrist Cathode at wrist: between tendons of palmaris longus (PL) and flexor carpi radialis (FCR). Anode is located more proximally	G1 ring or surface electrode placed on digit II[a] G2 is 3 cm distal to G1
Orthodromic	Ring or bar electrode(s) on digit II[a] Cathode located at crease of first MCP joint. Anode is distal (between PIP and DIP joint) Digit I can be studied, but distance must curve around thenar eminence to reflect course of nerve	G1 surface electrode placed at the wrist (crease between tendons of PL and FCR) G2 is 3 cm proximal to G1
Palmar study *Orthodromic*	Stimulator placed on palm. In adults, cathode is located at the mid-palm, 7 cm from recording electrodes in a line with the webspace of digits II and III.	G1 is placed at the middle of the proximal wrist (as above) G2 is 3 cm proximal to G1
Ulnar nerve		
Antidromic	Stimulator placed at the wrist Cathode at wrist: just lateral to flexi carpi ulnaris (FCU) tendon. Anode is located more proximally	G1 ring or surface electrode placed on digit V[b] G2 is 3 cm distal to G1
Orthodromic	Ring or bar electrode(s) on digit V[b] Cathode located at skin crease of digit V MCP joint. Anode is distal (between PIP-DIP joints)	G1 over the medial wrist (just lateral to FCU tendon) G2 is 3 cm proximal to G1
Palmar *Orthodromic*	Stimulator placed on palm. In adults, cathode is located at the mid-palm, 7 cm from recording electrodes in a line with the webspace of digits IV and V.	G1 over the medial wrist at the proximal wrist crease (just lateral to FCU tendon) G2 is 3 cm proximal to G1

Table 4.1 (continued)

Radial nerve		
Antidromic	Stimulator place on dorsolateral radius. Cathode is 8-10 cm proximal to G1 in adult limb	G1 over superficial radial nerve as it crosses extensor pollicis longus tendon (base of 'anatomical snuffbox'). G2 placed over dorsum of first MCP
Orthodromic	Stimulator placed at skin crease of Digit I MCP joint. Anode is distal (at DIP joint skin crease)	G1 over radial bone at same distance proximal to the anatomical snuffbox as the tip of thumb is distal to it. G2 is 3 cm proximal to G1
Medial antebrachial cutaneous nerve		
Antidromic	Stimulator placed over medial elbow at mid-point between medial epicondyle and biceps tendon.	G1 surface electrode place in adults, 12 cm distal to cathode (along line between cathode and medial wrist). G2 is 3 cm distal to G1
Lateral antebrachial cutaneous nerve		
Antidromic	Stimulator place in antecubital fossa, just lateral to biceps tendon. *Note: low stimulation intensity < 15 mA is required. Cathode must be manipulated to reduce concomitant stimulation of the median nerve which causes a motor twitch*	G1 surface electrode place in adults, 12 cm distal to cathode (along line between cathode and radial styloid / lateral wrist) G2 is 3 cm distal to G1

PL, palmaris longus; *FCR*, flexi carpi radialis; *FCU*, flexi carpi ulnaris; *MCP*, metacarpal-phalangeal; *PIP*, proximal interphalangeal; *DIP*, distal interphalangeal
Mid palm, mid-point of line between proximal wrist crease and the PIP-skin creases
[a]Digit III or IV can also be studied (digit IV can be used for a median-to-sensory comparison study to investigate possible carpal tunnel syndrome)
[b]Digit IV can also be studied (digit IV can be used for median-to-sensory comparison study to investigate possible carpal tunnel syndrome)

Other important membrane parameters, such as nerve excitability parameters are beyond the scope of this chapter (see [Bostock et al.] for detailed review) [11]. The key points to remember when determining how to calculate amplitude and velocity are to maintain consistency and to use reference ranges appropriate for the approach.

Common Pitfalls

Many of the pitfalls that may arise can be avoided by attention to the measures already discussed above, particularly in relation to stimulation or shock artifact. Some additional problems that can be encountered include underestimation or overestimation of conduction velocity, particularly in very young children and in

Table 4.2 Positioning of Electrodes for Lower Limb Sensory Nerve Conduction Studies

	Stimulation site	Recording site
Sural nerve		
Antidromic	Stimulator placed midline in dorsal, lower leg between heads of gastrocnemius. Cathode is at point below inferior belly of muscle with the cathode held firmly against the leg and angled slightly laterally	G1 posterior to lateral malleolus G2 is 3 cm distal to G1
Superficial peroneal nerve		
Antidromic	Stimulator placed 2/3 of the distance along a line drawn from the inferior patella to G1 (upper malleolus); this placement corresponds to 11–14 cm from G1 in adult limbs. Distance for optimal stimulation varies.	G1 upper level of lateral malleolus between the malleolus and tendon of the tibialis anterior. G2 is 3 cm distal to G1
Medial plantar		
Orthodromic	Stimulator placed such that the anode is proximal to the first metatarsal head (cathode is 3 cm more proximal almost at the mid-point of the sole). Stimulator should be held parallel and between first & second metatarsal bones. Alternatively, ring electrodes may be placed on Digit II	G1 placed posterior to medial malleolus; G2 is 3 cm proximal to G1
Lateral plantar		
Orthodromic	Stimulator placed such that the anode is proximal to the first metatarsal head (cathode is 3 cm more proximal almost at the mid-point of the sole). Stimulator should be held parallel and between fourth and fifth metatarsal bones. Alternatively, ring electrodes may be placed on Digit V	G1 placed posterior to medial malleolus; G2 is 3 cm proximal to G1

newborns. Notwithstanding the fact that newborns have slower conduction velocities because of incomplete myelination, the very small distances involved in testing young babies increases the margin of error in conduction velocity that can result from mismeasurement by even a few millimeters. This can produce erroneously slow or non-physiologically fast conduction velocities in this age group. Mismeasurement can be avoided by being consistent in the way that the limb is held and optimizing distances (gently stretching the ankle or wrist, or bending the elbow to maximize the distance between stimulation and recording) and more faithfully representing the actual course of the nerve.

Overstimulation is not tolerated by children. To insure acquisition of the most detailed study possible, it is important to start small and minimize the number of larger shocks. Conversely, it is important not to shirk from giving supramaximal stimulation sparingly since submaximal stimulation will falsely under-represent the nerve being studied and can lead to misdiagnosis.

Interpreting the Data

Understanding sensory conduction data can be challenging. Ideally each EMG laboratory should acquire its own normative data set over time. Despite standardization of technique and similarity of equipment, there will always be variations between different centers and different operators. Nevertheless, for those neurophysiologists who are establishing new laboratories, it seems sensible to suggest that they borrow established reference values from their training institution or alternatively they can refer judiciously to published datasets (see Chap. 24 for normal values). In such cases it is most important that they remain attentive to the techniques used (anti- or orthodromic) and to the age of the published population.

Sensory conduction velocities and sensory nerve action potentials (SNAPs) are significantly influenced by the age of the child: velocities effectively double from the time of birth to the age of 1–2 years, undergoing an especially sharp increase within the first 6 months of life. From 2 years of age onward a more modest increase will occur until adult velocities are achieved. A similar time-course and scale of maturation is also evident in SNAP amplitudes.

Understanding Abnormalities in Sensory NCS

Earlier it was indicated that when performing sensory nerve conduction studies, the neurophysiologist is interested primarily in two things: size (amplitude) and speed (onset latency or conduction velocity). This simplification holds true when it comes to interpreting the NCS data. Demyelinating nerve injury (acquired or hereditary) leads to slowing of nerve conduction velocities; it can also lead to conduction block which is discussed in more detail in the chapter on motor nerve conduction studies [12]. Demyelination will also produce changes in the duration and shape of the sensory nerve action potential (SNAP) since acquired as well as some inherited demyelinating neuropathies will affect some axons more than others giving rise to variable rates of demyelination which gives rise to a phenomenon of temporal dispersion. It can also increase the threshold for stimulation. However, these more subtle changes will not occur in isolation and therefore velocity reduction remains the primary parameter. Once again, it is stressed that temperature and age will both have independent effects on conduction velocity and must be taken into account.

Axonotmesis leads to a reduction in the SNAP amplitude due to the loss of sensory axons. In addition, the loss of axons will also result in a mild reduction (typically >75% lower limit of normal) of sensory conduction velocity.

Whilst the total number of nerves sampled in NCS in children may be less than a comparable study in an adult, it is nevertheless essential that sufficient data are gathered to answer the clinical question and to understand and characterize the pattern and distribution of any existing neuropathy.

Summary

Sensory nerve conduction studies in children are important in that they lay a platform for the rest of the electrodiagnostic study. Good technique and appreciation of the technical elements of the study are important and the challenges are undeniably greater than in adults. Reliable and accurate data can be obtained without undue discomfort or upset. The value of balanced information and establishing an early rapport with the child and parents cannot be overstated.

References

1. Kimura J. Electrodiagnosis in diseases of nerve and muscle: principles and practice. 4th ed. Oxford: Oxford University Press; 2013.
2. Preston DC, Shapiro BE. Electromyography and neuromuscular disorders: clinical-electrophysiologic correlations. 2nd ed. Philadelphia: Elsevier Butterworth-Heinemann; 2005.
3. Karakis I, Liew W, Darras BT, Jones HR, Kang PB. Referral and diagnostic trends in pediatric electromyography in the molecular era. Muscle Nerve. 2014;50(2):244–9.
4. Payan J. Clinical electromyography in infancy and childhood. In: Brett EM, editor. Paediatric neurology. 3rd ed. Great Britain: Churchill Livingstone; 1997. p. 823–54.
5. Mallik A, Weir AI. Nerve conduction studies: essentials and pitfalls in practice. J Neurol Neurosurg Psychiatry. 2005;76(Suppl 2):ii23–31.
6. Mchugh JC, Connolly S. Correction and transformation of normative neurophysiological data: is there added value in the diagnosis of distal symmetrical peripheral neuropathy? Muscle Nerve. 2011;44(6):890–6.
7. Denys EH. AAEM minimonograph #14: the influence of temperature in clinical neurophysiology. Muscle Nerve. 1991;14(9):795–811.
8. Franssen H, Wieneke GH. Nerve conduction and temperature: necessary warming time. Muscle Nerve. 1994;17(3):336–44.
9. Pitt MC. Nerve conduction studies and needle EMG in very small children. Eur J Paediatr Neurol. 2012;16(3):285–91.
10. Dumitru D, DeLisa JA. AAEM Minimonograph #10: volume conduction. Muscle Nerve. 1991;14(7):605–24.
11. Bostock H, Cikurel K, Burke D. Threshold tracking techniques in the study of human peripheral nerve. Muscle Nerve. 1998;21(2):137–58.
12. Miller RG, Gutmann L, Lewis RA, Sumner AJ. Acquired versus familial demyelinative neuropathies in children. Muscle Nerve. 1985;8(3):205–10.

Chapter 5
Motor Nerve Conduction Studies

John C. McHugh

Introduction

Motor nerve conduction studies (NCS), like their sensory counterparts are similarly well tolerated in children. Since motor studies are never conducted in isolation, it is intended that this chapter should be read in conjunction with Chap. 4, which describes sensory NCS. Chap. 4 also considers equipment, additional technical aspects, and the broader issue of the approach to pediatric patients and their parents or caregivers.

Differences Between Motor and Sensory NCS

The major physiological difference between sensory and motor NCS is that in motor studies, recordings are made from muscle and not from nerve. The measured potentials are therefore compound muscle action potentials (CMAPs), which represent the sum of stimulated motor unit potentials beneath the recording surface electrodes [1]. Unlike sensory nerve action potentials (SNAPs), which can be di- or triphasic, CMAP morphology should always be diphasic, featuring a sharp negative take-off which is generated by muscle fiber depolarizations immediately below the active recording electrode [2]. Additionally, the magnitude of the recorded signals is some thousand times greater than sensory or mixed nerve action potentials and is measured in millivolts (mV) rather than microvolts (μV). These aspects are routinely factored into the display and gain settings of the EMG machine.

J.C. McHugh, MB, BCh, BaO, M.D., M.R.C.P.I.
Department of Clinical Neurophysiology, Our Lady's Children's Hospital,
Crumlin and AMNCH; Academic Unit of Neurology, Trinity College, Dublin, Ireland
e-mail: John.McHugh@olchc.ie

© Springer International Publishing AG 2017

H.J. McMillan, P.B. Kang (eds.), *Pediatric Electromyography*,
DOI 10.1007/978-3-319-61361-1_5

A further physiological difference is that a synapse, the neuromuscular junction (NMJ), is interposed between the site of stimulation (nerve) and site of recording (muscle). This means that the latency between electrical stimulation and onset of the muscle action potential is accounted for not only by propagation of the action potential along the nerve, but also by the time required for neuromuscular transmission to occur and for conduction of the action potential along the muscle fiber. Therefore it is inaccurate to estimate motor conduction velocities on the basis of the distance between stimulation and muscle recording. This contrasts with the situation for sensory NCS, in which velocities are calculated more simply. Motor conduction velocities are instead calculated from the distances and latencies between different sites of stimulation along the same nerve. Distal motor latency (DML) and not velocity expresses the time required for conduction and neuromuscular transmission following stimulation at a distal site.

The motor unit is a basic but critically important concept for understanding the neurophysiology of the peripheral nervous system. The motor unit comprises an individual motor neuron and the collection of all the muscle fibers that it innervates [3]. The innervation ratio of each motor unit (number of muscle fibers controlled by a single motor neuron) varies from less than ten muscle fibers in extraocular muscles to almost 2000 muscle fibers per neuron in explosively strong voluntary muscles such as gastrocnemius [4].

Clarifying the Clinical Question

As mentioned in the previous chapter, the most common reasons for referral for NCS/EMG are evaluation of polyneuropathy or mononeuropathy followed by evaluations of symptoms affecting multiple limbs (e.g., weakness or pain) [5].

Evaluation of the floppy infant is a less frequent but very important indication for pediatric NCS/EMG. Such cases will always require a combination of NCS and needle EMG and may in rare cases benefit from other specialized neurophysiological techniques [6, 7].

Before starting EMG/NCS, it is essential to review the presenting history with parents and the child since it will often emerge that specific tests are necessary (e.g., repetitive nerve stimulation) or that particular emphasis is required in a certain limb or region. Equally, it may emerge that the presenting problem is less complicated than first anticipated and that a focused, minimal study may suffice to answer a specific question in a given child. It is also strongly advised to conduct at least a focused physical examination before any EMG study since EMG is rarely fruitful when the clinical examination gives normal results, especially when the only complaint is of pain [8]. Taking the opportunity to communicate with the parents and child before the test also affords a chance to establish rapport with the child and parents and minimize any apprehensions regarding the test [9].

Planning the Nerve Conduction Study

Strategic planning of the NCS has been dealt with in Chap. 4. To reiterate, it is always useful to plan the study in advance and to determine the nerves that are most important to study in order to answer the referring physician's clinical question. In some cases, the exact schedule of nerves to be tested will change iteratively as the study progresses. For example, in situations where a tibial CMAP may be unexpectedly small or un recordable, it is generally advisable to move immediately to testing another motor nerve in the same limb (e.g., peroneal motor study) or to examining the contralateral limb to establish whether the finding is due to a technical fault or whether it is a sign of true pathology. When CMAPs (or SNAPs for that matter) are bilaterally absent in the lower limbs, one should move immediately to the upper limbs to try to make an intact recording there. Of course, in most clinical cases, abnormalities of the NCS may be more or less anticipated from history and examination findings; however, there will always be cases in which the first recorded (or un recorded) potentials are a surprise. In these cases, it is helpful to anchor the study by establishing at least one normal or near-normal recording, whether that is sensory or motor, upper or lower limb.

Pre-test Measurements and Considerations

Height should be measured routinely in all children since F-wave latencies (see below) are directly related to height [10–12].

The effects of temperature on NCS were discussed in detail in Chap. 4. In summary, studies should ideally be carried out in warm limbs with a skin temperature ≥32 °C for the upper extremities and ≥30 °C for the lower extremities. Cooling is associated with slowing of motor conduction velocities and increases in DML and F-wave latency [13]. There is also a broadening of duration and an increase in CMAP area at low temperatures. Whilst such effects are rarely pronounced, it is important to be aware of temperature and to consider active limb warming in situations where slow conduction velocities may mimic a demyelinating nerve pathology [14].

As previously discussed, the age of the child or newborn is an important determinant of NCS latencies and peripheral nerve conduction velocity. Term neonates have conduction velocities that are roughly half of the adult range and these mature and begin to enter the lower reaches of the typical adult range by about the end of the second year of life. Thereafter, velocities begin to plateau within the typical range for adults from around 4 or 5 years of age (see Chap. 24 for a detailed discussion of normal values) [15, 16].

Getting Started

Motor nerve conduction studies are well tolerated by most children and can be accomplished in the waking state without sedation in all but extreme cases of anxiety or tactile aversion. It is my practice to introduce motor NCS by saying that this feeling is a little bit like banging your funny bone. As long as a calm and jocular rapport can be maintained, the experience of involuntary limb movements actually turns out to be an entertaining experience and often provokes giggles from children and their parents so long as the process does not become exhaustive. In general, supramaximal stimulation at distal motor sites can be achieved in children with stimuli below 20 mA (with stimulus duration up to 0.2 ms) and it is my practice to increment to this level in 3–4 steps as tolerated. More proximal sites such as the antecubital, popliteal fossa, and axilla can require higher stimulus intensities and/or prolonged stimulus duration in some instances.

Overview of Equipment and Physiology

Readers are again referred to Chap. 4 for a more detailed discussion of NCS/EMG equipment and the basic physiology of peripheral nerve stimulation.

Some essential terminology and concepts are briefly recapitulated here. Surface electrodes are used for recording motor nerve conduction studies in children. Recording with needle electrodes can be accomplished and was performed decades ago but is rarely ever indicated today and will not be discussed further. The recording electrodes are paired and referred to as the active and the reference electrode; the active is often referred to as electrode E1 and the reference (indifferent) E2, also known as G1 and G2 in other regions of the world such as North America on account of the grid-like materials employed in making early surface electrodes. It is customary to place the active electrode over the belly of the muscle and the reference electrode over the tendon, the so-called belly-tendon montage.

Stimulating electrodes (black-cathode-negative; red-anode-positive) induce localized changes in the distribution of charge across the underlying axonal membranes at specialized sites known as the nodes of Ranvier. When the membrane potential becomes sufficiently depolarized from its resting value (−70 mV), it reaches a threshold potential (typically −55 mv) that initiates an all-or-nothing event, the action potential, during which there is a cascading influx of sodium ions through voltage gated sodium channels (Nav1.1). The action potential is terminated by inactivation of Nav1.1 and resting membrane potential is restored by the efflux of potassium and through activity of the electrogenic sodium-potassium exchange pump. Rapid and efficient conduction of action potentials is facilitated in mammalian cells by the presence of myelin, which forms myelinated internodes (of high capacitance) and unmyelinated nodes at which action potentials are regenerated in a saltatory fashion [17–19]. Stimulus durations of up to 0.2 ms are typical for study of motor NCS.

The shape of the CMAP should be diphasic with a sharp negative take-off; the peak of the response may be a simple hump (e.g., median or peroneal motor) or may be bifid (seen typically in ulnar studies of ADM muscle). In mixed or sensory nerve action potential recordings, there is often an initial positive deflection, which is attributed to G1 (E1) seeing the nerve action potential, which is modelled as a dipole with an advancing positive edge, before G2 (E2) [2]. However, in CMAP recordings the action potential should arise directly beneath the G1 electrode, which is therefore immediately negative relative to G2 resulting in an initial upward deflection. At very high gain-settings, a very small positive pre-potential may be seen which precedes CMAP onset; this is an antidromically conducted nerve action potential within the muscle but close to the recording electrodes [20]. However, if a positive deflection is apparent at conventional screen settings (2–5 mV/division), it suggests mal-positioning of the recording electrodes or alternatively over-stimulation. These points are further discussed below.

There are a number of measures and indices that derive from NCS but the essential attributes that determine the presence of nerve health or disease are size and speed. Size is primarily described by the amplitude of the CMAP in millivolts (mV). This is an index of the number of healthy motor axons lying in proximity to the stimulating electrode. CMAP amplitude is typically measured as the difference between baseline and negative peak, although some centers prefer to measure negative to positive peak values, which are typically just under twice the size. The precise method is important if utilizing reference values from another laboratory.

Speed of conduction is an index of healthy myelination of peripheral nerve but is also influenced to a small extent by the number of large diameter axons within the motor nerve. Speed of conduction can be assessed at various points along a given nerve via a combination of distal motor latency (DML), segmental motor conduction velocity (MCV), and F-wave latency.

Duration and area of the CMAP are indices that are determined by the number of conducting motor axons and the range of conduction velocities within the conducting motor axonal pool. Area is usually calculated for the positive component of the CMAP between the first and second baseline crossings. Measures of duration are again most commonly made for the negative component of the CMAP waveform although there is evidence that total CMAP duration may be a better marker in acquired demyelinating neuropathies [21]. Increased variability in motor axonal conduction velocities within a nerve leads to broadening of the duration, a phenomenon known as temporal dispersion and is a common finding in demyelinating nerve pathologies. Physiological temporal dispersion is also seen and is length dependent [22].

Late Responses

F-waves are late motor responses that occur in response to peripheral electrical stimulation. F is derived from an abbreviation for foot, although F-waves are also measurable for motor nerves in the upper limbs as well as for cranial nerves. The same stimulus that produces the direct motor or M-response is conducted antidromically along the motor nerve and triggers an efferent volley from the anterior horn cells. The latency of these responses, which varies a little between consecutive stimuli, and the number of F-waves that appear for a given number of stimuli (referred to as F-wave persistence) are features that can detect potential pathology along the proximal course of the nerve, in particular demyelinating pathology [23]. The latency of the F-wave is determined by the conduction velocity along the motor nerve and by the distance between the nerve at the point of stimulation and the spinal cord. F-wave latencies are thus directly related to height. An F-wave estimate can be derived using the formula: F-wave latency estimate = (2D/CV)*10 + 1 ms + DML [D = distance from ankle to xiphisternum (lower limb studies) or wrist to C7 spinous process (upper limb studies); CV = conduction velocity; DML = distal motor latency; 10 is a conversion factor to generate an answer in milliseconds; 1 ms is an estimate of latency within the cord] [24]. F-responses will be covered in more detail in Chap. 7.

Unlike the non-physiologic F-wave which does not cross a synapse and is not a reflex, the H-reflex (named after Hoffman) is a true monosynaptic reflex that is the neurophysiological representation of the deep tendon stretch reflex. H-reflexes are evoked by low intensity stimuli that selectively activate large diameter, low threshold sensory Ia afferents, which is equivalent to mechanical activation of the muscle spindle during the deep tendon reflex. This leads to orthodromic sensory conduction, followed by reflex activation of motor efferent fibres, producing a late motor response, the H-reflex [25]. The H-reflex is elicited most commonly in the tibial nerve by incrementing low intensity stimuli. The H-reflex, appears, grows, then attenuates and disappears as progressively increasing stimuli evoke larger M-responses, which ultimately render the motor axon refractory to the passage of the late H-reflex. The clinical significance of the H-reflex is equivalent to the presence of the ankle jerk. It is not a routine component of pediatric NCS in most instances, as it is uncomfortable and is often best performed under sedation or general anesthesia. H-reflexes are covered in more detail in Chap. 7.

A-waves (or axonal waves) are late motor potentials that are uniform in their shape and latency, and can therefore be readily distinguished from F-waves whose consecutive latencies and morphologies vary within a typically narrow range. Axonal waves are seen in axonal and demyelinating pathologies, and are often an early clue in acute inflammatory demyelinating neuropathies. It is believed that A-waves are caused by proximal axonal sprouting in reinnervated motor nerve and that they represent antidromic spread of the distal stimulus then passage along the reinnervating collateral branch to the muscle. The presence of abundant A-waves early in Guillain Barre syndrome likely represents reproducible ephaptic transmission of peripheral nerve stimuli between demyelinated axons [26].

Nerve Selection

The most common indication for pediatric EMG/NCS in the author's center, and globally it appears, is the investigation of suspected neuropathy, especially as suspected muscular dystrophies are more typically investigated with prompt genetic

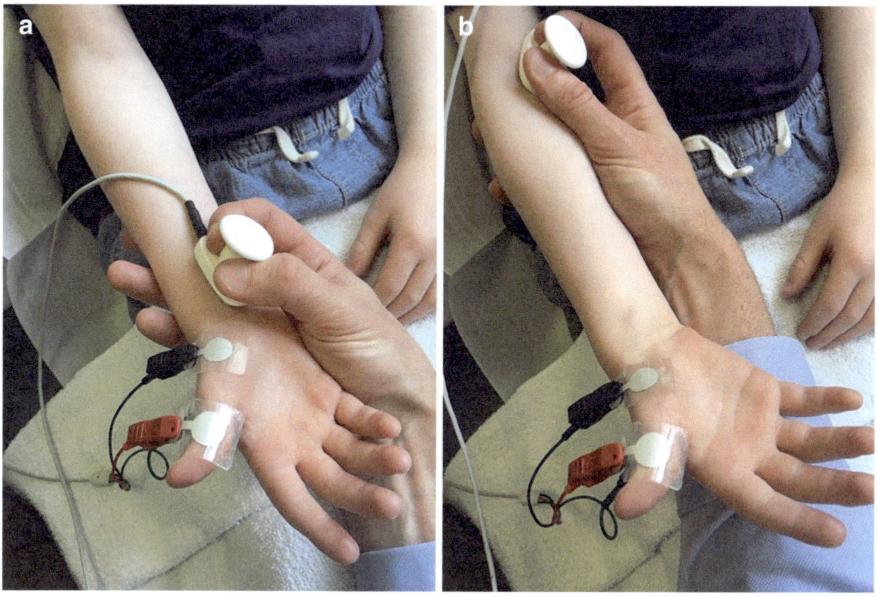

Fig. 5.1 Median motor study stimulating at the wrist (**a**) and at the antecubital fossa (**b**), recording abductor pollicis brevis (APB) muscle

testing. Ideally the study will involve sampling of sensory and motor nerves from both the upper and the lower limbs. However, if only a limited study is permissible then priority in most cases will be given to the lower limb for a question of polyneuropathy. Electrode placements for commonly studied motor nerves are illustrated in Figs. 5.1, 5.2, 5.3, 5.4, 5.5, 5.6 and 5.7 and are explained further in Table 5.1 (upper extremities and phrenic nerve) and Table 5.2 (lower extremities).

For upper limb motor NCS in babies or in older children who wriggle, my preference is to study the ulnar motor nerve (to abductor digiti minimi (ADM) or first dorsal interosseous (FDI)) instead of the median nerve when possible. This is because positioning of the recording electrodes over the thenar eminence for a median motor study is less secure and an unwilling or upset child can remove them easily by making a fist or flexing the fingers. The study can be achieved more quickly and efficiently in these cases by studying the ulnar nerve to FDI, in which the recording electrodes are located on the dorsum of the hand.

The peroneal motor study recording EDB muscle is a straightforward and easily recorded lower limb motor recording in most children. For children under 6 months it is my preference to sample the posterior tibial motor nerve to AHB; this is also a convenient choice for repetitive nerve stimulation in neonates, when required. An additional benefit of choosing the tibial motor in the very youngest and smallest of children is that it permits accurate confirmation of the course of the posterior tibial nerve behind the medial malleolus and can help to guide placement of the recording electrodes for the medial plantar sensory study. This is one situation in which I will often perform the technically easier motor study before carrying out the sensory study.

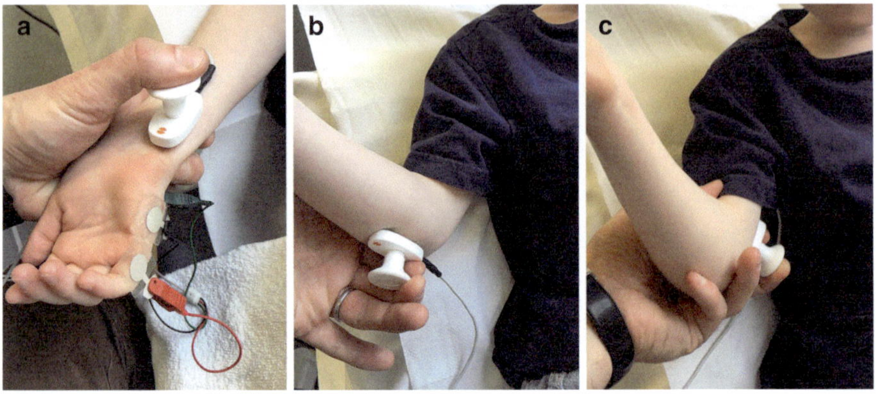

Fig. 5.2 Ulnar motor study stimulating at the wrist (**a**), below the elbow (**b**), and above the elbow (**c**), recording abductor digiti minimi (ADM) muscle

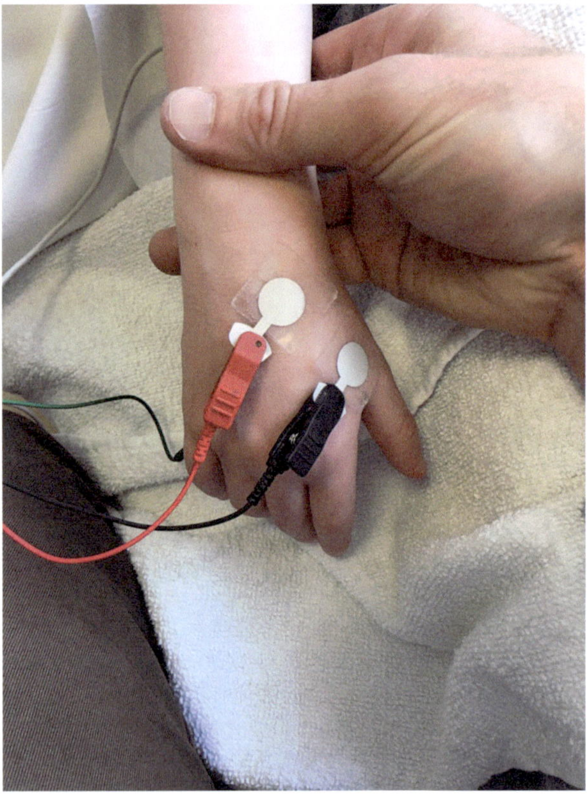

Fig. 5.3 Ulnar motor study illustrating electrode placement for recording of the first dorsal interosseous (FDI) muscle

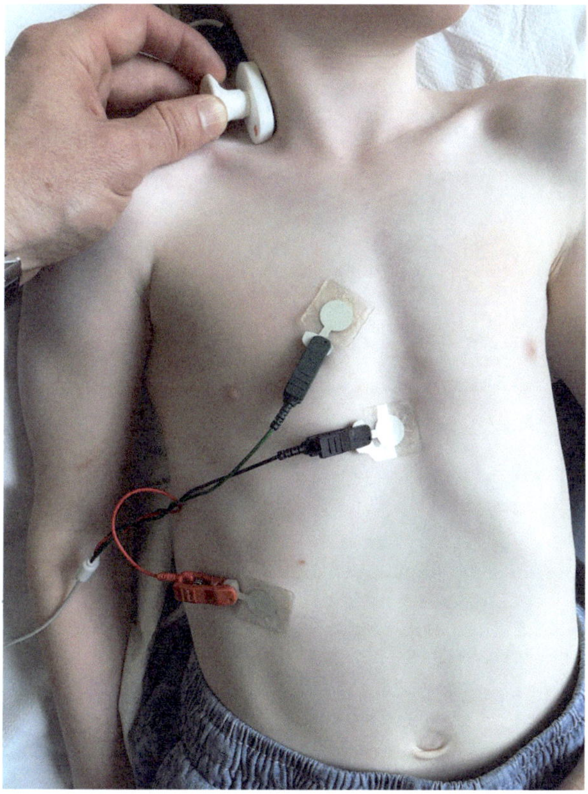

Fig. 5.4 Phrenic motor study stimulating at the neck, recording the diaphragm

Electrode Placement for Motor NCS

Recommended placements of stimulating and recording electrodes for routine pediatric studies of the limbs and trunk are presented in Table 5.1 and Figs. 5.1–5.7. In all cases an effort has been made to provide anatomical surface markings and distances to guide electrode placement. These are based on standard placement protocols in adults [27, 28]. However, the described positions utilize landmarks rather than fixed linear measures to allow for the size variability in children.

It is important to accord equal attention to placement of both the active (E1, also known as G1) and the reference (E2, also known as G2) electrodes. Although the reference is sometimes referred to as the "indifferent" electrode, it is well established that the tendon is not in fact electrically inactive. The placement of the reference has a major role in determining the morphology (whether bifid or simple) of the recorded CMAP [29].

As presented in Table 5.1, it is sometimes beneficial to choose an off-tendon site for the reference in order to achieve a sharp negative take-off for the

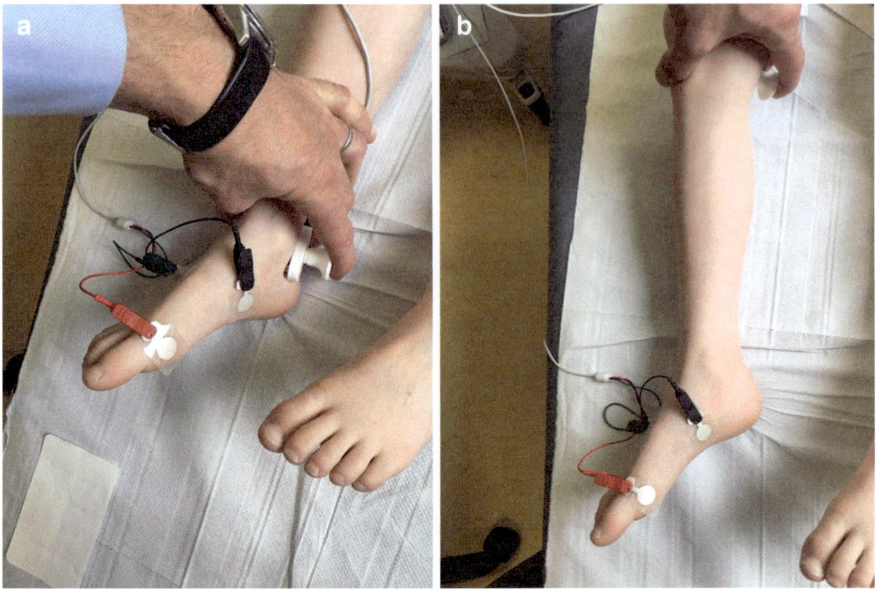

Fig. 5.5 Tibial motor study stimulating at the ankle (**a**) and popliteal fossa (**b**), recording abductor hallucis brevis (AHB) muscle

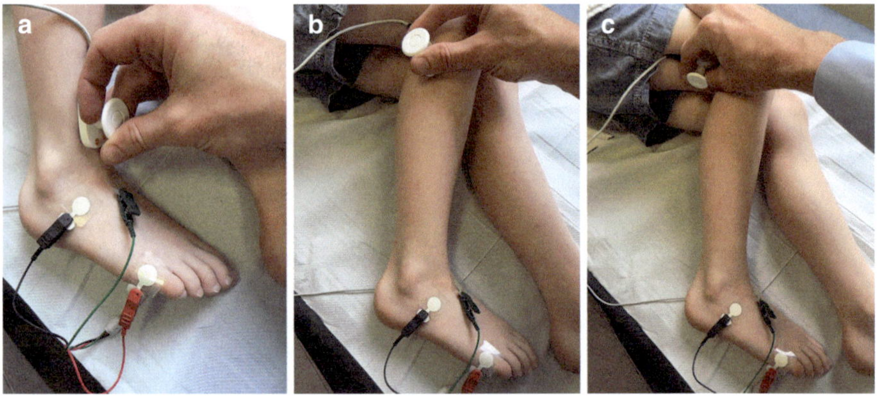

Fig. 5.6 Peroneal motor study stimulating at the ankle (**a**), below the fibular head (**b**), and popliteal fossa (**c**), recording extensor digitorum brevis (EDB) muscle

CMAP. This is notably the case for ulnar motor recording from the first dorsal interosseous muscle. It is not infrequent to observe a prominent positive deflection in FDI CMAP recordings, even when the reference is placed over the second and not the first MCP joint, which many authors report to be preferable [30]. In my experience the trapezoid bone, an off-tendon site proposed by Seror, produces sharper take off for FDI than either of the MCP sites and it is therefore my preference [31].

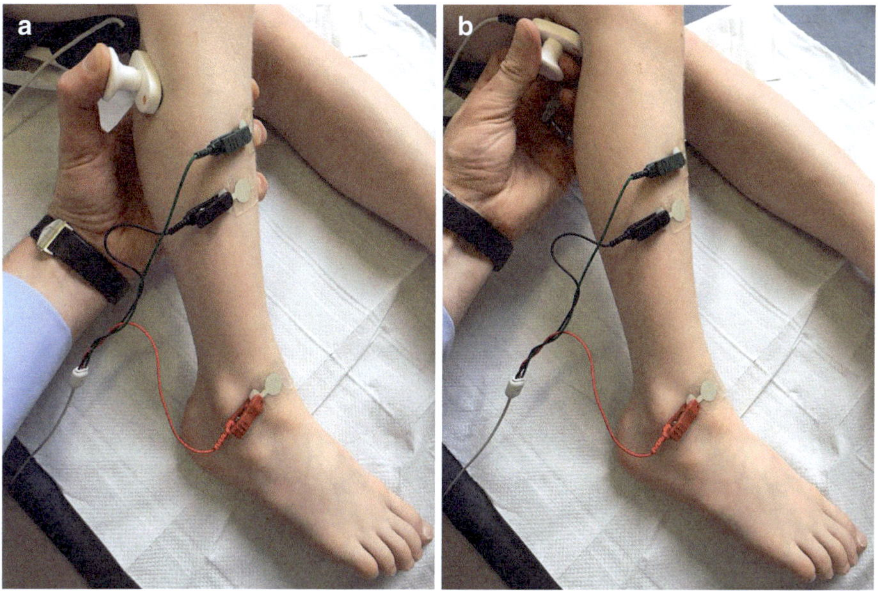

Fig. 5.7 Peroneal motor study stimulation below the fibular head (**a**) and popliteal fossa (**b**), recording tibialis anterior (TA) muscle

Table 5.1 Electrode Placement for Upper Limb and Phrenic Motor Nerve Conduction Studies

Stimulation site	Recording site
Median nerve (to abductor pollicis brevis)	
Distal stimulation site at wrist. Cathode placed at middle of proximal wrist crease (between tendons of palmaris longus and flexor carpi radialis). Proximal stimulation site at antecubital fossa. Cathode placed just medial to biceps tendon.	G1 placed over belly of APB muscle. This is midpoint of first metacarpal bone alone lateral edge of thenar eminence (care needed to ensure electrode not placed too medially or it will overlie flexor pollicis brevis). G2 is over first MCP joint.
Ulnar nerve (to abductor digiti minimi)	
Stimulator placed at the medial wrist. Cathode placed at proximal wrist crease just lateral to the flexor carpi ulnaris tendon. Proximal stimulation site (#1) on medial arm just about 5 cm distal to the ulnar styloid. Proximal stimulation site (#2) on medial, upper arm about 5 cm proximal to the ulnar styloid and in-between the belly of the biceps and triceps muscles.	G1 is placed over belly of ADM muscle which is located at the mid-point of the fifth metacarpal bone. G2 is over the fifth MCP joint.
Ulnar nerve (to first dorsal interosseous)	
Stimulator placed at the medial wrist. Cathode placed at proximal wrist crease just lateral to the flexor carpi ulnaris tendon. Proximal stimulation sites as above.	G1 is placed over belly of FDI muscle on the dorsal aspect of the first webspace. G2 is placed over the first MCP joint or alternatively over the trapezoid bone (palpable prominence proximal to the shaft of the second metacarpal).

(continued)

Table 5.1 (continued)

Stimulation site	Recording site
Radial nerve (to extensor indices proprius)	
Stimulator place on dorsolateral radius. Cathode is 8-10 cm proximal to G1 in adult limb.	G1 is placed on the belly of the EIP on the dorsal forearm, 5 cm proximal to the ulnar styloid. G2 is placed 4 cm distal to G1.
Phrenic nerve (to diaphragm)	
Stimulator is placed beneath the posterior border of the sternocleidomastoid muscle (in posterior triangle of the neck) just above the clavicle.	G1 is placed 1–2 finger breadths above the xiphisternium. G2 is placed along the anterior costal margin in a straight line above the iliac crest)[a].

[a]Distance corresponds to the 16 cm distance described in adult studies by Chen et al. (Muscle and Nerve 1995). Stimulation should be repeated if there is high amplitude ECG artifact; note that CMAP amplitude increases and duration decreases with inspiration and higher lung volumes.

Table 5.2 Electrode Placement for Lower Limb Motor Nerve Conduction Studies

Stimulation site	Recording site
Tibial nerve (to abductor hallucis)	
Distal stimulation site at ankle. Cathode placed posterior to medial malleolus. Proximal stimulation site at mid-popliteal fossa. Stimulator should be pressed firmly inward and not allowed to angle laterally so as to avoid co-stimulation of peroneal nerve.	G1 placed below navicular prominence at the mid-point between the metatarsal phalangeal (MTP) joint and heel along the medial arch of the foot. G2 is placed over the first MTP joint.
Common peroneal nerve (to extensor digitorum brevis)	
Distal stimulation site at ankle. Cathode placed over the anterior ankle, above the level of the malleoli and just lateral to the tibialis anterior tendon. Proximal stimulation site (#1) at fibular head. Cathode is placed just below the fibular head and pressed in ward such that the cathode and anode span the fibular head. Proximal stimulation site (#2) at knee. Cathode is placed laterally in the popliteal fossa so that it rests just medial to the hamstring tendon. If placed too medially and/or if high stimulation is used this can cause co-stimulation of the nearby tibial nerve.	G1 is placed over belly of EDB muscle which is usually a visible prominence in line with the inferior border of the lateral malleolus. G2 is over the fifth MCP joint.
Common peroneal nerve (to tibialis anterior)	
Stimulator sites at the fibular head and the knee as described above. In cases of suspected mononeuropathy it is particularly helpful to study contralateral side.	G1 is placed over belly of TA in the anterior-lateral leg at the junction of the upper and middle 1/3-of the leg (i.e. 1/3 of the distance between the tibial tuberosity and the inter-malleolar line). G2 is placed over the distal tibialis anterior tendon at the level of the malleoli)

The importance of standardizing placement of surface recording electrodes is emphasized by the work of Phongsamart and colleagues, which demonstrates that positioning of the reference influences not only CMAP morphology but also distal motor latencies [32].

Common Pitfalls in Stimulation and Recording

The presence of an initial positive deflection in the CMAP wave-form at conventional gain implies technical error and may be explained by one of two things. Firstly there may be mal positioning of either E1 (G1) relative to the motor-point (end-plate region) of the target muscle or there may be mal positioning of E2 (G2) leading to an abnormal electrical contribution from the reference. The second possibility is that positioning of the recording electrodes is accurate but that there is volume conduction from another source that is contaminating the recording; this occurs in situations of over-stimulation with subsequent radial spread of the stimulus to adjacent nerves (e.g., a median motor study causing co-excitation of ulnar-innervated thenar muscles because of spread of stimulus to the ulnar nerve at the wrist) [2].

Another effect of over-stimulation is longitudinal spread of the stimulus along the nerve beyond the site of the surface cathode. It is suggested that supramaximal stimulation of 15–20 mA results in longitudinal spread of stimulus current by some 3 mm, which produces depolarization at a more distal node of Ranvier. At stimuli of 60 mA (which may be required to elicit CMAPs in come demyelinating neuropathies), the extent of longitudinal spread can be as much as 12 mm; this affects latencies and alters calculations of motor conduction velocity [2].

The dangers of both radial and longitudinal spread of stimulus away from the site of the surface cathode are particularly real in children because of their smaller limbs. It is therefore required to strike a balance between using stimuli that are truly supramaximal and using stimuli that exceed this and which spread elsewhere. As a general rule, in the absence of demyelinating neuropathy, stimulus intensities of >50 mA can be avoided in almost all children unless it is required to stimulate very proximal sites such as Erb's point, or the phrenic nerve in the neck; neither is a routine site of stimulation in children.

The possibility of under-stimulation in pediatric NCS is another potential pitfall, as in adults, but the risk of this occurring is higher in some pediatric situations when the child becomes uncomfortable and the neurophysiologist is tempted to rush through the nerve conduction studies and avoid escalating the distress. Under-stimulation can occur when the given stimulus is too low or when it is off-target with respect to the underlying motor nerve as may happen, for example, if the child is moving during the test. The consequence of under-stimulation is to give the impression of abnormally low CMAP amplitudes or to create an impression of motor conduction block (see below).

As discussed in Chap. 4, the small distances involved in pediatric EMG will also increase the likelihood and scale of error related to over- or under-measurement of distances for calculation of velocities. For this reason, the examiner must be consistent with positioning of the limbs (e.g., right angled measurement of ulnar motor nerve conduction around the elbow) in all cases.

It is important to be aware that marked drops (21–43%) in tibial CMAP amplitude from abductor hallucis normally occur between distal and proximal stimulation sites of stimulation. This is a product of phase cancellation and physiological temporal dispersion and should not be misinterpreted as motor conduction block without evidence of demyelination from other nerves [33]. The phenomenon is less marked in children, particularly in the very young where the distances between proximal and distal stimulation are relatively short. The second point is that for lower limb F-wave measurement it is best to choose the tibial and not the peroneal motor nerve, in which F-waves are harder to elicit without recourse to very high supramaximal stimuli.

Interpreting the Data

Interpreting Low Amplitude CMAPs

Having excluded technical artifact, the finding of reduced CMAP amplitudes can imply a range of physiological causes, some common, some quite rare. For simplicity these can be divided into those that derive from nerve, from the NMJ or from the muscle.

The first, and commonest implication of low CMAP amplitude is the presence of motor axonal loss, which occurs in pathologies of the motor neuron such as the spinal muscular atrophies (SMA) and in pathologies affecting the peripheral nerve [34]. It should be noted that normality of strength and CMAP amplitude can be maintained in the setting of established denervation, so long as the processes of reinnervation and motor unit enlargement are sufficient to compensate for motor neuronal loss. Therefore, CMAP amplitude reductions are not as sensitive to the presence of denervating pathologies as is needle EMG examination (see Chap. 9 on muscle analysis).

Motor nerve conduction block is another nerve-mediated mechanism for pathologically diminished CMAP amplitudes. In this case, the motor neuronal number may be normal but a segmental peripheral myelinopathy produces conduction failure in a portion of stimulated fibres such that a significant proportion of single motor unit potentials fail to get through to the muscle [35, 36]. This leads to a drop in the CMAP amplitude upon proximal stimulation, with a 50% or greater reduction considered to be significant. A rare but related mechanism for low CMAP amplitudes is that seen in congenital hypomyelinating neuropathies in which severe failure of myelination can result in staggeringly high thresholds for peripheral nerve stimulation. In such situations, CMAPs may appear to be absent at conventional stimulus intensities but they are in fact present when stimulus intensity is increased.

Neuromuscular junction (NMJ) disorders are a comparatively less common cause of diminished CMAP amplitude. Pre-synaptic disorders including infantile botulism and (very rarely in children) Lambert Eaton syndrome are often associated with low amplitude CMAPs [37–39]. The cardinal neurophysiological feature of presynaptic NMJ disorders is the marked increment in CMAP amplitude (at least 200% increase) produced by high frequency (20–50 Hz) supramaximal repetitive stimulation. Post synaptic weakness can occur in the context of neuromuscular blocking agents (NMBAs) such as vecuronium. The scenario of sustained weakness attributable to NMBAs is most likely among neonates, in whom the drug effects can be prolonged, especially in the context of impaired renal clearance and/or co-administration of aminoglycosides [40].

Finally, CMAP amplitudes are often normal in early stages of primary muscle disease, but low amplitude CMAPs can be seen impressively in the context of episodic muscle weakness due to the muscle channelopathies such as the periodic paralyses [41, 42]. In these disorders, routine nerve conduction studies are normal between attacks but CMAPs can be low or even un-recordable during an acute attack.

Where CMAP amplitudes are pathologically reduced, the pattern of reduction and co-existing sensory abnormality are two important clues which guide accurate interpretation. Peripheral neuropathies of the axonal type generally affect sensory and motor nerve and cause a typically length dependent pattern of motor and sensory axonal loss such that CMAP and SNAP amplitude reductions will be first and most evident in the distal lower extremities [43]. Asymmetric, and or non-length dependent CMAP reductions (with co-existing SNAP abnormality) can be seen in the context of demyelinating neuropathies (e.g. hereditary neuropathy with liability to pressure palsies (HNPP) and chronic inflammatory demyelinating polyradiculoneuropathy (CIDP), in vincristine-related neuropathy in children and in mononeuritis multiplex attributable to vasculitic nerve injuries [44, 45]. Reductions in CMAP amplitudes accompanied by sparing of SNAP amplitudes represent the hallmark of pre-ganglionic motor neuronal or nerve root injuries. This pattern can be seen in widespread anterior horn cell disorders such as SMA or in regionalized variants such as Hirayama disease, monomelic amyotrophy, and Hopkin's syndrome [46–48].

Interpreting Abnormalities of Latency and Conduction Velocity

Minor reductions in MCV are typical in any cause of motor axonal loss. This is because when significant numbers of large diameter motor axons are lost, a proportion of the loss will affect the fastest conducting fibers and therefore the onset latency of the CMAP is likely to be marginally delayed. As a rule, however, motor conduction velocity slowing attributable to motor axonal loss should not exceed

130% of the upper range for DML and never fall below 75% of the lower limit of normal for conduction velocity. It is particularly important in cases of slowed conduction due to motor axonal loss to insure adequate warming of limbs, since the effect of cooling in such situations might result in velocities appearing to dip into the demyelinating range.

Demyelinating peripheral neuropathies classically cause slowing of motor conduction velocity (<90% of LLN), increase in DML (>115% ULN), and increased latency or absence of F-waves (>125% ULN) [49]. The degree of slowing varies with severity of the neuropathy and is further increased by co-existing motor axonal losses.

Increased duration of the CMAP is caused by the greater variability in individual motor axonal velocities within the demyelinated nerve and is referred to as temporal dispersion. Temporal dispersion results in an associated reduction in CMAP amplitude but not area and should not be confused with motor conduction block in which both area and amplitude are diminished without change in CMAP duration.

The distribution of slowing provides essential clues for determining the nature of nerve pathology. Mononeuropathies are typically isolated but may be multiple and if so should prompt consideration of HNPP. Acquired inflammatory demyelinating neuropathies usually have evidence of involvement in both the upper and lower limbs and often the face. Variants such as Lewis Sumner syndrome are more likely to be asymmetrical and upper limb predominant.

The distinction between uniform and non-uniform slowing of nerve conduction is an important one, though the concept has become more complex in recent years. Traditionally, uniform slowing was associated with inherited demyelinating neuropathies such as Charcot-Marie-Tooth disease (CMT) and non-uniform slowing with acquired demyelinating neuropathies such as chronic inflammatory demyelinating polyradiculoneuropathy (CIDP). For example, CMT type 1 will typically feature uniform motor conduction slowing; median MCV is less than 38 m/s by the time of presentation of classical CMT1A in late childhood or adolescence [50]. When the clinical presentation is at an earlier age, hereditary demyelinating neuropathies should be assessed cautiously and with reference to age-adjusted laboratory norms. In recent years, a number of cases of inherited diseases such as metachromatic leukodystrophy associated with non-uniform slowing have accumulated in the literature, suggesting a more nuanced interpretation of these features. A detailed review on this topic and on hereditary axonal neuropathies of early life is provided by Yiu and Ryan [51, 52].

Summary

In summary, motor NCS are technically straightforward if undertaken carefully in children and provide important information that is helpful in the diagnosis and delineation of axonal and demyelinating neuropathies.

Myelination of peripheral nerve is a progressive process in children and conduction velocities do not fully reach adult ranges until 4 or 5 years of age.

Most abnormalities of CMAP amplitude imply motor axonal loss or motor conduction block but rarely neuromuscular junction or muscle pathologies should be considered.

References

1. Kimura J. Facts, fallacies, and fancies of nerve conduction studies: twenty-first annual Edward H. Lambert Lecture. Muscle Nerve. 1997;20(7):777–87.
2. Dumitru D, DeLisa JA. AAEM Minimonograph #10: volume conduction. Muscle Nerve. 1991;14(7):605–24.
3. Eccles JC, Sherrington CS. Numbers and contraction values of individual motor-units examined in some muscles of the limb. Proceedings of The Royal Society. 1930;106: 326–57.
4. Feinstein B, Lindegard B, Nyman E, Wohlfart G. Morphologic studies of motor units in normal human muscles. Acta Anat (Basel). 1955;23(2):127–42.
5. Karakis I, Liew W, Darras BT, Jones HR, Kang PB. Referral and diagnostic trends in pediatric electromyography in the molecular era. Muscle Nerve. 2014;50(2):244–9.
6. Jones HR. EMG evaluation of the floppy infant: differential diagnosis and technical aspects. Muscle Nerve. 1990;13(4):338–47.
7. Bodensteiner JB. The evaluation of the hypotonic infant. Semin Pediatr Neurol. 2008;15(1): 10–20.
8. Payan J. Clinical electromyography in infancy and childhood. In: Brett EM, editor. Paediatric neurology. 3rd ed. Great Britain: Churchill Livingstone; 1997. p. 823–54.
9. Pitt MC. Nerve conduction studies and needle EMG in very small children. Eur J Paediatr Neurol. 2012;16(3):285–91.
10. Mchugh JC, Connolly S. Correction and transformation of normative neurophysiological data: is there added value in the diagnosis of distal symmetrical peripheral neuropathy? Muscle Nerve. 2011;44(6):890–6.
11. Miller RG, Kuntz NL. Nerve conduction studies in infants and children. J Child Neurol. 1986;1(1):19–26.
12. Puksa L, Eeg-Olofsson KE, Stålberg E, Falck B. Reference values for F wave parameters in healthy 3-20 year old subjects. Clin Neurophysiol. 2011;122(1):199–204.
13. Denys EH. AAEM minimonograph #14: the influence of temperature in clinical neurophysiology. Muscle Nerve. 1991;14(9):795–811.
14. Franssen H, Wieneke GH. Nerve conduction and temperature: necessary warming time. Muscle Nerve. 1994;17(3):336–44.
15. Gamstorp I. Conduction velocity of peripheral nerves and electromyography in infants and children. Psychiatr Neurol Med Psychol Beih. 1970;13-14:235–44.
16. Raimbault J. Les conductions nerveuses chez l'enfant normal. Paris: Expansion Scientifique Francaise; 1988.
17. Hodgkin AL, Huxley AF, Katz B. Measurement of current-voltage relations in the membrane of the giant axon of Loligo. J Physiol. 1952;116(4):424–48.
18. Hodgkin AL, Huxley AF. Movement of sodium and potassium ions during nervous activity. Cold Spring Harb Symp Quant Biol. 1952;17:43–52.
19. Burke D, Kiernan MC, Bostock H. Excitability of human axons. Clin Neurophysiol. 2001;112(9):1575–85.
20. Dumitru D, Walsh NE, Ramamurthy S. The premotor potential. Arch Phys Med Rehabil. 1989;70(7):537–40.

21. Lagarde J, Viala K, Fournier E. Is total duration of distal compound muscle action potential better than negative peak duration in the diagnosis of chronic inflammatory demyelinating polyneuropathy? Muscle Nerve. 2014;49(6):895–9.
22. Schulte-Mattler WJ, Müller T, Georgiadis D, Kornhuber ME, Zierz S. Length dependence of variables associated with temporal dispersion in human motor nerves. Muscle Nerve. 2001;24(4):527–33.
23. Kimura J. Current understanding of F-wave physiology in the clinical domain. Suppl Clin Neurophysiol. 2006;59:299–303.
24. Preston DC, Shapiro BE. Electromyography and neuromuscular disorders: clinical-electrophysiologic correlations. 2nd ed. Philadelphia: Elsevier Butterworth-Heinemann; 2005.
25. Misiaszek JE. The H-reflex as a tool in neurophysiology: its limitations and uses in understanding nervous system function. Muscle Nerve. 2003;28(2):144–60.
26. Kawakami S, Sonoo M, Kadoya A, Chiba A, Shimizu T. A-waves in Guillain-Barré syndrome: correlation with electrophysiological subtypes and antiganglioside antibodies. Clin Neurophysiol. 2012;123(6):1234–41.
27. Kimura J. Electrodiagnosis in diseases of nerve and muscle: principles and practice. 4th ed. Oxford: Oxford University Press; 2013.
28. Buschbacher RM, Kumbhare DA, Robinson LR. Buschbacher's manual of nerve conduction studies, vol. xiv. Third ed. New York: Demos Medical; 2016. p. 299.
29. Kincaid JC, Brashear A, Markand ON. The influence of the reference electrode on CMAP configuration. Muscle Nerve. 1993;16(4):392–6.
30. Kim DH. Ulnar nerve conduction study of the first dorsal interosseous muscle in korean subjects. Ann Rehabil Med. 2011;35(5):658–63.
31. Seror P, Maisonobe T, Bouche P. A new electrode placement for recording the compound motor action potential of the first dorsal interosseous muscle. Neurophysiol Clin. 2011;41(4):173–80.
32. Phongsamart G, Wertsch JJ, Ferdjallah M, King JC, Foster DT. Effect of reference electrode position on the compound muscle action potential (CMAP) onset latency. Muscle Nerve. 2002;25(6):816–21.
33. Barkhaus PE, Kincaid JC, Nandedkar SD. Tibial motor nerve conduction studies: an investigation into the mechanism for amplitude drop of the proximal evoked response. Muscle Nerve. 2011;44(5):776–82.
34. Bromberg MB, Swoboda KJ. Motor unit number estimation in infants and children with spinal muscular atrophy. Muscle Nerve. 2002;25(3):445–7.
35. Kokubun N, Nishibayashi M, Uncini A, Odaka M, Hirata K, Yuki N. Conduction block in acute motor axonal neuropathy. Brain. 2010;133(10):2897–908.
36. Olney RK, Medicine AAoE. Guidelines in electrodiagnostic medicine. Consensus criteria for the diagnosis of partial conduction block. Muscle Nerve Suppl. 1999;8:S225–9.
37. Morgan-Followell B, de Los Reyes E. Child neurology: diagnosis of Lambert-Eaton myasthenic syndrome in children. Neurology. 2013;80(21):e220–2.
38. Hajjar M, Markowitz J, Darras BT, Kissel JT, Srinivasan J, Jones HR. Lambert-Eaton syndrome, an unrecognized treatable pediatric neuromuscular disorder: three patients and literature review. Pediatr Neurol. 2014;50(1):11–7.
39. Tseng-Ong L, Mitchell WG. Infant botulism: 20 years' experience at a single institution. J Child Neurol. 2007;22(12):1333–7.
40. Sahni M, Richardson CJ, Jain SK. Sustained neuromuscular blockade after vecuronium use in a premature infant. AJP Rep. 2015;5(2):e121–3.
41. Tan SV, Matthews E, Barber M, Burge JA, Rajakulendran S, Fialho D, et al. Refined exercise testing can aid DNA-based diagnosis in muscle channelopathies. Ann Neurol. 2011;69(2):328–40.
42. Yoshinaga H, Sakoda S, Shibata T, Akiyama T, Oka M, Yuan JH, et al. Phenotypic variability in childhood of skeletal muscle sodium channelopathies. Pediatr Neurol. 2015;52(5):504–8.
43. Donofrio PD, Albers JW. AAEM minimonograph #34: polyneuropathy: classification by nerve conduction studies and electromyography. Muscle Nerve. 1990;13(10):889–903.

44. Courtemanche H, Magot A, Ollivier Y, Rialland F, Leclair-Visonneau L, Fayet G, et al. Vincristine-induced neuropathy: atypical electrophysiological patterns in children. Muscle Nerve. 2015;52(6):981–5.
45. McMillan HJ, Kang PB, Jones HR, Darras BT. Childhood chronic inflammatory demyelinating polyradiculoneuropathy: combined analysis of a large cohort and eleven published series. Neuromuscul Disord. 2013;23(2):103–11.
46. Cantarín-Extremera V, González-Gutiérrez-Solana L, Ramírez-Orellana M, López-Marín L, Duat-Rodríguez A, Ruíz-Falcó-Rojas ML. Immune-mediated mechanisms in the pathogenesis of Hopkins syndrome. Pediatr Neurol. 2012;47(5):373–4.
47. Yavuz H. A proposal for the definition of Hirayama disease and monomelic amyotrophy. J Child Neurol. 2012;27(6):815–6. author reply 7-8
48. McMillan HJ, Darras BT, Kang PB, Saleh F, Jones HR. Pediatric monomelic amyotrophy: evidence for poliomyelitis in vulnerable populations. Muscle Nerve. 2009;40(5):860–3.
49. Albers JW, Kelly JJ. Acquired inflammatory demyelinating polyneuropathies: clinical and electrodiagnostic features. Muscle Nerve. 1989;12(6):435–51.
50. Reilly MM, Hanna MG. Genetic neuromuscular disease. J Neurol Neurosurg Psychiatry. 2002;73(Suppl 2):II12–21.
51. Yiu EM, Ryan MM. Genetic axonal neuropathies and neuronopathies of pre-natal and infantile onset. J Peripher Nerv Syst. 2012;17(3):285–300.
52. Yiu EM, Ryan MM. Demyelinating prenatal and infantile developmental neuropathies. J Peripher Nerv Syst. 2012;17(1):32–52.

Chapter 6
Repetitive Nerve Stimulation, Short and Long Exercise Tests

Susana Quijano-Roy and Cyril Gitiaux

Introduction

Repetitive nerve stimulation and exercise testing are useful in the evaluation of patients with suspected disorders of the neuromuscular junction (NMJ) and muscle membrane excitability. They can be very helpful in the diagnosis of specific disorders such as myasthenia gravis, Lambert-Eaton myasthenic syndrome, and botulism, as well as congenital myasthenic syndromes and rare disorders of skeletal muscle membrane excitability, including paramyotonia congenita, myotonia congenita, and the periodic paralyses [1–6].

Disorders of the Neuromuscular Junction

Genetic or acquired disorders may impair neuromuscular junction (NMJ) transmission, leading to hypotonia, weakness and/or fatigability [1]. NMJ disorders, particularly those due to genetic causes, are probably underdiagnosed due to their clinical overlap with other more common neuromuscular disorders. Nevertheless, they constitute important causes of weakness, and accurate diagnosis is of extraordinary value because of the risk of life-threatening complications (primarily respiratory)

S. Quijano-Roy, M.D., Ph.D. (✉)
Unité de Maladies Neuromusculaires, Service de Neurologie,
Réeducation et Réanimation Pédiatriques, AP-HP, Hôpital R. Poincaré,
Hôpitaux Universitaires Paris-Ile-de-France-Ouest, (U1179- INSERM-UVSQ),
Université de Versailles, Garches, 92380 France
e-mail: susana.quijano-roy@aphp.fr

C. Gitiaux, M.D., Ph.D.
Department of Neurophysiology, Reference Center for Neuromuscular Diseases,
Paris Descartes University, Necker Enfants Malades Hospital, Paris, France

© Springer International Publishing AG 2017
H.J. McMillan, P.B. Kang (eds.), *Pediatric Electromyography*,
DOI 10.1007/978-3-319-61361-1_6

and the possibility of selecting specific drugs for specific diseases or even subtypes of diseases [7–10]. Whenever a peripheral nervous system disorder is suspected and other more common diseases of the motor unit (muscle, nerve, anterior horn) have been ruled out, consideration should be given to the exploration of potential disorders of the NMJ [11, 12].

Certain abnormalities, when found in standard nerve conduction studies (e.g., double motor responses, low motor amplitudes), may be of great value in narrowing the differential diagnosis to specific syndromes. For example, double motor responses are indicative of slow channel congenital myasthenic syndromes. Low compound motor action potential (CMAP) amplitudes showing facilitation after a short burst of exercise is indicative of pre-synaptic disorders such as Lambert-Eaton myasthenic syndrome (LEMS) [13–16]. Repetitive CMAPs are an electrophysiological feature of cholinergic toxicity that can be a seen with the use of acetylcholinesterase inhibitors in myasthenia gravis [17]. The neurophysiologist should take into account that although less frequent, myasthenic patients may mimic other motor unit disorders, in particular myopathies, and therefore NMJ tests should be considered during evaluations for possible myopathy, especially if studies such as muscle biopsy and muscle imaging reveal non-specific or non-contributory findings. Genetic advances in recent decades have revealed several neuromuscular disorders, originally believed to affect a single component of the motor unit such as the nerve or muscle, to also show abnormalities of the neuromuscular junction [18–21].

Electrodiagnostic studies may be particularly useful for exploring the neuromuscular junction, but it is important to remember that these tests sometimes have limited sensitivity and may present unique technical challenges in children. Stimulated single fibre EMG (SSFEMG) studies have shown a high sensitivity for detecting NMJ defects, and are relatively easy to perform across the entire range of the pediatric population in specialized laboratories that experience a high volume of such studies [22, 23]. Recent data suggest a role for SSFEMG studies in developing a prognosis for myasthenia gravis [24]. However, SSFEMG techniques are not specific for NMJ disorders and may be abnormal in other diseases, particularly those affecting the anterior horn cell [25].

More specific studies for NMJ disorders are based on the repetitive stimulation of motor nerves at supramaximal intensities, at variable frequencies, and when the occasion calls for it, after exercise as well. Low frequency repetitive stimulation (less than 10 Hz, but typically 2 or 3 Hz) may lead to a significant decrement of CMAP amplitudes, traditionally defined as a drop of at least 10% by the fourth or fifth stimulation in most types of myasthenic syndromes [4, 6, 26], while incremental responses may develop when high frequency (greater than 10 Hz, but typically 20–50 Hz) repetitive nerve stimulation is performed in presynaptic syndromes with low CMAPs [16]. Slow repetitive nerve stimulation after prolonged sub-tetanic repetitive nerve stimulation (rapid stimulation for several minutes) may elicit a "hidden" decremental response in certain forms of congenital myasthenic syndromes such as choline acetyltransferase deficiency in infants with episodic apnea [12, 27].

As results are highly influenced by factors such as patient positioning, pre- or post-exercise status, and temperature, accurate repetitive stimulation studies require excellent technical expertise. These factors, together with the relative discomfort associated with repetitive stimulation in an anxious child, make it often challenging to perform in young children. The neurophysiologist must pay particular attention to the way the examination is planned, maintain an empathic approach when working with children, and prioritize the specific tests and sites of study based upon information obtained from the clinical history and neurological examination [28]. The size of the electrodes has to be taken also into account in newborns or young infants as well as ensuring that limb temperature is monitored and controlled to avoid introducing artifacts. In some cases, sedation or anesthesia may be necessary to obtain interpretable data.

In summary, neurophysiology studies are useful to confirm or reject the clinical diagnosis, to exclude other concomitant neuromuscular diseases, to establish whether the process is pre- or post-synaptic, to monitor the clinical course of the disease (for both untreated cases and those that have been treated with specific medical or surgical interventions), to enable the physician to determine the status of neuromuscular transmission in cases of clinical remission, and to detect subclinical dysfunction of the neuromuscular junction.

Physiology of Neuromuscular Transmission

The main aspects of the complex ultra-structure, physiology and biochemical mechanisms of transmission within the neuromuscular junction have been elucidated (see Chap. 2). There are different elements and steps which play critical roles and their dysfunction may lead to neuromuscular disturbances that can be functionally studied by repetitive stimulation at different frequencies and by the responses after different exercise tests. These processes may be influenced by drugs and therefore the results of the EMG may have not only diagnostic implications but also guide the choice of medications.

Globally, the action potential arrives at the terminal bouton from the axon (presynaptic region) and triggers, via voltage gated calcium channels, the release of acetylcholine (ACh) into the synaptic space. ACh then diffuses across the synaptic cleft and binds to ACh receptors (AChRs) on the postsynaptic muscle membrane. The postsynaptic membrane is composed of numerous junctional folds, dramatically increasing the effective surface area of the membrane, with AChRs clustered on the crests of the folds. Subsequently, binding of ACh to these receptors leads to the generation of a new action potential within the end plate that propagates through the muscle fiber to trigger excitation-contraction coupling via changes in intracellular calcium concentrations and changes in the configuration of the contractile filaments. Therefore, the NMJ essentially forms an electrical–chemical–electrical link between nerve and muscle, where the chemical neurotransmitter at the NMJ is ACh.

In the synaptic cleft, ACh is broken down by the enzyme acetylcholinesterase, and the choline subsequently is taken up into the presynaptic terminal to be repackaged into ACh. Acetylcholine is stored in units known as 'quanta', within vesicles in the terminal bouton. There are 10,000 molecules of ACh per quanta. The vesicles

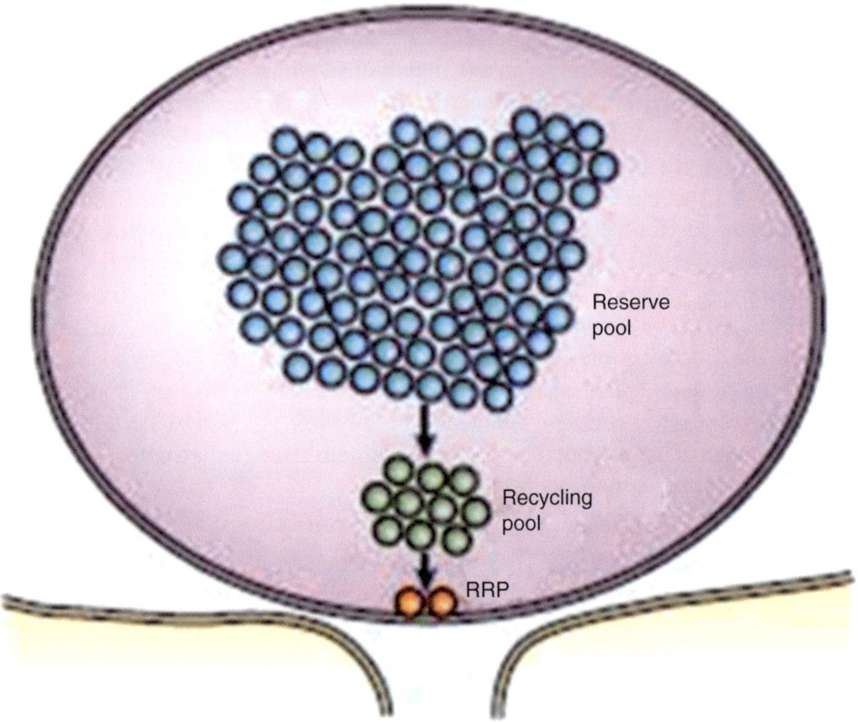

Fig. 6.1 Populations of ACh vesicles in the terminal nerve space (RRP: rapid release pool, recycling pool, reserve pool)

localize at different distances from the synaptic space (Fig. 6.1). Those vesicles that are immediately accessible beneath the presynaptic nerve terminal membrane constitute the readily releasable primary store, containing approximately 1000 quanta. Those that are mobilizable number approximately 10,000 quanta and can replenish the primary store within a few seconds. Finally, there is a reserve store of more than 100,000 quanta, which are found far from the NMJ in the axon and cell body [6, 29].

Released ACh binds to receptors (AChRs) on the post-synaptic membrane (two molecules can bind to each receptor). AChRs are sodium channels, and ACh binding produces a local depolarization or change in conductance of the postsynaptic membrane. This local depolarization of the muscle membrane is referred to as an excitatory postsynaptic potential or an *endplate potential (EPP)*. The depolarization of one AChR does not generate a sufficient EPP to generate a postsyaptic action potential. This is important since, even in the absence of synaptic transmission there is a baseline spontaneous release of a small number of vesicles (1–5/s) which leads to tiny postsynaptic depolarizations called miniature endplate potentials that are of no physiologic significance.

The change in membrane potential associated with each EPP will decrease with time and distance. Just like the ripples caused by a stone dropped into water the size of each ripple decreases as it spreads outwards until it eventually disappears. However adjacent EPPs are additive or summative when they occur simultaneously. The larger the number of ACh-bound receptors the greater the total EPP. Eventually a critical level of depolarization is reached, known as the *threshold potential*. When the threshold is surpassed at the endplate, an action potential is triggered in the muscle fiber.

To ensure that NM transmission occurs reliably, the endplate depolarization that is typically induced is usually much higher than this threshold. The excess of amplitude is called the *safety factor*. This amplitude depends on the quantity of synthesis and exocytosis of ACh and on the state of the ACh receptors. In newborns and premature infants, the safety factor of the endplate is reduced due to immaturity of the NMJ. They generate fewer endplate potentials, less quanta inside the vesicles, and prolonged durations of the individual endplate potentials and of the total endplate potential [29].

Repetitive Nerve Stimulation (RNS) Tests

Repetitive stimulation (RNS) of a nerve mimics certain types of exercise and modifies the safety factor of the NMJ. This phenomenon can be used to explore different types of abnormalities affecting the NMJ. In the setting of disorders of the neuromuscular junction, repetitive stimulation of a motor nerve may trigger a decrement or facilitation in the amplitudes of successive compound motor action potentials, the exact response depending in large part on the frequency of the stimulations [26, 30]. RNS may be performed at low frequencies (2–3 Hz) for a train of 6–10 supramaximal responses or at high frequencies (20–50 Hz) for a few seconds or minutes; 10 Hz is generally regarded as the boundary between low and high frequency, but to avoid ambiguity regarding the expected response, repetitive stimulation is rarely performed at 10 Hz. The results of RNS may be influenced by short (10 s) or long (1 or more minutes) exercise. It is difficult to elicit satisfactory voluntary sustained muscle contraction in infants and younger children. In children with suspected MG, RNS at rest is usually sufficient and any tolerance a child may have for additional testing should be used to examine other muscle-nerve combinations rather than post-exercise testing of a limited selection [31]. A short train of high frequency (20-50 Hz) repetitive stimulation for 1–2 s is generally regarded as mimicking brief maximal exercise and is typically followed by a standard train of low-frequency repetitive stimulation at 2–3 Hz; however, even a short duration of high frequency stimulation is quite uncomfortable, and in children conscious sedation or general anesthesia is generally regarded as being required for any high-frequency repetitive stimulation.

The choice of the sites examined is a key factor, and it is important to explore a broad range of anatomical sites, bilaterally when possible [32]. Examining those muscles that are clinically weak at the time of testing should be prioritized as that strategy will increase the yield of testing. The most accessible nerve-muscle pairs to study are in the limbs, including ulnar nerve recording abductor digiti minimi (ADM), the most commonly studied extremity site; median nerve to abductor pollicis brevis (APB); and peroneal nerve to extensor digitorum brevis (EDB) or tibialis anterior (TA). However, these sites may be less sensitive to abnormalities due to the topography of the symptoms or to the lower temperature of the limbs compared to more proximal muscles. To increase the yield, the neurophysiologist should ensure that the limbs have been adequately warmed prior to testing. Movement artifacts are also more likely to happen in the limbs and therefore a gentle stabilization of the extremity with reassurance and distraction are usually necessary to reduce the chances of the child introducing artifact by pulling away or flinching. Standardized stabilization bands for the stimulation electrode may be used to prevent slippage of the stimulator. Certain muscles sometimes studied in adults are too small to be examined in young children (e.g., anconeus) [28, 32]. Ulnar nerve studies recording ADM are less technically challenging and less prone to the introduction of artifact, particularly in a cooperative patient.

Examination of more proximal nerve-muscle pairs such as spinal accessory nerve recording trapezius and facial nerve recording nasalis, frontalis, or orbicularis oculi often will have a higher yield and should be included in the set of repetitive nerve stimulation studies whenever possible. Spinal accessory nerve stimulation to the trapezius is best performed by placing the recording (G1) electrode on the thicker bulk of the muscle (half way between the neck and the acromion process). This is a simple and useful test because the nerve is very accessible in the upper border of the sternocleidomastoid muscle in the neck and supramaximal stimulation can typically be reached at low stimulation intensities. A comfortable position may be obtained if the child is lying supine, with a slight elevation of the head on a pillow and the neck turned towards the contralateral side facing a parent, who may help distract and calm the child while stabilizing the head. Gentle stabilization of the shoulders and trunk may also be necessary. For facial nerve recordings, stimulation is performed in the pre-auricular area and the recording electrode may be placed on the nasal muscles (lateral to the nose), on the lateral orbicularis oculi muscle, or sometimes frontalis. Facial nerve studies may be difficult to interpret in children as compound motor amplitude potentials (CMAPs) tend to be quite small (sometimes well below 1 mV), which can present technical challenges when attempting to track CMAP amplitudes serially. Younger children may not tolerate repetitive stimulation at these sites as well as the extremity sites. However, since proximal muscles are often involved early and more severely in some disorders of neuromuscular transmission (e.g., juvenile myasthenia gravis), proximal sites are often important to check, especially if bulbar or facial symptoms are present [26].

Other recording sites may be of particular interest in certain settings, including the phrenic nerve in the ICU or in mechanically ventilated patients [33], and the hypoglossal nerve [34]. In addition to temperature and movement artifacts, other technical factors should be considered. Treatments that enhance the function of the neuromuscular junction, in particular acetylcholinesterase inhibitors, should be held for at least 6 h prior to RNS testing to maximize the potential diagnostic yield. It is important to remember that normal RNS does not always exclude a NMJ disorder, especially for specific subcategories such as ocular juvenile myasthenia gravis. Single fiber EMG is more sensitive for some disorders of neuromuscular transmission and will be discussed in Chap. 10.

Low Frequency (Slow) Repetitive Nerve Stimulation

Low frequency (also known as slow) RNS is performed at 2 or 3 Hz. The amplitudes of the negative phase of the first and fourth compound motor action potentials (CMAP) are measured from baseline to negative peak, and the percent change of the fourth response compared with the first is defined as the decrement or increment. A CMAP decrement of greater than 10% is accepted as abnormal, assuming that a smooth progression of the response amplitude train and reproducibility are present. Children may tolerate the studies better when the number of stimuli per train are limited. One popular protocol consists of trains of 6 stimuli at 2 Hz.

A normal recording without artifact will show little variation in CMAP amplitudes throughout the train. Low frequency RNS at 2–3 Hz will progressively deplete the primary store of ACh quanta, and fewer quanta will be released with each consecutive stimulation. The corresponding total EPP will fall in amplitude, but in a healthy individual the large safety factor ensures that even the reduced EPPs are larger than threshold, thus the resulting muscle fiber action potential is preserved throughout the recording. Within seconds, the secondary stores will be mobilized to replenish the primary ones, thus ensuring that the threshold potential is always surpassed. In pathologic conditions of the neuromuscular junction, the safety factor is reduced, so that normally tolerated drops in the EPP will fall below the required threshold potential, thus leading to failure of synaptic transmission and the absence of the expected muscle fiber action potential in some muscle fibers. This development gives rise to the decrement that is observed when looking at the overall CMAP amplitude generated by that muscle (Fig. 6.2). These concepts form the basis of the decrements with slow RNS that are seen in NMJ disorders.

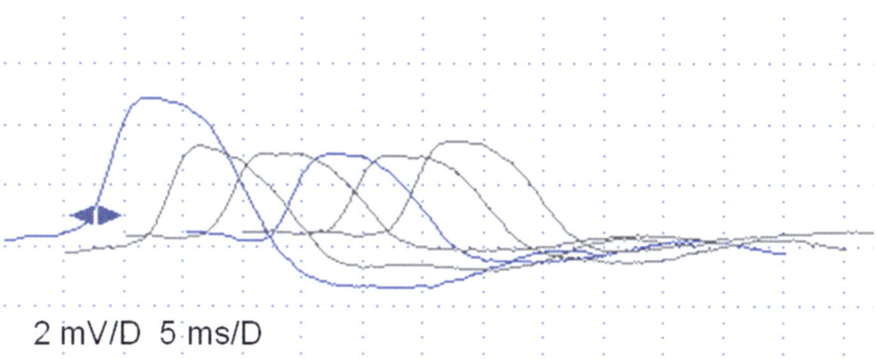

Fig. 6.2 RNS at 2 Hz in a 6 year–old girl with a congenital myasthenic syndrome (de novo mutation in *CHRND*). The child was mechanically ventilated via tracheostomy and fed by gastrostomy and suffered severe muscle weakness from the first months of life. RNS shows an abnormal decrement (30%) observed between the first and fourth stimulations in the phrenic nerve. The study was performed under sedation and the mechanical ventilation was stopped for a few seconds during the test to prevent ventilation artifact

High Frequency (Rapid) Repetitive Nerve Stimulation Tests

High frequency (also known as rapid) RNS (10–50 Hz) is particularly valuable for detecting disorders affecting the pre synaptic processes of neuromuscular transmission. After release of quanta from the presynaptic terminal, mobilization of additional quanta from the secondary store is the primary physiologic means of replenishing presynaptic acetylcholine stores. In the setting of high frequency repetitive stimulation, which is non-physiologic (i.e., does not occur in the setting of natural neuromuscular transmission), the mobilization of additional quanta is complemented by the accumulation of intracellular calcium. At frequencies over 10 Hz, the calcium pump is not able to pump calcium ions back into the extracellular synapse before the next stimulation, and thus abnormally high intracellular calcium concentrations occur, leading to increased release of quanta and a correspondingly higher EPP. In normal individuals, higher EPPs are non-consequential, as the same all-or-none muscle fiber action potentials are generated. In pathologic conditions where the baseline EPP is below threshold for some muscle fibers and a muscle fiber action potential is not generated for affected muscle fibers, the baseline CMAP amplitude is reduced. In those circumstances, the higher presynaptic intracellular calcium concentrations associated with rapid RNS (20–50 Hz) increases the number of muscle fibers that reach threshold, resulting in a higher CMAP amplitude and the phenomenon of facilitation associated with presynaptic disorders of neuromuscular transmission (Fig. 6.3).

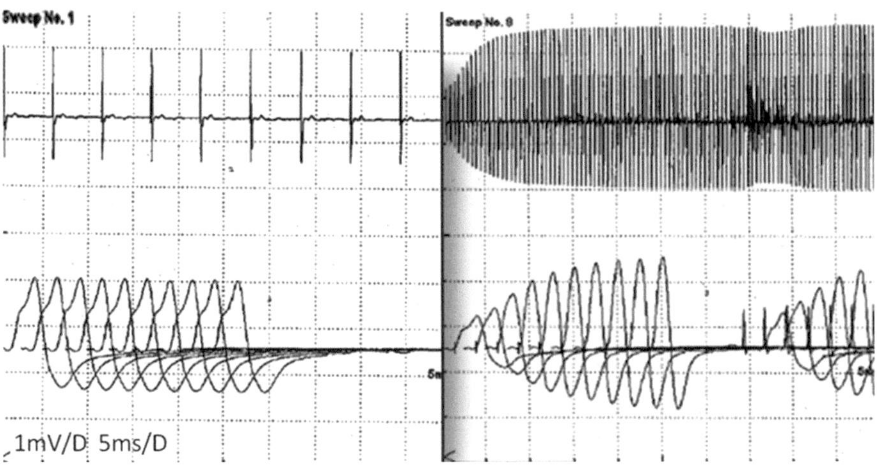

Fig. 6.3 Slow RNS (3 Hz) (**a**) and Rapid RNS (30 Hz) (**b**) in a 3-year-old boy with severe congenital hypotonia, intellectual disability, epilepsy, and low-amplitude CMAPs on standard nerve conduction studies (setting 2 mV/5 ms). No significant decrement is observed at 3 Hz (**a**), but 30 Hz stimulation is associated with a striking increment (+154% from first to tenth CMAP) indicating a dysfunction of the NMJ, probably pre-synaptic. This patient's clinical diagnosis was Lambert-Eaton like syndrome, with an unknown etiology

Presynaptic disorders that display facilitation on high frequency RNS include botulism and presynaptic variants of congenital myasthenic syndrome [4, 6]. These disorders are discussed in greater detail in Chap. 21.

Disorders of Membrane Excitability (Muscle Channelopathies) and Exercise Tests

Familial periodic paralyses and non-dystrophic myotonias are disorders of skeletal muscle excitability caused by mutations in genes coding for voltage-gated ion channels (so called "channelopathies"). These channels involve various cations (sodium, potassium, calcium) or anion (chloride) channels which play an important role in depolarizing the muscle membrane. Muscle channelopathies are characterized by episodic failure of motor activity due to muscle weakness (paralysis) or stiffness (myotonia). Clinical studies have identified three distinct forms of myotonias: recessive and dominant forms of myotonia congenita (MC), paramyotonia congenita (PC), and potassium-aggravated myotonia (PAM); and two forms of periodic paralyses: hyperkalemic (hyperPP) and hypokalemic (hypoPP) periodic paralyses, based on changes in blood potassium levels during the attacks. Both the recessive and dominant forms of myotonia congenita arise from mutations in *CLCN1*, which encodes a chloride channel that is found in skeletal muscle. Paramyotonia congenita (PC) and potassium-aggravated myotonia (PAM) are associated with mutations in *SCN4A*. Two genes have been implicated in periodic paralysis, *SCN4A* and *CACNA1S*. There are several factors that can make diagnosis difficult. Some affected patients will display no symptoms aside from myotonia. Clinical signs could also be transient, and influenced by various environmental variables such as temperature, exercise, and potassium ingestion. Furthermore, multiple clinical phenotypes (PC + hyperPP for example) may be observed in the same patient [4, 35, 36].

Neurophysiological studies play an important role in cases of suspected muscle channelopathies as they may substantiate aberrant membrane excitability, which will help guide genetic testing and the selection of a therapeutic regimen. Standardized protocols comprising short and long exercise tests have been developed to differentiate among these disorders during neurophysiologic testing [2]. However, these tests may be difficult to perform and to analyze in children for two major reasons: (i) articulation displacements and changes in muscle during the exercise tests due to movements; and (ii) some of the protocols may be associated with discomfort and anxiety in the child. Furthermore, younger children often do not cooperate with the exercise tests. The number of muscles examined may be limited, and long exercise tests should be restricted to cases when periodic paralysis is suspected. However, a careful and thorough examination is feasible in most infants when the study is performed by a neurophysiologist experienced with children.

Neurophysiological Tests for Muscle Excitability Disorders

(1) "*Myotonic discharges*" are sought using concentric needle EMG, ideally recording from several representative muscles. Myotonic discharges, the electrophysiologic correlate of clinical myotonia, regardless of the type of channel affected, are due to involuntary repetitive firing of muscle fiber action potentials. Needle insertion by itself will elicit myotonic bursts when a patient is susceptible to muscle excitability. These are bursts of fibrillation potentials and positive sharp waves with amplitudes typically ranging from 10 μV to 1 mV and frequencies of 50–150 Hz. Both parameters are expected to vary significantly in a single burst, classically resembling the sound of a "dive-bomber" on acoustic recordings. In pseudomyotonia or complex repetitive discharges, the frequency and amplitude will not change and thus careful assessment of these bursts is needed to distinguish between the different patterns.

(2) *Short exercise test*: The CMAP is recorded from the abductor digiti minimi (ADM) muscle after stimulation of the ulnar nerve at the wrist. Skin temperature must be measured and maintained between 32 and 34 °C at the wrist, thereby preventing artificially low CMAP amplitudes due to excessive warmth, or artificially high CMAP amplitudes due to excessive cooling.

    The short exercise test consists of maximal contraction of the ADM for 15 seconds (sec). CMAPs are recorded 2 sec immediately after the end of the exercise and then every 10 sec for 60 sec. The whole process is repeated three times with 60 sec between the beginnings of two trials.

(3) *Long exercise test:* On practical grounds, is it important not to perform this test on the same hand as the short exercise test in case there are some residual effects. Long exercise lasts 5 minutes (min) with brief (3–4 sec) rest periods every 30–45 sec to prevent ischemia. CMAPs are recorded 2 sec immediately after cessation of exercise and then every minute for 5 min, and finally every 5 min for a total of 40 min. If the response changes, the position of the electrodes should be checked, and maintenance of supramaximal stimulation should be verified. Due to its duration, this long exercice test is more technically challenging in younger children than the short exercise test.

(4) Fournier et al. [2] has proposed a standardized testing protocol for patients who are suspected to have a disorder of skeletal membrane excitability. We find this protocol useful and would recommend it be considered particularly for older children. Overall, in the setting of unexplained transient muscle stiffness or weakness in childhood, exercise tests are a very useful tool to accurately determine different patterns of abnormalities that may guide further genetic testing and treatment (Figs. 6.4 and 6.5).

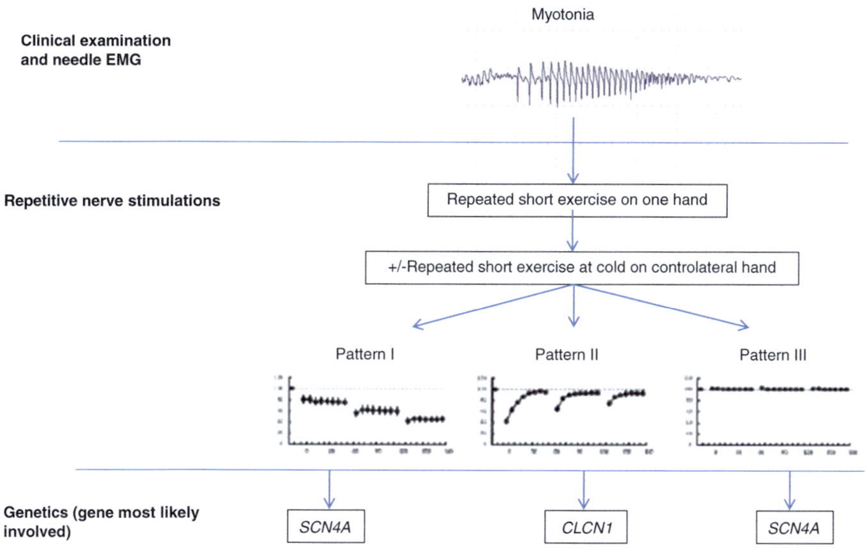

Fig. 6.4 Genetic guidelines based on ElectroNeuroMyography(ENMG) screening in myotonia/ paramyotonia congenita (adapted from [2, 37])

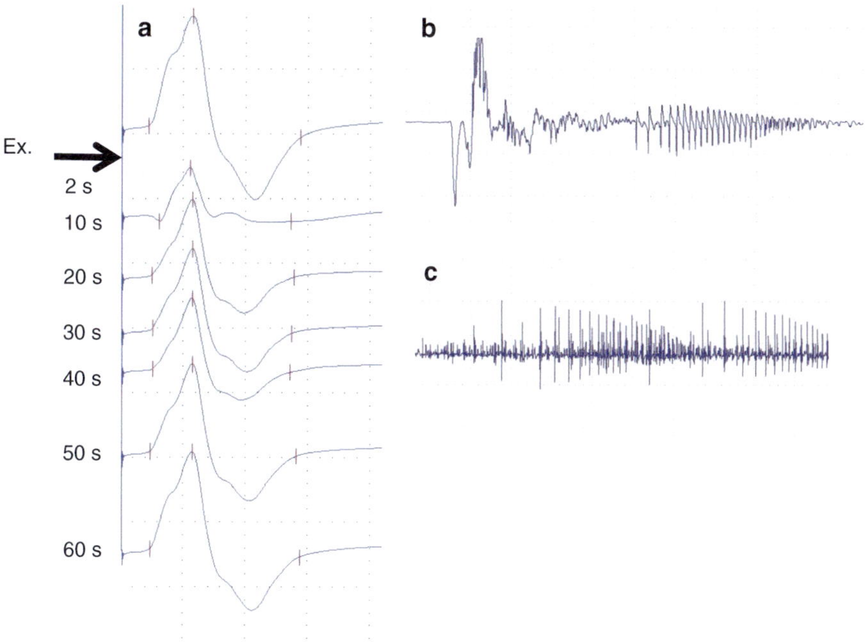

Fig. 6.5 Neurophysiological findings in a patient harboring *CLCN1* mutations: (**a**) Short exercise test showing a transient decrease of compound muscle action potential (CMAP) amplitude (pattern II). Pre-exercise trace (top trace) and post exercise recordings (bottom trace) after the trial (Ex.) 5 ms/5 mV/D; (**b**) Myotonic discharge (deltoid muscle 100μV/100 ms/D); (**c**) Myotonic discharge (first interosseous muscle 100μV/100 ms/D)

References

1. Verschuuren J, Strijbos E, Vincent A. Neuromuscular junction disorders. Handb Clin Neurol. 2016;133:447–66.
2. Fournier E, Arzel M, Sternberg D, Vicart S, Laforet P, Eymard B, et al. Electromyography guides toward subgroups of mutations in muscle channelopathies. Ann Neurol. 2004;56(5):650–61.
3. Michel P, Sternberg D, Jeannet PY, Dunand M, Thonney F, Kress W, et al. Comparative efficacy of repetitive nerve stimulation, exercise, and cold in differentiating myotonic disorders. Muscle Nerve. 2007;36(5):643–50.
4. Darras BT, Jones HR Jr, Ryan MM, De Vivo DC, editors. Neuromuscular disorders of infancy, childhood, and adolescence: a clinician's approach. 2nd ed. London: Elsevier; 2015. p. 1123.
5. Amato AA, Russell JA. Neuromuscular disorders. 2nd ed. New York: McGraw-Hill; 2016. p. 788.
6. Preston DC, Shapiro BE, editors. Electromyography and neuromuscular disorders: clinical-electrophysiologic correlations. 3rd ed. London: Elsevier; 2013.
7. Gilhus NE. Myasthenia gravis. N Engl J med. 2016;375(26):2570–81.
8. Beeson D. Congenital myasthenic syndromes: recent advances. Curr Opin Neurol. 2016;29(5):565–71.
9. Engel AG, Shen XM, Selcen D, Sine SM. Congenital myasthenic syndromes: pathogenesis, diagnosis, and treatment. Lancet Neurol. 2015;14(4):420–34.
10. Abicht A, Muller JS, Lochmuller H. Congenital myasthenic syndromes. In: Pagon RA, Adam MP, Ardinger HH, Wallace SE, Amemiya A, LJH B, et al., editors. GeneReviews(R). Seattle; 1993.
11. Juel VC. Evaluation of neuromuscular junction disorders in the electromyography laboratory. Neurol Clin. 2012;30(2):621–39.
12. Gurnett CA, Bodnar JA, Neil J, Connolly AM. Congenital myasthenic syndrome: presentation, electrodiagnosis, and muscle biopsy. J Child Neurol. 2004;19(3):175–82.
13. van Dijk JG, Lammers GJ, Wintzen AR, Molenaar PC. Repetitive CMAPs: mechanisms of neural and synaptic genesis. Muscle Nerve. 1996;19(9):1127–33.
14. Kumar RS, Kuruvilla A. Repetitive compound muscle action potentials in electrophysiological diagnosis of congenital myasthenic syndromes: a case report and review of literature. Ann Indian Acad Neurol. 2010;13(2):139–41.
15. Wintzen AR, Plomp JJ, Molenaar PC, van Dijk JG, van Kempen GT, Vos RM, et al. Acquired slow-channel syndrome: a form of myasthenia gravis with prolonged open time of the acetylcholine receptor channel. Ann Neurol. 1998;44(4):657–64.
16. Zambelis T, Foutsitzi A, Giannakopoulou A, Poulopoulou K, Karandreas N. Lambert-Eaton myasthenic syndrome. Clinical and electrophysiological findings in seven cases. Electromyogr Clin Neurophysiol. 2004;44(5):289–92.
17. Lee HE, Kim YH, Kim SM, Shin HY. Clinical significance of repetitive compound muscle action potentials in patients with myasthenia gravis: a predictor for cholinergic side effects of acetylcholinesterase inhibitors. J Clin Neurol. 2016;12(4):482–8.
18. Kariya S, Park GH, Maeno-Hikichi Y, Leykekhman O, Lutz C, Arkovitz MS, et al. Reduced SMN protein impairs maturation of the neuromuscular junctions in mouse models of spinal muscular atrophy. Hum Mol Genet. 2008;17(16):2552–69.
19. Kim JY, Park KD, Kim SM, Sunwoo IN. Decremental responses to repetitive nerve stimulation in x-linked bulbospinal muscular atrophy. J Clin Neurol. 2013;9(1):32–5.
20. Belaya K, Rodriguez Cruz PM, Liu WW, Maxwell S, McGowan S, Farrugia ME, et al. Mutations in GMPPB cause congenital myasthenic syndrome and bridge myasthenic disorders with dystroglycanopathies. Brain. 2015;138(Pt 9):2493–504.
21. Rodriguez Cruz PM, Sewry C, Beeson D, Jayawant S, Squier W, McWilliam R, et al. Congenital myopathies with secondary neuromuscular transmission defects; a case report and review of the literature. Neuromuscul Disord. 2014;24(12):1103–10.

22. Pitt MC, Jabre JF. Determining jitter values in the very young by use of the e-norms methodology. Muscle Nerve. 2017;55(1):51–4.
23. Pitt MC, McHugh JC, Deeb J, Smith RA. Assessing neuromuscular junction stability from stimulated EMG in children. Clin Neurophysiol. 2017;128(2):290–6.
24. Baruca M, Leonardis L, Podnar S, Hojs-Fabjan T, Grad A, Jerin A, et al. Single fiber EMG as a prognostic tool in myasthenia gravis. Muscle Nerve. 2016;54(6):1034–40.
25. Stalberg E, Schwartz MS, Trontelj JV. Single fibre electromyography in various processes affecting the anterior horn cell. J Neurol Sci. 1975;24(4):403–15.
26. Abraham A, Alabdali M, Alsulaiman A, Breiner A, Barnett C, Katzberg HD, et al. Repetitive nerve stimulation cutoff values for the diagnosis of myasthenia gravis. Muscle Nerve. 2017;55(2):166–70.
27. Dilena R, Abicht A, Sergi P, Comi GP, Di Fonzo A, Chidini G, et al. Congenital myasthenic syndrome due to choline acetyltransferase mutations in infants: clinical suspicion and comprehensive electrophysiological assessment are important for early diagnosis. J Child Neurol. 2014;29(3):389–93.
28. Jones HR Jr, Bolton CF, Harper CM Jr. Pediatric clinical electromyography. Philadelphia: Lippincott-Raven; 1996. p. 487.
29. Shapiro BE, Preston DC. Repetitive nerve stimulation and exercise testing. Phys med Rehabil Clin N am. 2003;14(2):185–206.
30. Chiou-Tan FY, Gilchrist JM. Repetitive nerve stimulation and single-fiber electromyography in the evaluation of patients with suspected myasthenia gravis or Lambert-Eaton myasthenic syndrome: review of recent literature. Muscle Nerve. 2015;52(3):455–62.
31. Rubin DI, Hentschel K. Is exercise necessary with repetitive nerve stimulation in evaluating patients with suspected myasthenia gravis? Muscle Nerve. 2007;35(1):103–6.
32. Bou Ali H, Salort-Campana E, Grapperon AM, Gallard J, Franques J, Sevy A, et al. New strategy for improving the diagnostic sensitivity of repetitive nerve stimulation in myasthenia gravis. Muscle Nerve. 2017;55(4):532–8.
33. Zhuang L, Tang X, Fan D, Xu X, Wang X, Jiang J. Phrenic and intercostal repetitive nerve stimulation: a useful electroneurophysiological method to detect the respiratory status of myasthenia gravis patients. Electromyogr Clin Neurophysiol. 2003;43(1):9–16.
34. Lo YL, Leoh TH, Tan YE, Foo ML, Dan YF, Ratnagopal P. Repetitive hypoglossal nerve stimulation in myasthenia gravis. Clin Neurophysiol. 2002;113(8):1227–30.
35. Quinn C, Salajegheh MK. Myotonic disorders and channelopathies. Semin Neurol. 2015;35(4):360–8.
36. Al-Ghamdi et al. Spectrum of non dystrophic skeletal muscle channelopathies in children. Pediatr Neurol. 2017;70:26–33. doi: 10.1016/j.pediatrneurol.2017.02.006. Epub 2017 Feb 16.
37. Fournier E, Viala K, Gervais H, Sternberg D, Arzel-Hezode M, Laforet P, et al. Cold extends electromyography distinction between ion channel mutations causing myotonia. Ann Neurol. 2006;60(3):356–65.

Chapter 7
Late Responses

Karin Edebol Eeg-Olofsson

F Waves (F Responses)

Background

More than 65 years ago Magladery and McDougal first described F waves [1]. When a motor nerve is given supramaximal stimulation, an action potential travels orthodromically directly to the muscle and evokes the M-response. Simultaneously, an antidromic action potential travels proximally to anterior horn cells in the spinal cord resulting in a delayed orthodromic response that travels back down, past the stimulation point, to the muscle where it generates an F wave. Since a different population of anterior horn cells is activated with each stimulus, the number of reactivated axons will vary from one stimulation to the next. As a result, when a series of F-waves is obtained for a specific nerve, each individual F-wave will vary slightly in shape, amplitude and latency (Fig. 7.1). For a given motor nerve, recurrent potentials are generated by only 0–5% of motor units with each stimulation [1, 2]. Accordingly, the amplitude of the F-wave usually is less than 5% of the maximal CMAP amplitude, i.e., only a few motor units contribute to each response. The frequency of occurrence of F-waves is 70–100% depending on applied stimuli and nerve.

Minimum F-wave latency is the most commonly measured F-wave parameter, and reflects propagation of the fastest conducting motor axons (Fig. 7.2). Maximum F wave latency and mean F wave latency have also been studied, but are not widely used in isolation. The *F-wave amplitude* reflects the excitability of motor neurons, and correlates with the size compound motor action potential (CMAP) amplitude that is generated. *Chronodispersion* is a measurement of the dispersion of F-waves

K.E. Eeg-Olofsson, M.D., Ph.D.
University of Uppsala, Uppsala, Sweden

Department of Clinical Neurophysiology, University Hospital Uppsala,
Uppsala S-751 85, Sweden
e-mail: karin.edebol.eeg-olofsson@akademiska.se

© Springer International Publishing AG 2017

H.J. McMillan, P.B. Kang (eds.), *Pediatric Electromyography*,
DOI 10.1007/978-3-319-61361-1_7

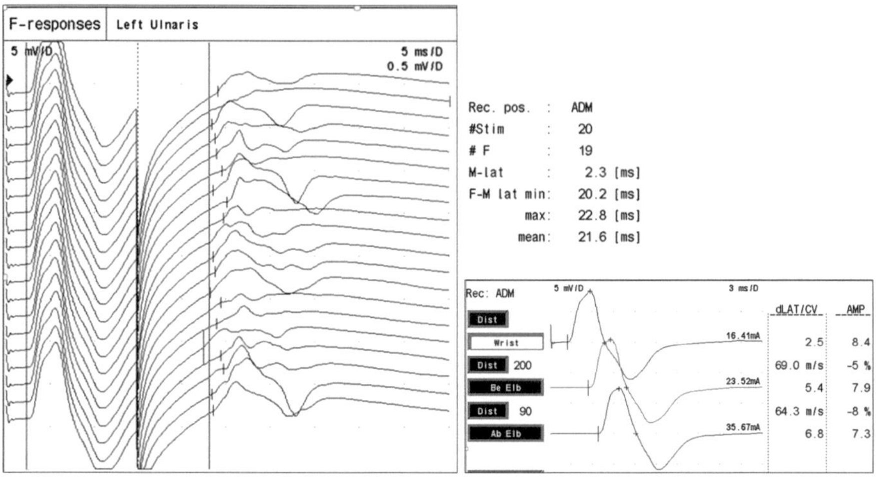

Fig. 7.1 F waves from *left ulnar nerve* in a healthy teenager. M-waves (*left*) exhibit higher amplitude and similar morphology with each stimulation; they occur first due to the proximity of the recording site and the stimulator. F-waves (*left*) in contrast, show variation in shape, amplitude and latency. The minimum F-wave latency is 20.2 msec for this patient. The ulnar nerve motor study (*right*) shows compound motor action potential (CMAP) morphology which appear similar at each stimulation site and resemble M-waves

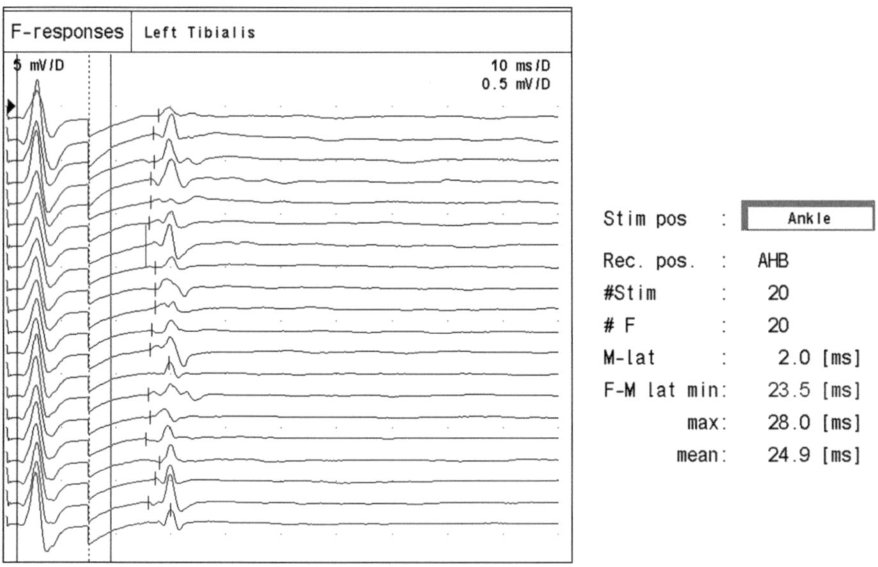

Fig. 7.2 Normal F wave study in the left tibial nerve in a boy 2.5 years of age. Minimum F wave latency is 23.5 ms

and is calculated by F maximum latency minus F minimum latency [1–6]. *Persistence* is a measurement of number of traces with F-waves out of 20 stimuli [7, 8]. Persistence together with amplitude reflect the excitability of the motor neurons.

In adults, the F wave latency depends upon a patient's height (i.e., limb length), as well as factors that can influence conduction velocity and distal motor latency. As such, an F-estimate can be calculated using the formula:

$$\text{F estimate} = (2D/CV) \times 10 + 1\ \text{ms} + DL$$

In this calculation: D = distance from the stimulation site to the spinal cord (where F-wave must travel to and from); CV = conduction velocity (m/sec); DL = distal motor latency (msec). Multiplying the product of the distance and conduction velocity by 10 thereby converts the time units into milliseconds.

Except perhaps for tall adolescent patients, F estimates are not routinely used in pediatric studies and will not be discussed further.

Chronodispersion and F wave persistence are not dependent on age or height.

F Waves in Disease

Nerve conduction studies including F wave studies are used in daily clinical practice. F wave latency is the most sensitive nerve conduction parameter in patients with diabetic neuropathy [9, 10] and F wave abnormalities are often seen early on in neuropathies of other origins as well. In demyelinating polyneuropathy, the F waves are delayed, (i.e., the latencies are increased), and in proximal conduction block they are few in number and delayed. In severe axonal loss with reduced compound muscle action potential (CMAP) amplitudes, the number of F waves is reduced but the F wave amplitudes may be normal. The F waves are also affected by a myopathy with reduced CMAP, where the number of F waves is normal but the F wave amplitudes are reduced. In spastic conditions such as cerebral palsy, F wave amplitudes may be increased, along with the number of F waves showing prolonged duration [11]. The increased F wave amplitude in spasticity was described as early as 1979 [12], and has been observed in patients with konzo which is a progressive spastic disorder that results from consuming bitter (high cyanide) cassava flour (Fig. 7.3) [13].

F Waves and Age

In the peripheral nervous system, nerve conduction velocities are slow at birth due to immature myelination patterns. The velocities increase as myelination progresses (Fig. 7.4). The conduction velocity varies with the length of the nerve, thickness of the myelin sheath, diameter of the nerve and distance between nodes of Ranvier. Reference studies with nerve conduction velocities from pediatric populations have been performed, and some early studies were published from 1960 to 1993 [14–22]. A comprehensive overview of results of different studies was published in 2002 [23].

In the 1980s, two studies of F waves in children were published [24, 25]. Reference values in healthy children 6 weeks to 14 years of age ($n = 49$) were collected by the author for use in daily neurophysiological work (Fig. 7.4) [26]. The *minimum F-wave latency* in children up to 1 year of age correlates more with age

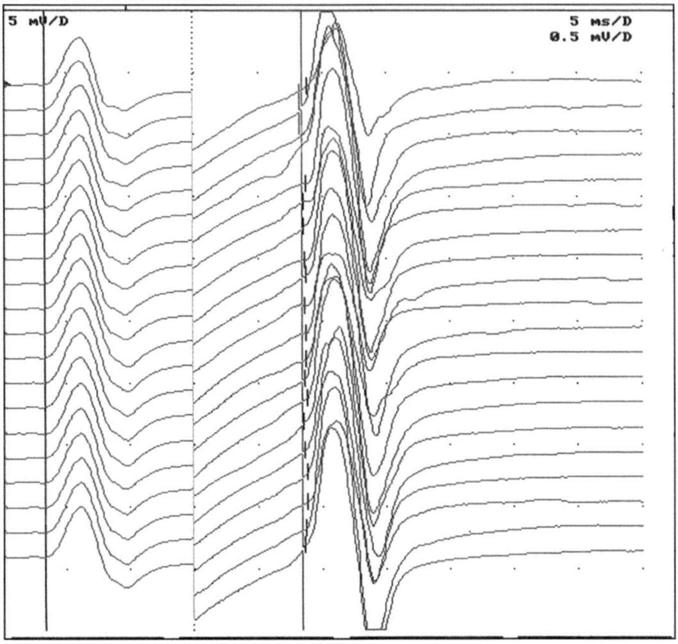

Fig. 7.3 High amplitude F waves in *right median nerve* in a young woman with konzo complicated by spastic tetraparesis

than height; between 1 and 2 years of age the reverse becomes true, with height becoming more important than age. Table 7.1 shows minimum F wave latencies in young children. The *number of F-waves* varies between young individuals (Table 7.2), however, the median values for each age group do not differ significantly from those in older children.

F-wave parameters were studied with linear regression analysis in order to obtain reference values in healthy children and adolescents aged 3–20 years [27]. In 175 subjects (91 boys, 84 girls) 410 nerves were studied (117 median, 102 ulnar, 114 peroneal, 77 tibial). All subjects were studied unilaterally. Linear regression with height as an independent variable generated the best model for the study of minimum F wave latency. The F wave latency increased with height, with 0.12 ms/cm in arm nerves and 0.28 ms/cm in the motor nerves of lower extremity. Height explained 86–93% of the variability of the minimum F wave latency, and age explained 71–87% of the variability. Age and height are closely interrelated in children. There was no correlation between the number of F waves versus height or age. Dispersion of F wave latencies did not correlate with age, height or gender.

Maturation of the nervous system depends heavily on myelination, although several other developmental processes make major contributions as well. The continuous progress and developmental milestones are reflected in the findings of various neurophysiological studies. Knowledge of normality is a prerequisite for identifying abnormalities, rendering diagnostic studies possible, paving the way for adequate care and treatment.

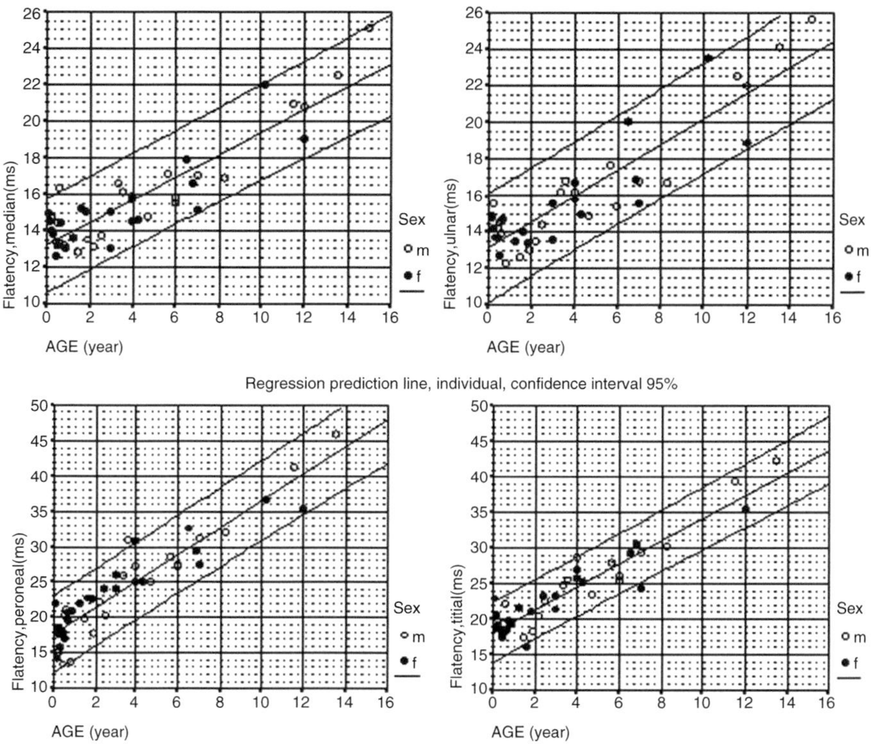

Fig. 7.4 Development of F wave latencies. Minimum F-wave latency (ms) in median (*upper left*), ulnar (*upper right*), peroneal (*lower left*) and tibial (*lower right*) nerves of healthy children 6 weeks to 14 years of age. *White dots* are males, *black dots* females. Regression prediction line, individual; confidence interval 95%. Courtesy Karin Edebol Eeg-Olofsson, reference study for the Neurophysiological Laboratory, Uppsala, Sweden

Table 7.1 Minimum F wave latencies in young healthy children

Investigated nerves				
Age	Median	Ulnar	Peroneal	Tibial
1.5–4.5 months (*n* = 7)	13.8–14.9 (14.6)	13.7–15.6 (14.8)	14.3–22.0 (17.1)	18.6–22.9 (19.0)
>4.5 months–1 yearr (*n* = 10)	13.0–16.3 (13.3)	12.3–14.7 (14.1)	14.4–20.9 (19.5)	17.3–22.1 (18.9)
>1–2 years (*n* = 6)	12.8–15.2 (13.6)	12.6–14.0 (13.4)	18.8–22.8 (22.0)	16.0–21.6 (18.1)
>2–3 years (*n* = 5)	13.0–15.0 (13.4)	13.5–15.6 (14.0)	20.3–26.0 (24.0)	20.5–23.34 (22.5)

Range and (median) values; ms
Courtesy Karin Edebol Eeg-Olofsson, reference study for the Neurophysiological Laboratory, Uppsala, Sweden

Table 7.2 Number of F-waves after 20 stimulations in young healthy children

Investigated nerves				
Age	Median	Ulnar	Peroneal	Tibial
1.5–4.5 months ($n = 7$)	10–19 (15)	4–13 (11)	2–19 (4)	12–20 (19)
>4.5 months–1 year ($n = 10$)	3–20 (17)	5–20 (11)	3–16 (6)	5–20 (17)
>1–2 years ($n = 6$)	4–18 (11)	1–19 (16)	6–12 (10)	10–20 (16)
>2–3 years ($n = 5$)	15–18 (17)	14–17 (15)	3–10 (9)	15–20 (17)

Range and (median) values
Courtesy Karin Edebol Eeg-Olofsson, reference study for the Neurophysiological Laboratory, Uppsala, Sweden

Method

As a motor nerve is stimulated 15–20% above the level for obtaining maximal muscle response (M wave), F responses (F waves) can be obtained, using a sweep speed of 5 ms/D up to 10 ms/D. F waves are action potentials of at least 20 μV. The gain should be set at 0.2–0.5 mV/D for F waves and 2 or 5 mV/D for M responses. By stimulating at 1 Hz for 20 times, the number of F responses from different nerves vary, with the highest number of responses typically obtained from the tibial nerve.

Axon Reflex, A Waves

Background

A comprehensive paper on the axon reflex was published 50 years ago involving 25 adult subjects with lower motor neuron lesions in the hand [28]. Several of these subjects were found to have a small potential between the M wave (direct muscle response) and the F wave that was named the axon reflex, with a latency intermediate between those of the M and F waves. The term axon reflex indicates the conduction of an impulse antidromically up one branch of a motor axon to a branch point, where it changes direction and propagates orthodromically down another branch to the muscle. In no case was the axon reflex seen with a stimulus too weak to produce an M response, and it was only with higher stimulation intensities that the potentials would appear. In contrast to F waves, the morphology, amplitude and latency of the axon reflexes were constant, though their latencies shortened when the stimulating cathode was moved in a proximal direction. When the stimulus intensity is increased beyond a certain point, they convert into M responses. Axonal branching may occur proximal to the muscles but below the level of a lesion. Motor nerve fibers in young healthy subjects were found to demonstrate axon reflexes [29]. In the early 1980s "peripheral late waves" were recorded from foot muscles of patients with neuropathy, after stimulation of the posterior tibial nerve at the ankle [30]. In contrast to the

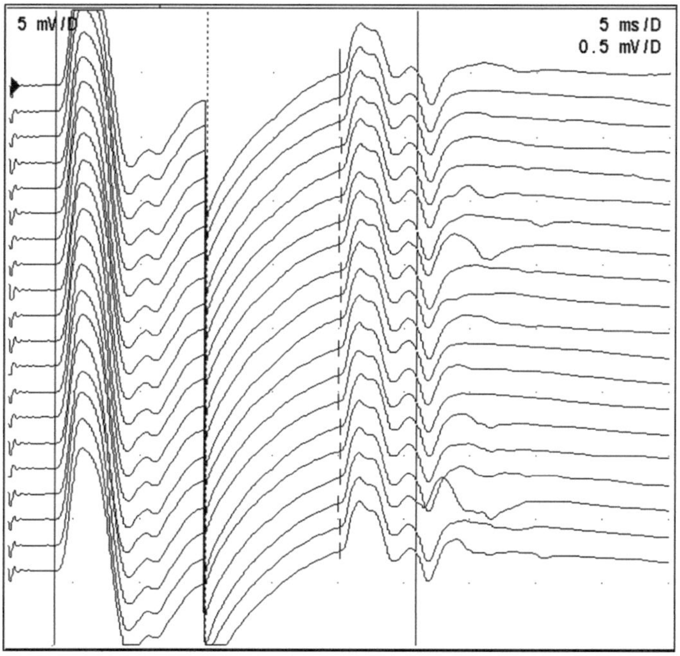

Fig. 7.5 A-waves in the right peroneal nerve of a patient undergoing investigation for lower back pain. A-waves should not be confused with F-waves. An important distinguishing features is the similar morphology and latency of each A-wave which is not seen with F-waves

described axon reflexes, these late responses did not disappear on supramaximal stimulation. Later on, axon reflexes and peripheral late waves were grouped together as A waves (Fig. 7.5).

A Waves in Disease

Originally, A-waves were regarded as a pathological finding (except in the tibial nerve), however they are now recognized to occur in many young healthy patients as well as in certain diseases. The occurrence of A waves was studied in 2367 nerves from 556 consecutive patients at the Department of Clinical Neurophysiology at the University Hospital in Uppsala [31]. On consecutive nerve fibre stimulations, A waves could be recorded with a nearly constant latency and uniform morphology in 124 of those patients (and 184 nerves, constituting 7.8% of the total). A waves may be found in polyneuropathy or focal nerve lesions. Of patients with polyneuropathy, 65% had at least one nerve with A waves. In motor neuron disease, A waves were present in six out of ten patients.

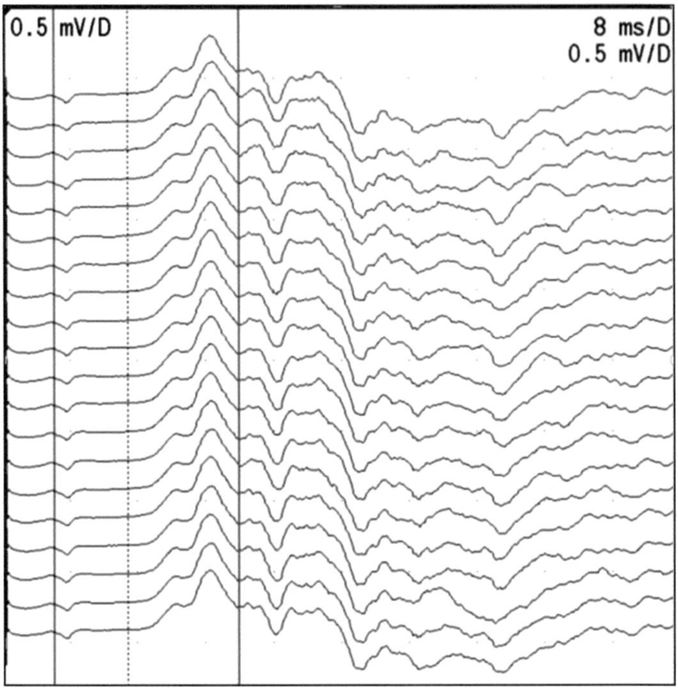

Fig. 7.6 A waves noted when testing late responses in the left median nerve of a boy who suffered a left arm fracture with resulting left median nerve injury. His left median nerve compound motor action potential (CMAP) was very low amplitude (0.5 mV) with temporal dispersion evident

In radiculopathies, A waves were seen less frequently. There was no correlation between the number of A waves and the etiology or severity of the disease.

In Guillain-Barré syndrome (GBS) it is well-known that A waves may occur. Multiple A waves were found in at least one limb on routine nerve conduction studies within seven days after onset of GBS symptoms in 14 patients [32]. The existence of A waves soon after onset of symptoms seems to be a sensitive sign of GBS. Multiple A waves may also occur in a mononeuropathy (Fig. 7.6).

H Reflex

Background

The H reflex is named after the first initial of the last name of the investigator, Hoffman, who described an elicited muscle response reflecting spinal excitability in 1910 [33]. The H reflex is an electrophysiologically recorded gastrocnemius/soleus

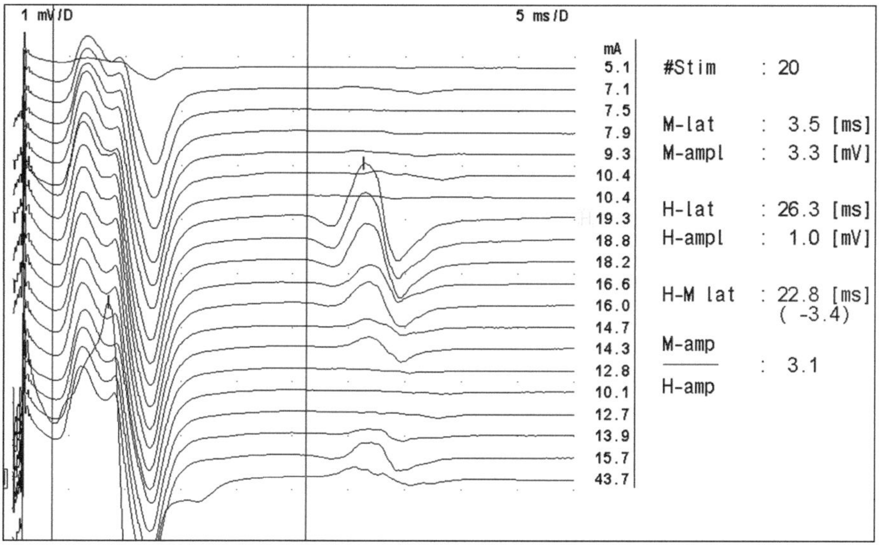

Fig. 7.7 Normal H reflex from the *right tibial nerve* in a young woman investigated for pain in the dorsal aspect of the proximal and distal lower limbs

muscle stretch reflex. It is performed by stimulating the tibial nerve at the popliteal fossa. From there, the action potential propagates proximally through the reflex arc at that spinal segment, synapsing with the anterior horn cell that in turn propagates an action potential down through the motor nerve to the soleus and gastrocnemius muscles, where the motor action potential is recorded. The H reflex is mostly used to evaluate for an S1 radiculopathy or to distinguish more distal lesions from an L5 radiculopathy.

The H reflex most commonly is recorded from the soleus muscle, and is an illustration of the combined effects of a mixed nerve. At low stimulations, the 1a fibers innervating the muscle spindles are activated and a long-latency muscle response is elicited (H-reflex) (Fig. 7.7). As stimulation strength increases the H response becomes smaller and a response with short latency is elicited due to direct activation of the motor nerve (M response). As the stimulation strength is further increased the H-reflex disappears.

Diurnal variation in the amplitude of the H reflex has been found in the human soleus muscle, with increasing amplitude from morning to evening [34]. The same measures did not change for the flexor carpi radialis muscle. A difference in diurnal CNS function between the lower and upper body may be due to the bipedal nature of humans, with possibly different CNS activity in the lower versus upper limbs. Diurnal variation in the rat H reflex has been described, suggesting that the pacemaker responsible for diurnal variations in H reflex amplitude likely exerts its influence presynaptically on the 1a synaptic connection and/or postsynaptically on the α-motorneuron [35].

Method

In contrast to F waves, the H reflexes are elicited with a low stimulation intensity. Configuration and amplitude are stimulus dependent. The latency of the H-reflex is constant. The persistence is 100%. In clinical practise the H reflex may be examined in the tibial nerve as well as the median nerve, although the latter is less commonly performed.

H Reflex of Tibial Nerve

Position of patient and limb: Patient prone or reclining. Legs extended.
Type of recording electrodes: Surface plate electrodes.
Position of recording electrodes: Over medial soleus muscle halfway between the knee and ankle.
Position of the reference electrode: Over the Achilles tendon.
Type of stimulating electrodes: Surface electrodes on a fixed bar.
Stimulation site: Knee, in the popliteal fossa.

H Reflex of Median Nerve

Position of limb: Patient supine, sitting or reclining. Elbow slightly extended or slightly flexed, forearm supinated.
Type of recording electrodes: Surface plate electrodes.
Placement of recording electrode: Over flexor carpi radialis muscle 6–8 cm distal to the medial epicondyle of the humerus.
Placement of reference electrode: Over the lateral epicondyle of the humerus.
Type of stimulating electrodes: Surface electrodes on a fixed bar.
Stimulation site: Elbow.

References

1. Magladery JW, McDougal DD. Electrophysiological studies of nerve and reflex activity in normal man. Identification of certain reflexes in the electromyogram and the conduction velocity of peripheral nerve fibres. Bull Johns Hopkins Hosp. 1950;86:265–90.
2. Trontelj JV, Trontelj M. F-responses of human facial muscles. A single motoneurone study. J Neurol Sci. 1973;20:211–22.
3. Schiller HH, Stålberg E. F responses studied with single fibre EMG in normal subjects and spastic patients. J Neurol Neurosurg Psychiatry. 1978;41:45–53.

4. Panayiotopoulos CP. F chronodispersion: a new electrophysiologic method. Muscle Nerve. 1979;2:68–72.
5. Chroni E, Panayiotopoulos CP. F Tacheodispersion. J Neurol Neurosurg Psychiatry. 1993a;56:1103–8.
6. Chroni E, Panayiotopoulos CP. F Tacheodispersion: quantitative analysis of motor fiber conduction velocities in patients with polyneuropathy. Muscle Nerve. 1993b;16:1302–9.
7. Panayiotopoulos CP, Scarpalezos S, Nastas PE. F wave studies on the deep peroneus nerve. Part 1: control subjects. J Neurol Sci. 1977;31:319–29.
8. Zappia M, Valentino P, Marchello LP, Paniccia M, Montagna P. F-wave normative studies in different nerves of healthy subjects. Electroencephalogr Clin Neurophysiol. 1993;89:67–72.
9. Andersen H, Stålberg E, Falck B. F-wave latency, the most sensitive conduction parameter in patients with diabetes mellitus. Muscle Nerve. 1997;20:1296–302.
10. Kohara N, Kimura J, Koji R, Goto Y, Ishii J, Tahiguchi M, Nakai M. F-wave latency serves as the most reproducible measure in nerve conduction studies of diabetic polyneuropathy: muticore analysis in healthy subjects and patients with diabetic polyneuropathy. Diabetologia. 2000;43:915–21.
11. Bischoff C, Schoenie PW, Conrad B. Increased F-wave duration in patients with spasticity. Electromyogr Clin Neurophysiol. 1992;32:449–53.
12. Eisen A, Odusote K. Amplitude of the F-wave: a potential means of documenting spasticity. Neurology. 1979;29:1306–9.
13. Edebol Eeg-Olofsson K, Tshala-Katumbay D. In: Eisen A, editor. Clinical neurophysiology of motor neuron diseases. Amsterdam: Elsevier; 2004. p. 675–86.
14. Thomas JE, Lambert EH. Ulnar nerve conduction velocity and H-reflex in infants and children. J Appl Physiol. 1960;15:1–9.
15. Gamstorp I. Normal conduction velocity of ulnar, median and peroneal nerves in infancy childhood and adolescence. Acta Paediatr Scand Suppl. 1963;146(suppl):68–76.
16. Gamstorp I, Shelburne SA Jr. Peripheral sensory conduction in ulnar and median nerves of normal infants, children and adolescents. Acta Paediatr Scand. 1965;54:309–13.
17. Baer RD, Johnson EW. Motor nerve conduction velocities in normal children. Arch Phys Med Rehabil. 1965;46:698–704.
18. Wagner AL, Buchtal F. Motor and sensory conduction in infancy and childhood: reappraisal. Dev Med Child Neurol. 1972;14:189–216.
19. Cruz Martinez A, Perez Conde ML, Ferrer MT. Motor conduction velocity and H-reflex in infancy and childhood: I. Study in newborns, twins, and small-for-dates. Electromyogr Clin Neurophysiol. 1977;17:493–505.
20. Cruz Martinez A, Ferrer MT, Perez Conde M, Bernacer M. Motor conduction velocity and H-reflex in infancy and childhood: 11-intra and extrauterine maturation of the nerve fibers: development of the peripheral nerve from 1 month to 11 years of age. Electromyogr Clin Neurophysiol. 1978;18:11–27.
21. Miller RG, Kuntz NL. Nerve conduction studies in infants and children. J Child Neurol. 1986;1:19–26.
22. Parano E, Uncini A, De Vivo DC, Lovelace RE. Electrophysiologic correlates of peripheral nervous system maturation in infancy and childhood. J Child Neurol. 1993;8:336–8.
23. Swoboda K, Edebol Eeg-Olofsson K, Harmon R, Bolton C, Harper M, Pitt M, Darras B, Jones R. Pediatric electromyography. In: Jones R, De Vivo D, Darras B, editors. Neuromuscular disorders of infancy, childhood and adolescence, vol. 2002. USA: Elsevier Science; 2002. p. 35–75.
24. Kwast O, Krajewska G, Kozlowski K. Analysis of F wave parameters in median and ulnar nerves in healthy infants and children: age related changes. Electromyogr Clin Neurophysiol. 1984;24:439–56.
25. Misra UK, Tiwari S, Shukla N, et al. F-response studies in neonates, infants and children. Electromyogr Clin Neurophysiol. 1989;29:251–4.

26. Edebol Eeg-Olofsson K. Nerve conduction studies in children. In: Edebol Eeg-Olofsson K, editor. Pediatric clinical neurophysiology. London: Mac Keith Press; 2007. p. 18–46.
27. Puksa L, Edebol Eeg-Olofsson K, Stålberg E, Falck B. Reference values for F-wave parameters in healthy 3-20 year old subjects. Clin Neurophysiol. 2011;122(1):199–204.
28. Fullerton PM, Gilliatt RW. Axon reflexes in human motor nerve fibres. J Neurol Neurosurg Psychiatry. 1965;28:1–11.
29. Stålberg E, Trontelj JV. Demonstration of axon reflexes in human motor nerve fibres. J Neurol Neurosurg Psychiatry. 1970;33:571–9.
30. Tomasulo RA. Aberrant conduction in human peripheral nerve: ephaptic transmission? Neurology. 1982 Jul;32(7):712–9.
31. Bischoff C, Stålberg E, Falck B, Puksa L. Significance of A-waves recorded in routine motor nerve conduction studies. Electroencephalogr Clin Neurophysiol. 1996;101(6):528–33.
32. Kornhuber ME, Bischoff C, Mentrup H, Conrad B. Multiple A waves in Guillain-Barré syndrome. Muscle Nerve. 1999;22(3):394–9.
33. Hoffman P. Beiträge zur Kenntnis der menschlichen Reflexe mit besonder Berücksichtigung der elektrischen Erscheinungen (Contributions to the knowledge of human reflexes with particular reference to electrical phenomena). Arch Anat Physiol Wissenschaft Med. 1910: 223–46.
34. Lagerquist O, Zehr P, Baldwin E, Klakowicz P, Collins D. Diurnal changes in the amplitude of the Hoffman reflex in the human soleus but not in the flexor carpi radialis muscle. Exp Brain Res. 2006;170:1–6.
35. Chen XY, Wolpaw JR. Circadian rhythm in rat H-reflex. Brain Res. 1994;648:167–70.

Chapter 8
Pediatric Intraoperative Neuromonitoring

Kerry A. Vaughan, Alier J. Franco, and Gregory G. Heuer

Introduction

Intraoperative neuromonitoring (IONM) has transformed the fields of pediatric surgery and anesthesia since its introduction in 1979, and is an important diagnostic and preventative tool to potentially decrease neurological complications in children after surgical procedures [1]. Its value in minimizing neurological injury during surgery has been well established in adults, with a 10–30% difference in injury rates in neurosurgical historical cohorts, but this risk reduction has yet to be systematically studied in children [2–4]. The goal of neuromonitoring during surgery is to detect changes in neural signaling as early as possible, allow surgical teams to prevent further injury by monitoring for and potentially reversing the electrophysiological changes that are detected. The adaptation of various neuromonitoring techniques from the adult population to pediatrics has proved crucial in assessing and optimizing surgical outcomes across numerous subspecialty fields. Early uses of IONM included the use of brainstem auditory evoked potentials (BAERs) and monitoring effects on the spinal cord during spine deformity correction [5]. These early applications demonstrated the powerful utility of IONM and its applicability to children.

These early adopters proved crucial in defining the nuances of pediatric monitoring and developing its modalities [6]. Complex spine operations were an ideal setting in which to develop and solidify the role of neurophysiologic monitoring in

K.A. Vaughan, M.D. • G.G. Heuer, M.D., Ph.D. (✉)
Division of Neurosurgery, Children's Hospital of Philadelphia, Philadelphia, PA, USA

Department of Neurosurgery, University of Pennsylvania Healthcare System, Philadelphia, PA, USA
e-mail: heuerg@email.chop.edu

A.J. Franco, Ph.D., C.N.I.M.
Division of Neurosurgery, Children's Hospital of Philadelphia, Philadelphia, PA, USA

Intraoperative Neuromonitoring Division, SpecialtyCare, Nashville, TN, USA

© Springer International Publishing AG 2017

H.J. McMillan, P.B. Kang (eds.), *Pediatric Electromyography*,
DOI 10.1007/978-3-319-61361-1_8

children. The goal of intraoperative monitoring is to improve the surgical safety profile by minimizing the risk of neurological injury in the operating room. It can provide not only important insights into the pathophysiology of intraoperative neurological injury, but also aid in identifying neural structures and detect injury early. A multimodal approach allows for safe, continuous neuromonitoring throughout procedures. Although IONM is most commonly used in neurosurgical, orthopedic, and cardiac procedures, it has broad applications ranging across nearly all pediatric surgical domains.

Neurophysiology of Monitoring

The basis of all neurophysiologic monitoring lies in recording either passive or active electrophysiological potentials within the neural pathway(s) at risk for intraoperative injury. Conduction of signals across neural pathways is dictated by a combination of intrinsic and extrinsic factors. An understanding of these factors and how they may affect the data being analyzed is important to assure that the interpretation of the data is accurate. Neuroanatomical considerations are paramount, whether the tissue at risk is in the immediate surgical field or is subject to other manipulations such as traction or compression due to positioning. For example, brain and spine operations are both typically amenable to monitoring via somatosensory evoked potentials (SSEPs) due to the long pathways involved in SSEP measurements, while brainstem procedures specifically may benefit from brainstem auditory evoked potentials (BAERs), and spine procedures in which lower motor neuron pathways may be injured may benefit from electromyography (EMG) monitoring.

Signal conduction is the primary endpoint evaluated in intraoperative modalities. The primary factors that can affect signal conduction are the physical properties of the neuron itself. Intrinsic properties of neurons, such as axonal caliber, neuronal health, and extent of myelination, dictate conduction velocity. Some of these properties have unique challenges in children. In particular, the developmental stage of a child will determine the extent of myelination of neurons. Also, genetic or degenerative health conditions may negatively impact the health of neurons and their signal conduction.

In addition to intrinsic neuronal properties, neuronal environment can also affect the neurophysiologic monitoring data. Physiological factors affecting neurotransmission include any changes that affect the biochemical or mechanical environment of neuronal pathways. Systemic parameters including temperature, acid-base status, perfusion, and pharmacological or anesthetic agents can alter or even abolish the ability to monitor neuronal signaling. Localized changes such as mechanical compression or surgical disruption of pathways can be reflected in the signal data acquired. Many of these factors are related to physiologic parameters controlled or affected by anesthesia or medical treatment.

The interplay of intrinsic and extrinsic factors regulating neural signaling creates a complex background for intraoperative neuromonitoring. These parameters represent both numerous possible barriers to effective monitoring, but also provide the surgical and anesthetic teams with a highly controlled environment in which to optimize safety and diminish the risk of neurological injury. There remains an uncertainty with IONM, as not all injuries to the nervous system may be reflected in real-time data and post-operative neurological deficits may occur even with adequate neuromonitoring [7, 8]. Undetected neurological injuries have become less prevalent as our understanding of pediatric IONM and related anesthetic and surgical management has expanded.

Pediatric Specific Considerations for Intraoperative Monitoring and Anesthesia

Pediatric patients pose a particular challenge for IONM based on their age and neurodevelopmental status, and require a well-versed neurophysiology, anesthesia, and surgical team in order to perform successful monitoring during a procedure. Understanding the differential maturation of both the peripheral and central nervous system is crucial in selecting appropriate pediatric patients for monitoring and subsequently delivering appropriate monitoring.

Normative data are available in the literature for evoked potentials in healthy children, but are highly dependent on recording techniques that vary significantly from neonates and infants to children and adults [9]. As neural responses to stimuli evolve with nervous system maturation, so must the neurophysiologist carefully select modalities, stimulation, recording, and filter settings tailored to the age and physical characteristics of the patient. Somatosensory evoked potentials (SSEPs) and transcranial motor evoked potentials (tcMEPs) have age-dependent latency differences in childhood relative to adulthood, and age, gender, and height can help predict peak latencies [10]. Both of these evoked potential signals demonstrate increasing latencies after approximately age four, which may be primarily related to increasing height. In children younger than 4 years old, height and maturation of the nervous system appear to have similar contrasting effects on latencies. Latencies decrease as the nervous system matures, while a child's growth may lengthen latencies even at young ages [11]. These variations do not preclude safe and effective IONM in the very young patient.

Certain populations have confounding factors that must be considered in interpretation of IONM. Patients with Down syndrome may be at higher risk of unreliable evoked potential monitoring intraoperatively or of baseline pathologic changes in monitoring that can obscure the interpretation of intraoperative monitoring changes [12]. Modalities such as tcMEPs involving a cortical stimulus must be carefully administered in patients with a seizure history or with prior cochlear implants to avoid seizures or unwanted complications. In our experience, successful, seizure-free tcMEPs have been reported in pediatric patients, even in children with cochlear implants and in those with seizure disorders, but tcMEPs should be used with caution in such patients [13, 14]. The last consideration is the baseline function of the pediatric patient. Monitoring can be complicated or even precluded if there are weak or absent baseline signals. This is encountered in patients with pre-existing neurological conditions such as cerebral palsy, severe myelopathy, or new onset significant weakness. For these reasons, it is important to understand the preoperative function of a patient, consider their neurophysiologic status, and order appropriate imaging studies to help predict which of these patients may still undergo successful IONM [15].

Pediatric anesthesia represents a particular challenge, especially in the context of monitoring, given the differential response of the pediatric patient to anesthetic agents compared to adults. The various monitoring modalities are sensitive to the type, dose, and timing of anesthetic agents employed. For example, inhalational agents depress motor-evoked potential (MEP) amplitude in children in a dose-dependent manner [16, 17]. However, a propofol-based total intravenous anesthesia (TIVA) protocol has largely supplanted halogenated agents as it allows for improved optimization of MEPs over a mixed inhalational/propofol-based anesthetic protocol [18]. SSEPs, including central sulcus and dorsal column mapping in the cord, are less sensitive to inhalational agents but are nonetheless more reliable with TIVA. Anesthesiologists may use adjuncts to TIVA judiciously, to balance adequate anesthesia with optimal IONM recording. Both MEP and electromyography (EMG) recordings are impaired by neuromuscular blockade, which conversely may improve SSEP recordings by decreasing background noise. TIVA may also be supplemented with ketamine for pediatric spine surgery, with successful maintenance of IONM [19].

Dexmedetomidine, an α-2 agonist, can supplement TIVA in order to reduce the total propofol load during surgery. Successful monitoring of MEPs and SSEPs has been published in pediatric spine procedures when using dexmedetomidine [20–22]. When considering dexmedetomidine as an adjunct to propofol in a TIVA protocol, care must be exercised to consider the type of surgical procedure and corresponding IONM technique employed. Spine procedures typically employ a suprathreshold technique in obtaining tcMEPs. There are reports of progressive decreases in tcMEPs during cases performed under TIVA with dexmedetomidine, which improved following cessation of dexmedetomidine infusion [23]. Perhaps more important than the anesthetic itself is the close relationship between the surgeon, anesthesiologist, and the neuromonitoring team to maintain adequate anesthesia while allowing for proper monitoring.

Neurosurgical procedures, and in particular intracranial procedures, often employ a threshold-based technique when obtaining tcMEPs. These neurosurgical procedures place greater emphasis on a more stable anesthetic background with limits on TIVA adjuncts that may increase the activation threshold of the corticospinal pathway that can lead to false positive intraoperative neuromonitoring changes. However, even non-sedative medications can significantly alter neuromonitoring signals, potentially leading to unnecessary changes in operative or anesthetic management in response to medication-induced changes in signaling. Commonly used anticonvulsant medications such as levetiracetam can reproducibly suppress tcMEPs during craniotomies [24]. Again, the necessity and timing of both anesthetic and adjunct medications should be discussed amongst the anesthesia, surgical, and monitoring teams to avoid potentially preventable anesthesia-related changes in monitoring.

Although complications of neuromonitoring in the operating room are few and far, they can be more frequent in pediatric patients. Dermal sequelae of monitoring electrodes and pads such as burns (<1%) and discolorations (16%) are noticeable but transient [25]. Stimulation pulses carry a small but non-zero risk of systemic effects, including seizures via tcMEPs or even transient hypotension via transcervical MEPs [26]. A well-prepared surgical, neurophysiological, and neuroanesthesia team should always be on alert for these complications and be ready for rapid management changes to maintain patient safety during IONM.

Significant changes in the signals observed during IONM should elicit an immediate and careful evaluation of the patient's status from all teams involved in order to interpret the changes and adjust management strategies as needed. The first step is to establish what constitutes a significant change in signals that would require evaluation, or a negligible change that may be artifact. This often varies by institution; common thresholds reported including a greater than 50% decrease in amplitude for SSEPs or MEPs, or a greater than 10% increase in latency as a positive signal change requiring notification of the anesthetic and surgical teams by the neurophysiologists [27, 28] (Fig. 8.1).

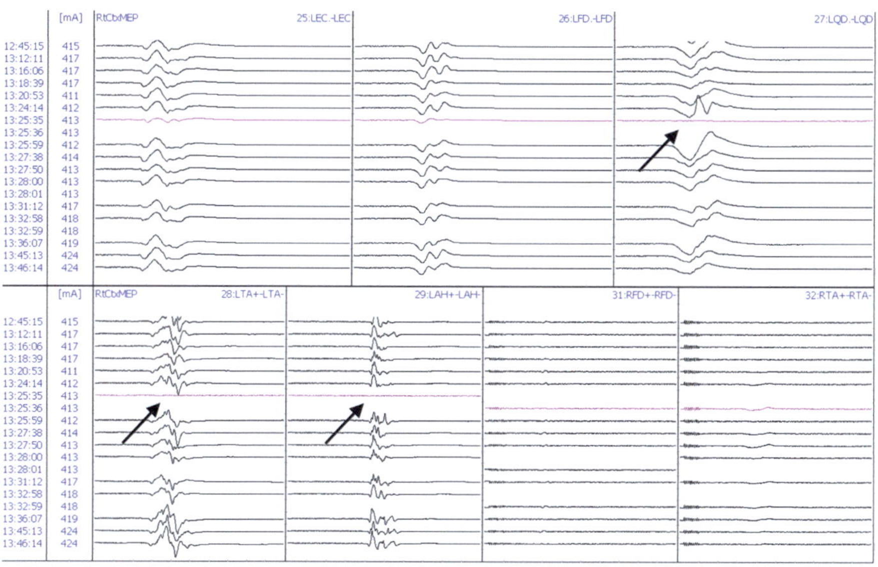

Fig. 8.1 Changes to motor evoked potentials (MEPs) during corpus callosotomy following placement of interhemispheric retractor resulting in loss of MEPs to lower extremities (*arrow*). Note changes recorded primarily from lower extremity myotomes. Following immediate discussion with surgical and anesthesia teams, retractors were repositioned with subsequent rapid recovery of all motor evoked potentials. Timebase 10 ms/division, amplitudes varying with no less than 100 μV/division, *RtCtxMEP* stimulation of right cortical hemisphere, *LEC* left extensor carpi radialis muscle, *LFD* left first dorsal interosseous muscle, *LQD* left quadriceps muscle, *LTA* left tibialis anterior muscle, *LAH* left abductor hallucis muscle, *RFD* right first dorsal interosseous muscle, *RTA* right tibialis anterior muscle (right-sided myotomes utilized to assess extent of contralateral current spread)

Once the neurophysiology team has observed changes, these should be communicated immediately to the surgical and anesthetic teams so that they may respond appropriately to the signal changes. The patient's hemodynamic parameters and anesthetic agents may require rapid adjustments in response to a change or loss of signals, especially if the patient is in relative hypotension with subsequent hypoperfusion to the nervous system. Positioning should also be re-evaluated, especially in the setting of focal IONM changes. The surgeon should pause and consider any recent changes in the surgical field that can be reversed or mitigated to return to their prior state [29, 30]. This could include releasing distracting forces slowly during spinal procedures or removing clips during vascular procedures. Repeat evaluations and further modification of surgical and anesthetic techniques should continue until IONM signals have returned to their baseline; if it is felt the risk of proceeding is unacceptably high given the changes in monitoring signals, the procedure may need to be aborted until the patient is stabilized and evaluated post-operatively.

Cerebral Monitoring

The success of cortical monitoring in children is dependent on brain maturation and optimizing monitoring and stimulation parameters based on age and pathology. Long tract monitoring (SSEPs and tcMEPs) is the mainstay of cortical monitoring, with direct mapping (motor, somatosensory, and verbal) as powerful adjuncts for a select group of patients. Cortical regions associated with long tracts, including somatosensory and motor cortex, myelinate earlier—usually wholly so by 1 year of age—than other regions such as fronto-temporal cortex, and therefore can be monitored in very young patients [31].

Modalities such as SSEPs and tcMEPs allow for early detection of changes during positioning as well as intra-operatively for nearly all intracranial pathologies. The pediatric cranial IONM experience is most firmly established in epilepsy and tumor surgery, and SSEP/MEP-based IONM is recognized as a gold standard for these surgeries. The goal of this type of monitoring is to improve surgical safety by alerting the surgeon to early signs of ischemia and allow management changes ideally prior to permanent ischemic/hypoxic injury [32]. An important adjunct to traditional long tract monitoring within the brainstem is the use of BAERs to provide additional information on global cerebral changes such as temperature and ischemia [33]. Cranio-cervical junction pathology, such as Chiari malformations and skull base lesions, also benefits from monitoring to reduce the risk of injury to the junction while the head is fixed in the cranial frame and during decompression [34–36]. Outside of the realm of neurosurgery, cranial monitoring with SSEPs and electroencephalography (EEG) has been widely documented in cardiac surgery [37, 38]. Although changes from baseline trigger intra-operative interventions, evidence to support improved outcomes after pediatric cardiac surgery is still limited [38].

Cortical mapping has evolved into a standard technique for supratentorial pediatric surgery in regions of eloquent cortex—the most common form being direct motor cortex mapping. Traditionally, motor mapping has been performed via a bipolar handheld probe with low frequency sustained stimulation, known as the Penfield technique since its development in the 1930s [4, 39]. Monopolar electrical stimulation can also be reliably used to map primary motor cortex [40]. Its thresholds in pediatric cortical mapping may be more consistent in certain areas of motor cortex such as the upper extremities compared to face and lower extremities [41]. Cortical lesions including those found in tuberous sclerosis or cortical dysplasia can also alter monitoring considerations and exhibit higher stimulation thresholds [41].

Surgeons can more precisely delineate eloquent territories intraoperatively based on function rather than imaging alone, and thus guide their cortical entry point and subcortical path to the targeted lesion [4, 41, 42]. Direct identification of primary somatosensory cortex as well as probable location of the central sulcus utilizes recording the location of the SSEP phase reversal to contralateral peripheral nerve stimulation [43, 44] (Fig. 8.2). This technique often employs a strip electrode containing at least two and often four or more electrodes in a straight line placed perpendicular to the orientation of the putative central sulcus straddling both the primary motor and primary sensory cortices. Typically, half the electrodes on the strip are placed pre-centrally with remaining half post-centrally. The recorded SSEP

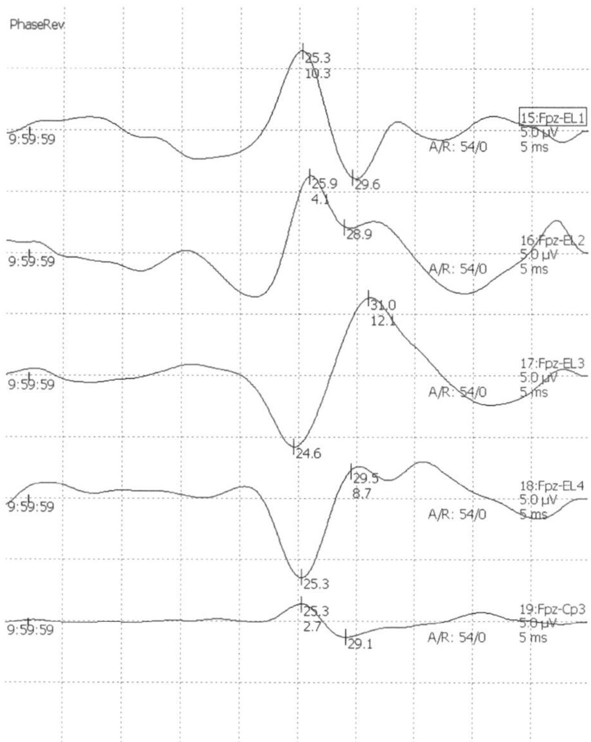

Fig. 8.2 Somatosensory evoked potentials (SSEPs) with right ulnar nerve stimulation, recording electrodes 1 and 2 placed post-centrally, and recording electrodes 3 and 4 placed pre-centrally. Note that the fifth tracing represents a transcranial control electrode placed posterior to the sensory cortex to allow the neurophysiologist to rapidly identify the sensory side. A phase reversal was recorded between electrodes 2 and 3, confirming the locations of the physiologic motor and sensory cortical regions

will appear "in phase" when recorded over primary sensory cortex and appear "reversed" in phase when recorded from the electrode placed over the motor cortex leading to the technique being termed phase reversal.

Technical considerations to this technique should include possible distortion of parenchyma by a lesion. Distortion can affect both the amplitude and phase of the SSEP precluding strict identification of a phase reversal. In these scenarios, it's important to recognize that the technique will most reliably identify primary somatosensory cortex even without a phase reversal. We routinely include a positive control transcranial recording of the expected SSEP when employing the phase reversal technique to guide "in phase" identification and therefore primary sensory cortex mediated responses. Thus, localization of the central sulcus, primary motor cortex, and primary somatosensory cortex is one of the primary indications for phase reversal and motor mapping. These techniques should be considered complementary and performed together in order to provide the most accurate mapping data to the surgeon.

Awake craniotomies have been adapted from adult neurosurgery to the pediatric population with awake mapping, and can allow for resection in eloquent territories previously deemed too risky for operative intervention. There is no established minimum age for participating in awake craniotomies, but a successful awake procedure hinges on the child's cooperation. The patient must be able to cooperate while moderately sedated and secured on the operating table in an unfamiliar and overwhelming environment [4]. This requires a mature child or adolescent, without cognitive or developmental delays, and cooperation and consent from the parents to optimize pre-operative psychological patient preparation. Based on our institutional experience, we would suggest that mature pre-adolescents and adolescents may be candidates for awake monitoring. Younger children may not tolerate these procedures well and more likely to be unable to cooperate with testing. Cognitive, language, motor and somatosensory systems can be assessed via awake intraoperative mapping. Careful patient selection and precise neuroanesthesia are crucial in ensuring a calm, comfortable, and cooperative patient during this mapping process. Complications from awake mapping are both rare and similar to direct cortical mapping, including seizures, and additionally can include language or cognition-specific deficits such as transient dysphasias [45].

Spinal Cord Monitoring

Intraoperative neuromonitoring is especially important in pediatric spinal surgeries as they are associated with a higher risk of new neurologic deficits than in a similar adult population—1.3% vs 0.8%—and even more so in the setting of instrumentation [46, 47]. There is extensive literature on IONM in pediatric spinal deformity correction and its utility in detecting early neurological injuries, such that some advocate its use in every case [48]. Somatosensory and motor evoked potentials are regarded as the building blocks of successful neuromonitoring for spinal procedures—for both spine and nervous system procedures.

A multimodal approach with SSEPs, tcMEPs, and EMG can be 99.6% sensitive at detecting permanent neurological injuries during pediatric spinal procedures, even if lower thresholds increase the risk of false-positive monitoring alerts [49–51]. A base of SSEP and MEP monitoring can be effectively supplemented by indirect stimulation with transduced EMG during instrumentation placement, proven to be as safe as image-based navigation for instrumentation in pediatric deformity cases [52]. Alerts can lead to effective changes in surgical and anesthetic management in order to reduce the risk of permanent neurological deficits to 1% or less [50, 51]. Although changes in neuromonitoring are seen in up to 10% of spinal deformity cases, only 1% of pediatric patients will emerge with a permanent neurological deficit [53].

IONM is feasible in spine patients even at a very young age. In children less than 6 years old, MEP reliability in spine surgery only decreases to 86%, compared to 98% in older children and can still be safely and reliably utilized for very young patients [19, 54]. TcMEPs are exquisitely sensitive to altered spinal cord perfusion secondary to hypotension, ischemia or direct vascular injury, and can detect changes earlier than SSEPs in scoliosis surgery [55]. However if MEPs are not detectable or feasible in certain pediatric spine patients, SSEPs alone can safely be used for scoliosis surgery [56]. Somatosensory monitoring is flexible, and can be performed with epidural electrodes if needed [57]. If underlying diseases introduce risk factors that preclude reliable MEP evaluation and only SSEPs are utilized, it's important to highlight that changes to both anterior spinal artery perfusion of the ventral two thirds of the spinal cord and the corticospinal motor tracts will not be detected. The use of somatosensory evoked potentials for spinal cord monitoring is not an adequate proxy for assessing the long tract motor pathways. Alternatively, preoperative neurophysiologic evaluation may help identify which patients could reasonably be monitored using combined MEPs and SSEPs [58].

Monitoring has become standard of care for surgery for intramedullary spinal cord lesions and has been recognized as a neurosurgical guideline [59]. Changes in IONM, especially SSEPs and tcMEPs, during resection of intramedullary spinal cord tumors can predict the severity of postoperative motor deficits in pediatric patients [60]. Though monitoring is widely utilized for intramedullary spinal cord operations, there is also evidence that it may mitigate the risk of neurological injury for intradural extramedullary tumor resection and syringomyelia procedures [61, 62]. Tethered cord procedures have also been improved by the addition of multimodal monitoring, including MEPs/SSEPs, as well as direct stimulation for tether and sacral root identification, and even reflex testing [63]. EMG has also been reported as a valuable supplemental modality for conus medullaris and cauda equina mapping in conjunction with MEPs/SSEPs [64].

Transcranial electrical stimulation activates fast conducting axons in descending motor pathways via both direct and indirect means. Direct activation can be recorded as a D-wave over the spinal cord utilizing either an epidural or subdural recording electrode, which is more reliable through all depths of anesthesia than its indirectly activated counterpart, the I-wave (Fig. 8.3). This technique, first described in 1954, can often be employed for spinal cord monitoring even when MEPs and SSEPs are not recordable and provides a robust general sense of spinal cord health intraoperatively [65]. It does not provide nearly the granularity of mapping compared to standard evoked potentials nor the sensitivity to cord ischemic insults of MEPs [66]. D-wave signals may become minimal below T11-12 when corticospinal motor

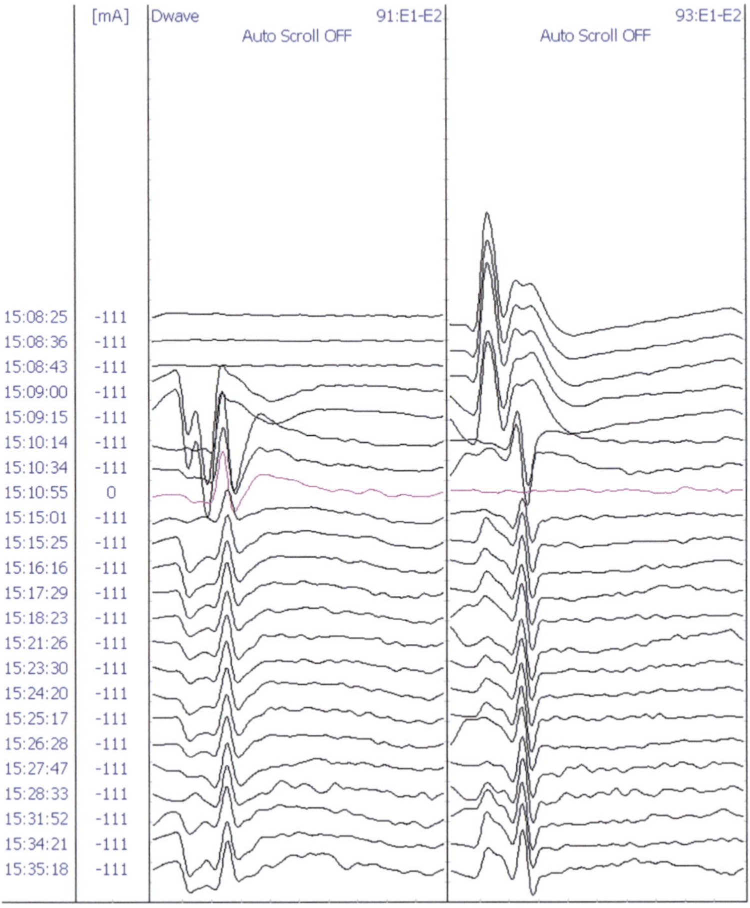

Fig. 8.3 Recording of transcranial electrical stimulation. D-wave: timebase 2 ms/division, amplitude 5 μV/division. *Left column* represents right cortical stimulation and recording of *left corticospinal* tract D wave, *right column* represents *left cortical* stimulation and recording of *right corticospinal* tract D wave. First eight traces represent placement of subdural electrode rostral to the lesion and is considered a positive control recording normal D wave. Subsequent traces show recorded D wave following placement of subdural electrode caudal to lesion and throughout resection. *Flat lines* noted in the initial traces and again on eighth trace highlight unilateral stimulation. Remaining traces obtained via interleaved stimulation for lateral spinal cord specificity

fibers have already exited the cord towards the periphery, and may not be present at baseline with prior spinal cord pathology or secondary to age [66–68]. It is essentially absent in children younger than 21 months, and in older pediatric patients may only be present in 30–50% of patients, compared to up to 80% of adult patients with similar neurological status [66, 69]. If utilized, a 50% decrease from its baseline amplitude should be considered a critical threshold to alert the surgical and anesthetic teams in order to pause and alter management [66]. Perhaps the strongest case in adding D-wave to a multimodal IONM battery is that loss of the MEP during resection of intramedullary spinal cord lesions precedes loss of the D-wave. Finally, preservation of at least 50% of the D-wave supports a positive prognostic outcome for patients regaining motor function following surgery [67, 70].

Dorsal column mapping to identify the midline of the spinal cord can be utilized prior to performing a midline myelotomy for resection of an intramedullary lesion [71]. This is a general application of the phase reversal technique described above whereby instead of peripheral nerve stimulation, stimulation of the gracile fasciculus is performed directly, typically via placing a bipolar electrode over the spinal cord starting in a lateral position and walking the stimulation across midline. The neurophysiologist will subsequently record the phase reversal of the gracile fasciculus stimulated SSEP from the scalp and guide the surgeon in identifying the neurophysiological midline of the dorsal column of the spinal cord (Fig. 8.4).

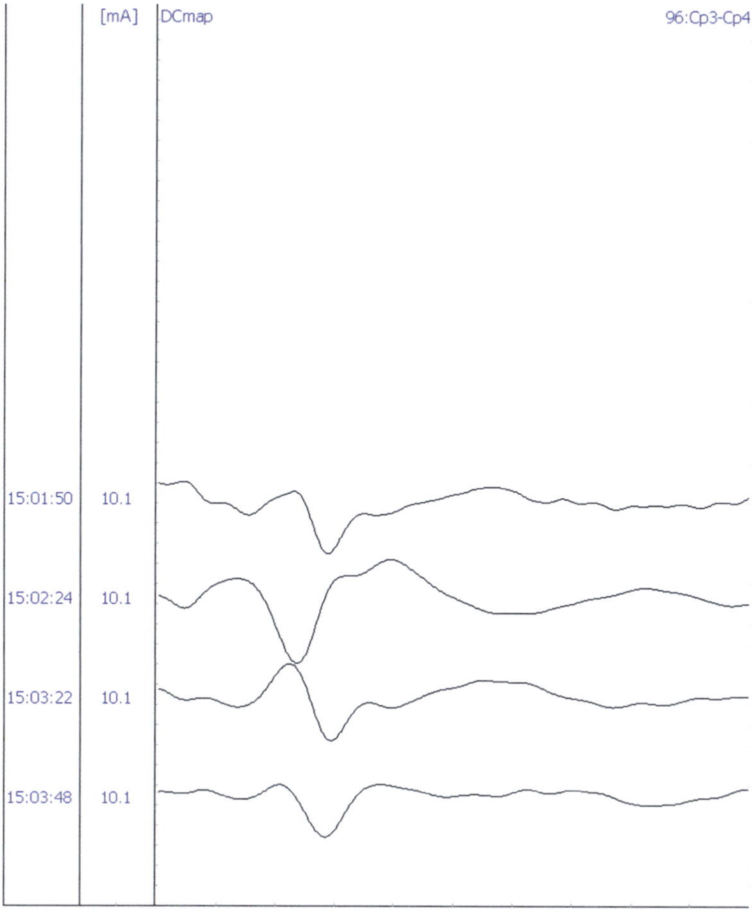

Fig. 8.4 Dorsal column mapping: Phase reversal of scalp-recorded gracile-mediated SSEPs (Cp3–Cp4) responding to direct stimulation of the dorsal columns using a concentric bipolar electrode. *Top to bottom*: the first trial was performed on the *left lateral dorsal column*, the second trial was on the *left medial dorsal column*, the third trial was on the *right medial dorsal column*, and the fourth trial was on the *right lateral dorsal column*. Note the phase reversal to gracile fasciculus stimulation occurring between the second and third trials. Timebase 5 ms/division, amplitude 0.5 μV/division

Some of the challenges of performing IONM in children include pre-existing conditions and the dynamic nature of nervous system development, which can lead to abnormal baseline neurophysiology. Cardiopulmonary co-morbidities in these patients can increase the risk of neuromonitoring changes intraoperatively, which may require more frequent or escalated interventions [49]. In those patients with pre-existing spinal cord pathology, IONM may be slightly less consistent—more so for MEPs than SSEPs—and need to be more frequently supplemented with other confirmatory testing such as a wake-up test [72].

Peripheral Nerve Monitoring

Monitoring for the peripheral nervous system is an important adjunct for many pediatric procedures, especially in the extremities. Tissue handling and dissection alone can directly or indirectly injure peripheral nerves, and the safety profile of pediatric operations can be enhanced by IONM. Modalities discussed earlier in this chapter such as SSEPs and tcMEPs can be of great value in monitoring the health of long tracts. These can reflect neurological injuries both in the surgical field, as well as distant changes in conduction. Children at high risk of neurological deterioration from hemodynamic changes and positioning, such as scoliosis patients and those with genetic or metabolic disorders should be considered for IONM during extremity surgery that may either be lengthy or require special positioning. Specifically, patients with Morquio syndrome highlight the importance of not only a multimodal IONM approach, but a multidisciplinary approach to their surgical care [73]. These patients are at high risk of cervical myelopathy secondary to atlantoaxial instability, which may be precipitated or aggravated during routine surgical care without significant precautions. Spinal cord injury has been documented following pediatric extremity orthopedic surgery, thought to be due to relative hypotension and positioning in the setting of severe kyphosis and scoliosis [74].

Along with long tract monitoring, local testing in the surgical field can be employed for monitoring peripheral nerve pathways. EMG and direct nerve conduction studies can aid the surgeon in identifying segments of injured nerve, and guide surgical decision-making in order to minimize the risk of any further injury [75].

Peripheral nerves can be distinguished from nearby lesions such as neurofibromas using direct stimulation. These can provide a better understanding of local nerve health than a purely visual inspection of a nerve, as immediate feedback of their function instead of waiting to examine the patient post-operatively. EMG may also be useful for non-extremity procedures, such as recurrent laryngeal nerve monitoring for pediatric anterior cervical surgery, or even cranial nerve monitoring during endonasal procedures [36, 76, 77]. More specifically, facial nerve IONM via EMG and nerve conduction studies, which is commonly performed in adult patients, is both safe and feasible in the pediatric population [78].

Conclusion

Neuromonitoring plays a major role in detecting and minimizing neurological injuries and thus maximizing safety during procedures that put nervous system structures at risk, and has become a significant presence in many pediatric operating rooms. It allows for real-time feedback of nervous system tissue health to the surgical and anesthesia teams in order to minimize the risk of neurological injury and guide further management. This immediate feedback reduces the surgeon's dependence on the Stagnara wake up test, especially beneficial in the pediatric population where a wake up test may often be unfeasible. Further studies are needed to fully evaluate the risk reduction and cost effectiveness of IONM. Although limited by some anesthetic and age-related physiological considerations, a multimodal IONM approach provides detailed insight into conduction from the cerebrum out to dermatomes and myotomes. It is both safe and feasible to employ neurophysiologic monitoring for pediatric patients with appropriate adjustments in monitoring parameters to take into account the child's age, health, and developmental status. Intraoperative neuromonitoring can be tailored to the individual child's needs, and thus integrates well into the era of personalized medicine.

References

1. Fasano VA, Barolat-Romana G, Zeme S, Squazzi A. Electrophysiological assessment of spinal circuits in spasticity by direct dorsal root stimulation. Neurosurgery. 1979;4:146–51.
2. Duffau H, Lopes M, Arthuis F, Bitar A, Sichez J-P, van Effenterre R, et al. Contribution of intraoperative electrical stimulations in surgery of low grade gliomas: a comparative study between two series without (1985-96) and with (1996-2003) functional mapping in the same institution. J Neurol Neurosurg Psychiatry. 2005;76:845–51.
3. Harner SG, Daube JR, Ebersold MJ, Beatty CW. Improved preservation of facial nerve function with use of electrical monitoring during removal of acoustic neuromas. Mayo Clin Proc. 1987;62:92–102.
4. Coppola A, Tramontano V, Basaldella F, Arcaro C, Squintani G, Sala F. Intra-operative neurophysiological mapping and monitoring during brain tumour surgery in children: an update. Childs Nerv Syst. 2016;32:1849–59.
5. Hall JW, Brown DP, Mackey-Hargadine JR. Pediatric applications of serial auditory brainstem and middle-latency evoked response recordings. Int J Pediatr Otorhinolaryngol. 1985;9:201–18.
6. Helmers SL, Hall JE. Intraoperative somatosensory evoked potential monitoring in pediatrics. J Pediatr Orthop. 1994;14:592–8.
7. Lesser RP, Raudzens P, Lüders H, Nuwer MR, Goldie WD, Morris HH, et al. Postoperative neurological deficits may occur despite unchanged intraoperative somatosensory evoked potentials. Ann Neurol. 1986;19:22–5.
8. Molaie M. False negative intraoperative somatosensory evoked potentials with simultaneous bilateral stimulation. Clin Electroencephalogr. 1986;17:6–9.
9. Trollmann R, Nüsken E, Wenzel D. Neonatal somatosensory evoked potentials: maturational aspects and prognostic value. Pediatr Neurol. 2010;42:427–33.

10. Allison T, Wood CC, Goff WR. Brain stem auditory, pattern-reversal visual, and short-latency somatosensory evoked potentials: latencies in relation to age, sex, and brain and body size. Electroencephalogr Clin Neurophysiol. 1983;55:619–36.
11. Gavaret M, Trébuchon A, Aubert S, Jacopin S, Blondel B, Glard Y, et al. Intraoperative monitoring in pediatric orthopedic spinal surgery: three hundred consecutive monitoring cases of which 10% of patients were younger than 4 years of age. Spine. 2011;36:1855–63.
12. Patel AJ, Agadi S, Thomas JG, Schmidt RJ, Hwang SW, Fulkerson DH, et al. Neurophysiologic intraoperative monitoring in children with down syndrome. Childs Nerv Syst. 2013;29:281–7.
13. Yellin JL, Wiggins CR, Franco AJ, Sankar WN. Safe transcranial electric stimulation motor evoked potential monitoring during posterior spinal fusion in two patients with cochlear implants. J Clin Monit Comput. 2016;30:503–6.
14. Master DL, Thompson GH, Poe-Kochert C, Biro C. Spinal cord monitoring for scoliosis surgery in Rett syndrome: can these patients be accurately monitored? J Pediatr Orthop. 2008;28:342–6.
15. Mo AZ, Asemota AO, Venkatesan A, Ritzl EK, Njoku DB, Sponseller PD. Why no signals? Cerebral anatomy predicts success of intraoperative neuromonitoring during correction of scoliosis secondary to cerebral palsy. J Pediatr Orthop. 2015:1.
16. Lieberman JA, Lyon R, Feiner J, Diab M, Gregory GA. The effect of age on motor evoked potentials in children under propofol/isoflurane anesthesia. Anesth Analg. 2006;103:316–21–tableofcontents.
17. Lo Y-L, Dan Y-F, Tan YE, Nurjannah S, Tan S-B, Tan C-T, et al. Intraoperative motor-evoked potential monitoring in scoliosis surgery: comparison of desflurane/nitrous oxide with propofol total intravenous anesthetic regimens. J Neurosurg Anesthesiol. 2006;18:211–4.
18. DiCindio S, Schwartz DM. Anesthetic management for pediatric spinal fusion: implications of advances in spinal cord monitoring. Anesthesiol Clin North Am. 2005;23:765–87–x.
19. Frei FJ, Ryhult SE, Duitmann E, Hasler CC, Luetschg J, Erb TO. Intraoperative monitoring of motor-evoked potentials in children undergoing spinal surgery. Spine. 2007;32:911–7.
20. Tobias JD, Goble TJ, Bates G, Anderson JT, Hoernschemeyer DG. Effects of dexmedetomidine on intraoperative motor and somatosensory evoked potential monitoring during spinal surgery in adolescents. Paediatr Anaesth. 2008;18:1082–8.
21. Busso VO, McAuliffe JJ. Intraoperative neurophysiological monitoring in pediatric neurosurgery. Paediatr Anaesth. 2014;24:690–7.
22. Anschel DJ, Aherne A, Soto RG, Carrion W, Hoegerl C, Nori P, et al. Successful intraoperative spinal cord monitoring during scoliosis surgery using a total intravenous anesthetic regimen including dexmedetomidine. J Clin Neurophysiol. 2008;25:56–61.
23. Mahmoud M, Sadhasivam S, Sestokas AK, Samuels P, McAuliffe J. Loss of transcranial electric motor evoked potentials during pediatric spine surgery with dexmedetomidine. Anesthesiology. 2007;106:393–6.
24. Simpao AF, Janik LS, Hsu G, Schwartz AJ, Heuer GG, Warrington AP, et al. Transient and reproducible loss of motor-evoked potential signals after intravenous levetiracetam in a child undergoing craniotomy for resection of astrocytoma. A A Case Rep. 2015;4:26–8.
25. Sanders A, Andras L, Lehman A, Bridges N, Skaggs DL. Dermal discolorations and burns at neuromonitoring electrodes in pediatric spine surgery. Spine. 2016;42:20–4.
26. Hays SR, Schwengel DA. Transient hypotension as a complication of monitoring transcervical motor evoked potentials. Anesthesiology. 1999;90:314–7.
27. Nandyala SV, Hassanzadeh H, Jain A, Sponseller PD. Neuromonitoring in pediatric spine surgery. Seminars in Spine Surgery. 2015;27:201–8.
28. Ferguson J, Hwang SW, Tataryn Z, Samdani AF. Neuromonitoring changes in pediatric spinal deformity surgery: a single-institution experience. J Neurosurg Pediatr. 2014;13:247–54.
29. Jain A, Khanna AJ, Hassanzadeh H. Management of intraoperative neuromonitoring signal loss. Semin Spine Surg. 2015;27:229–32.

30. Cheh G, Lenke LG, Padberg AM, Kim YJ, Daubs MD, Kuhns C, et al. Loss of spinal cord monitoring signals in children during thoracic kyphosis correction with spinal osteotomy: why does it occur and what should you do? Spine. 2008;33:1093–9.
31. Deoni SCL, Dean DC, Remer J, Dirks H, O'Muircheartaigh J. Cortical maturation and myelination in healthy toddlers and young children. NeuroImage. 2015;115:147–61.
32. Lopez JR. Neurophysiologic intraoperative monitoring of pediatric cerebrovascular surgery. J Clin Neurophysiol. 2009;26:85–94.
33. Rodriguez RA, Edmonds HL, Auden SM, Austin EH. Auditory brainstem evoked responses and temperature monitoring during pediatric cardiopulmonary bypass. Can J Anaesth. 1999;46:832–9.
34. Barzilai O, Roth J, Korn A, Constantini S. The value of multimodality intraoperative neurophysiological monitoring in treating pediatric Chiari malformation type I. Acta Neurochir. 2016;158:335–40.
35. Anderson RCE, Dowling KC, Feldstein NA, Emerson RG. Chiari I malformation: potential role for intraoperative electrophysiologic monitoring. J Clin Neurophysiol. 2003;20:65–72.
36. Elangovan C, Singh SP, Gardner P, Snyderman C, Tyler-Kabara EC, Habeych M, et al. Intraoperative neurophysiological monitoring during endoscopic endonasal surgery for pediatric skull base tumors. J Neurosurg Pediatr. 2015;17:1–9.
37. Chang T, Jonas RA. Neurologic complications of cardiovascular surgery. Curr Neurol Neurosci Rep. 2006;6:121–6.
38. Clark JB, Barnes ML, Undar A, Myers JL. Multimodality neuromonitoring for pediatric cardiac surgery: our approach and a critical appraisal of the available evidence. World J Pediatr Congenit Heart Surg. 2012;3:87–95.
39. Penfield W, Boldrey E. Somatic motor and sensory representation in the cerebral cortex of man as studied by electrical stimulation. Brain. 1937;60:389–443.
40. Kombos T, Suess O, Kern BC, Funk T, Hoell T, Kopetsch O, et al. Comparison between monopolar and bipolar electrical stimulation of the motor cortex. Acta Neurochir. 1999;141:1295–301.
41. Ng WH, Ochi A, Rutka JT, Strantzas S, Holmes L, Otsubo H. Stimulation threshold potentials of intraoperative cortical motor mapping using monopolar trains of five in pediatric epilepsy surgery. Childs Nerv Syst. 2010;26:675–9.
42. Noh J-H, Cho KR, Yeon JY, Seol HJ, Shin HJ. Microsurgical treatment and outcome of pediatric supratentorial cerebral cavernous malformation. J Korean Neurosurg Soc. 2014;56:237–42.
43. Goldring S. A method for surgical management of focal epilepsy, especially as it relates to children. J Neurosurg. 1978;49:344–56.
44. Goldring S, Gregorie EM. Surgical management of epilepsy using epidural recordings to localize the seizure focus. Review of 100 cases. J Neurosurg. 1984;60:457–66.
45. Balogun JA, Khan OH, Taylor M, Dirks P, Der T, Carter Snead Iii O, et al. Pediatric awake craniotomy and intra-operative stimulation mapping. J Clin Neurosci. 2014;21:1891–4.
46. Eccher M. Intraoperative neurophysiologic monitoring: are we really that bad? J Clin Neurophysiol. 2012;29:157–9.
47. Hamilton DK, Smith JS, Sansur CA, Glassman SD, Ames CP, Berven SH, et al. Rates of new neurological deficit associated with spine surgery based on 108,419 procedures: a report of the scoliosis research society morbidity and mortality committee. Spine. 2011;36:1218–28.
48. Drake J, Zeller R, Kulkarni AV, Strantzas S, Holmes L. Intraoperative neurophysiological monitoring during complex spinal deformity cases in pediatric patients: methodology, utility, prognostication, and outcome. Childs Nerv Syst. 2010;26:523–44.
49. Vitale MG, Moore DW, Matsumoto H, Emerson RG, Booker WA, Gomez JA, et al. Risk factors for spinal cord injury during surgery for spinal deformity. J Bone Joint Surg Am. 2010;92:64–71.
50. Emerson RG. NIOM for spinal deformity surgery: there's more than one way to skin a cat. J Clin Neurophysiol. 2012;29:149–50.

51. Thuet ED, Winscher JC, Padberg AM, Bridwell KH, Lenke LG, Dobbs MB, et al. Validity and reliability of intraoperative monitoring in pediatric spinal deformity surgery: a 23-year experience of 3436 surgical cases. Spine. 2010;35:1880–6.
52. Duffy MF, Phillips JH, Knapp DR, Herrera-Soto JA. Usefulness of electromyography compared to computed tomography scans in pedicle screw placement. Spine. 2010;35:E43–8.
53. Kamerlink JR, Errico T, Xavier S, Patel A, Patel A, Cohen A, et al. Major intraoperative neurologic monitoring deficits in consecutive pediatric and adult spinal deformity patients at one institution. Spine. 2010;35:240–5.
54. Fulkerson DH, Satyan KB, Wilder LM, Riviello JJ, Stayer SA, Whitehead WE, et al. Intraoperative monitoring of motor evoked potentials in very young children. J Neurosurg Pediatr. 2011;7:331–7.
55. Schwartz DM, Auerbach JD, Dormans JP, Flynn J, Drummond DS, Bowe JA, et al. Neurophysiological detection of impending spinal cord injury during scoliosis surgery. J Bone Joint Surg Am. 2007;89:2440–9.
56. Thirumala PD, Bodily L, Tint D, Ward WT, Deeney VF, Crammond DJ, et al. Somatosensory-evoked potential monitoring during instrumented scoliosis corrective procedures: validity revisited. Spine J. 2014;14:1572–80.
57. Accadbled F, Henry P, de Gauzy JS, Cahuzac JP. Spinal cord monitoring in scoliosis surgery using an epidural electrode. Results of a prospective, consecutive series of 191 cases. Spine. 2006;31:2614–23.
58. Azabou E, Manel V, Abelin-Genevois K, Andre-Obadia N, Cunin V, Garin C, et al. Predicting intraoperative feasibility of combined TES-mMEP and cSSEP monitoring during scoliosis surgery based on preoperative neurophysiological assessment. Spine J. 2014;14:1214–20.
59. Nadkarni TD, Rekate HL. Pediatric intramedullary spinal cord tumors. Critical review of the literature. Childs Nerv Syst. 1999;15:17–28.
60. Cheng JS, Ivan ME, Stapleton CJ, Quinones-Hinojosa A, Gupta N, Auguste KI. Intraoperative changes in transcranial motor evoked potentials and somatosensory evoked potentials predicting outcome in children with intramedullary spinal cord tumors. J Neurosurg Pediatr. 2014;13:591–9.
61. Ghadirpour R, Nasi D, Iaccarino C, Giraldi D, Sabadini R, Motti L, et al. Intraoperative neurophysiological monitoring for intradural extramedullary tumors: why not? Clin Neurol Neurosurg. 2015;130:140–9.
62. Pencovich N, Korn A, Constantini S. Intraoperative neurophysiologic monitoring during syringomyelia surgery: lessons from a series of 13 patients. Acta Neurochir. 2013;155:785–91: discussion 791
63. Kothbauer KF, Novak K. Intraoperative monitoring for tethered cord surgery: an update. Neurosurg Focus. 2004;16:E8.
64. Kothbauer KF, Deletis V. Intraoperative neurophysiology of the conus medullaris and cauda equina. Childs Nerv Syst. 2010;26:247–53.
65. Patton HD, Amassian VE. Single and multiple-unit analysis of cortical stage of pyramidal tract activation. J Neurophysiol. 1954;17:345–63.
66. Sala F, Manganotti P, Grossauer S, Tramontanto V, Mazza C, Gerosa M. Intraoperative neurophysiology of the motor system in children: a tailored approach. Childs Nerv Syst. 2010;26:473–90.
67. Deletis V, Sala F. Intraoperative neurophysiological monitoring of the spinal cord during spinal cord and spine surgery: a review focus on the corticospinal tracts. Clin Neurophysiol. 2008;119:248–64.
68. Szelenyi A, Bueno de Camargo A, Deletis V. Neurophysiological evaluation of the corticospinal tract by D-wave recordings in young children. Childs Nerv Syst. 2003;19:30–4.
69. Kothbauer KF, Deletis V, Epstein FJ. Motor-evoked potential monitoring for intramedullary spinal cord tumor surgery: correlation of clinical and neurophysiological data in a series of 100 consecutive procedures. Neurosurg Focus. 1998;4:e1.

70. Deletis V, Kothbauer K. Intraoperative neurophysiology of the corticospinal tract. Spinal Cord Monitoring. 1998:421–44.
71. Simon MV, Chiappa KH, Borges LF. Phase reversal of somatosensory evoked potentials triggered by gracilis tract stimulation: case report of a new technique for neurophysiologic dorsal column mapping. Neurosurgery. 2012;70:E783–8.
72. Wilson-Holden TJ, Padberg AM, Lenke LG, Larson BJ, Bridwell KH, Bassett GS. Efficacy of intraoperative monitoring for pediatric patients with spinal cord pathology undergoing spinal deformity surgery. Spine. 1999;24:1685–92.
73. Charrow J, Alden TD, Breathnach CAR, Frawley GP, Hendriksz CJ, Link B, et al. Diagnostic evaluation, monitoring, and perioperative management of spinal cord compression in patients with Morquio syndrome. Mol Genet. 2015:11–8.
74. Pruszczynski B, Mackenzie WG, Rogers K, White KK. Spinal cord injury after extremity surgery in children with thoracic kyphosis. Clin Orthop Relat Res. 2015;473:3315–20.
75. Jahangiri FR. Multimodality neurophysiological monitoring during tibial/fibular osteotomies for preventing peripheral nerve injuries. Neurodiagn J. 2013;53:153–68.
76. White WM, Randolph GW, Hartnick CJ, Cunningham MJ. Recurrent laryngeal nerve monitoring during thyroidectomy and related cervical procedures in the pediatric population. Arch Otolaryngol Head Neck Surg. 2009;135:88–94.
77. Maturo SC, Braun N, Brown DJ, Chong PST, Kerschner JE, Hartnick CJ. Intraoperative laryngeal electromyography in children with vocal fold immobility: results of a multicenter longitudinal study. Arch Otolaryngol Head Neck Surg. 2011;137:1251–7.
78. Bozinov O, Grotzer MA, Sarnthein J. Intraoperative monitoring of facial nerve motor-evoked potentials in children. World Neurosurg. 2015;84:786–94.

Part III
Needle Electromyography

Chapter 9
Muscle Analysis

Peter B. Kang

The overall goal of needle electromyography (EMG) is to evaluate the electrical field potentials of selected portions of the skeletal muscle at rest and during active voluntary muscle contraction. While the technical aspects of EMG are similar in children compared to adults, there are many details regarding the approach and data interpretation in pediatric studies that differ from those in adults. The general approach to the needle examination is well described in the literature [1, 2]. It is important to remember that EMG is intended to investigate lower motor neuron diseases. It can provide important diagnostic information that can help localize lesions within the peripheral nervous system. Although poor activation may indicate an upper motor neuron lesion, EMG should not be used to diagnose and/or localize lesions within the central nervous system. Needle EMG examination is typically normal or shows decreased activation in central nervous system diseases such as cerebral palsy.

Prior to the start of a needle examination, it is important to ask the patient and the family about potential contraindications to that portion of the study. Two major considerations are: (1) coagulopathies, whether endogenous or pharmacologically-induced, and; (2) the presence of any implanted surgical hardware near sites of anticipated examination. With respect to coagulopathies, it is usually sufficient to ask the family if the child is known to have a bleeding disorder or if he or she is receiving anticoagulation therapy. Intramuscular hematomas and other bleeding complications have been documented in the literature, though such complications are rare [3]. The needle examination in a child may need to be deferred if the family reports any such risk factors. With respect to surgical hardware, there is a small risk of iatrogenic infection if the needle electrode comes in contact with such hardware. Thus neurophysiologists must balance the potential risks versus benefits of performing this

P.B. Kang, M.D., F.A.A.N., F.A.A.P.
Division of Pediatric Neurology, Shands Children's Hospital, University of Florida College of Medicine, Gainesville, FL, USA
e-mail: pbkang@ufl.edu

© Springer International Publishing AG 2017

H.J. McMillan, P.B. Kang (eds.), *Pediatric Electromyography*,
DOI 10.1007/978-3-319-61361-1_9

study and avoid inserting needle electrodes near such areas. Similarly, the needle electrode should not penetrate any areas of skin that are infected in any way.

Concentric needles are the most convenient to use, and modern concentric needles provide excellent signal quality in children as well as in adults. As mentioned in Chap. 3, it is critical to use the thinnest concentric needle electrode commercially available, unless sampling a deep muscle such as the gluteus medius in an older child or adolescent. Full-sized ground electrodes may be used in all but the smallest infants where it may be necessary to trim the leads. Even more important than in adults, the neurophysiologist should counsel and explain to the patient prior to the needle examination that the goal is to "listen to the noise and crackling" that the muscle will make when the muscle is "resting" versus when the muscle is "moving". It helps for the child to practice the muscle contraction for at least the first muscle to be sampled prior to initiation of the study.

Many older children and adolescents will tolerate full examination of a muscle that includes sampling of multiple insertions in multiple quadrants at rest, mild activation to evaluate motor unit morphology (the standard for adults is 20 distinct motor units) [2], and full activation to evaluate recruitment and interference patterns. However, it is important to remember that even an older child or adolescent who appears to be tolerating a study well may abruptly decompensate with little warning, thus even in those patients the number of insertions performed to assess spontaneous activity and the number of different motor units examined during activation should be the minimum needed for a full appraisal of the electrophysiologic data. Also, the muscles examined first should be the ones that are most likely to answer the electrophysiologic question, in case the child does not tolerate the examination of as many muscles as originally planned. Muscles in the hand and foot are more sensitive and unless they are deemed the most important muscles for diagnostic purposes they should be studied last.

The thought process required for the selection of muscles to sample in infants and some toddlers is quite different from that in older children and adolescents. Infants and some toddlers cannot relax their muscles and activate them on command as older patients are expected to do. This may also be true of older children and adolescents who have intellectual disabilities. In such patients, the usual response to the mild prick of the needle electrode is to withdraw, i.e., flex their muscles. Thus, motor unit morphology and recruitment patterns may only be adequately assessed in flexor muscles. Examples of flexor muscles include the biceps, iliopsoas and tibialis anterior. Similarly, spontaneous activity may better assessed in extensor muscles, since children are less likely to extend their limbs during a needle EMG. Examples of extensor muscles include the triceps, quadriceps, and gastrocnemius muscles. The movements that occur while examining muscles that are not strictly flexor or extensor, such as the deltoid and first dorsal interosseous muscles, are variable but may be sampled if additional data are needed. The genioglossus muscle is particularly useful to examine when evaluating an infant for spinal muscular atrophy, and may be approached through the underside of the chin, slightly to the left or right of midline.

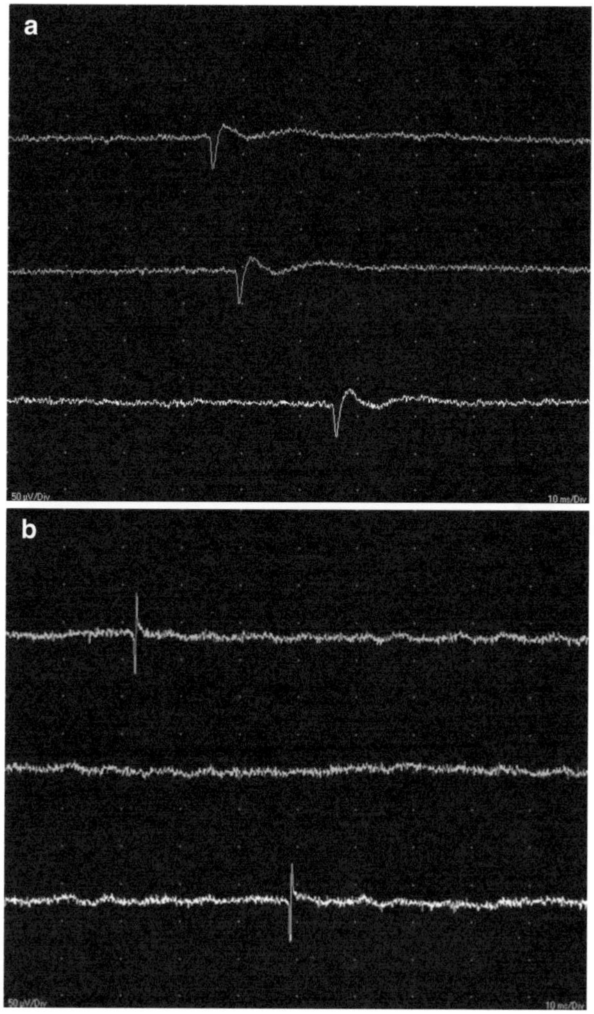

Fig. 9.1 Positive sharp waves (**a**) and fibrillation potentials (**b**). Note the initial positive (downward) deflection of both types of potentials. Courtesy Hugh J. McMillan, MD

As in other age groups, pediatric patients should not display any spontaneous activity beyond the burst of insertional discharges that occur with movement of the needle electrode. The interpretation of classic positive sharp waves (Fig. 9.1a) and fibrillation potentials (Fig. 9.1b) (also known as "denervating findings") is also not age-dependent, as these findings indicate the presence of a peripheral nervous system disorder but are not specific regarding exact localization, having been observed in motor neuron disease, axonal neuropathies, presynaptic disorders of the neuromuscular junction, and generalized myopathies. As in adults, fibrillations and positive sharp waves tend to have a positive, or downward, orientation on the screen, and also tend to occur at regular intervals, in contrast with the irregular firing rates of voluntary motor units. Fasciculation potentials, which in adults raise concerns for motor neuron disease such as amyotrophic lateral sclerosis, are rarely seen in children, even those who have motor neuron disease such as spinal muscular atrophy. Myotonic discharges at any age are often associated with diagnoses such as myotonia congenita, paramyotonia congenita, congenital myopathy, and Pompe disease (also known as glycogen storage disorder type II, or acid maltase deficiency). It is important to note that myotonic discharges are most consistently present in older children, adolescents, and adults with myotonic dystrophy; infants and young children with myotonic dystrophy do not consistently display this finding, even when they are affected by the congenital form of the disease [4]. It is notable that myotonic discharges are not commonly seen in the muscular dystrophies [5], especially in childhood [4].

The analysis of motor unit morphology in the pediatric age group is dependent on the ability of the child to activate a muscle in a controlled fashion, or in the case of an infant, the ability of the neurophysiologist to capture and interpret motor unit action potentials with practiced eyes and ears when they may only be present fleetingly. In both cases, the number of distinct action potentials available for viewing and analysis may be less than would be expected in a typical adult needle examination. In most situations, a skilled neurophysiologist will still be able to assess patterns of amplitudes, durations, and phases of the motor units that present themselves (Fig. 9.2). As in adults, high amplitudes and long durations are suggestive of a neurogenic injury, which can be focal (Fig. 9.3) or generalized (Fig. 9.4) depending on the pattern of abnormalities seen. Low amplitudes and short durations are suggestive of myopathic disease (Fig. 9.5). However, the amplitudes and durations of normal motor unit action potentials may be smaller in younger children and especially in infants. Thus, there is a dual risk of missing neurogenic motor units and "overcalling" myopathic motor units in this age group particularly when studying facial muscles. It is also important to remember that the duration is often more informative than the

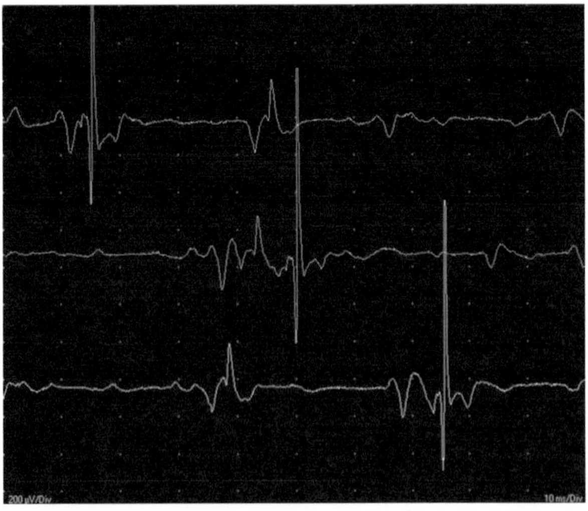

Fig. 9.2 Normal voluntary motor units and recruitment pattern observed upon needle examination in a 16-year-old adolescent male. Courtesy Hugh J. McMillan, MD

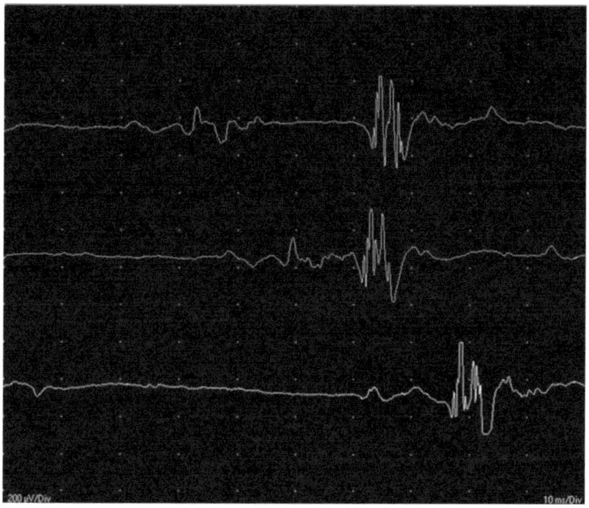

Fig. 9.3 Polyphasic, rapidly firing motor unit action potentials in a 14-year-old with radial neuropathy. Courtesy Hugh J. McMillan, MD

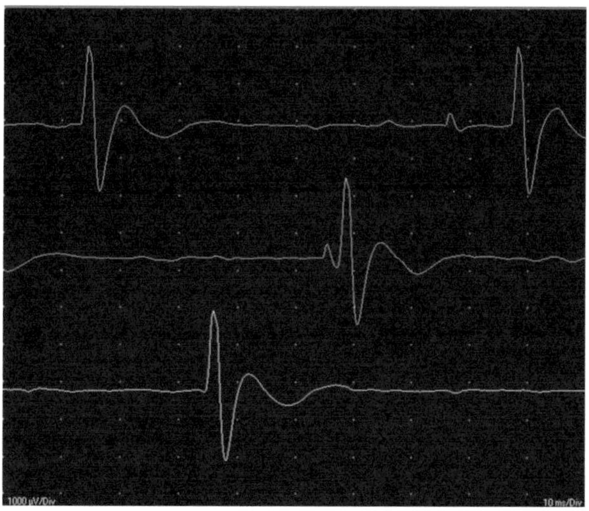

Fig. 9.4 Large amplitude (4 mV) rapidly firing motor unit action potentials in a 5 month old infant with spinal muscular atrophy. Courtesy Hugh J. McMillan, MD

amplitude with respect to sensitivity and specificity, though the measurement of duration may be confounded when the recorded motor units are distant from the recording electrode.

Recruitment patterns are often critical in distinguishing between normal motor units versus those that are large for age, as well as between smaller motor unit action potentials that are actually normal for age versus motor unit action potentials that are truly myopathic. Normal firing rates are similar at all ages including infants, children, and adults. In a normal muscle, additional motor units are recruited once the initial motor unit begins to fire faster than ~10 Hz [2]. Rapidly firing motor units indicate the presence of a neurogenic process (Figs. 9.3 and 9.4). Early recruitment

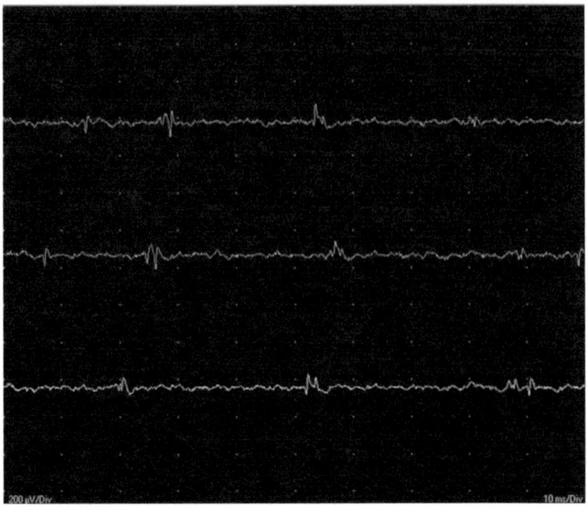

Fig. 9.5 Polyphasic, low-amplitude motor unit action potentials in a 1-month-old infant with myotubular myopathy. Courtesy Hugh J. McMillan, MD

patterns are discernable with a combined assessment of force generation by the muscle and the variety of different motor units observed. A finding that sometimes occurs is poor activation, where the patient does not activate the array of different motor units needed to assess recruitment patterns effectively. Poor activation may arise from a number of possible causes, including poor cooperation (due to pain, anxiety), upper motor neuron lesions as well as psychiatric diagnoses such as conversion disorder. Poor motor unit activation on needle examination should not be relied upon in isolation to support a psychiatric diagnosis such as conversion disorder.

The approach to the needle examination differs substantially when a child is sedated or anesthetized for the procedure. Clinicians should ensure that the use of neuromuscular blocking medications is avoided. One advantage of performing a sedated study is that the assessment of spontaneous activity is easier than in the awake patient. Under such conditions a full sampling of insertions in a broad array of muscles may be performed. However, elicitation of muscle activation is more difficult in a sedated or anesthetized patient.

Depending on the level of conscious sedation, a child may feel pain enough to withdraw during needle insertion as an infant does, and some motor unit activity may be detected and analyzed. Under general anesthesia, a patient would ideally not feel or react to pain at all, thus obviating the ability to perform motor unit analysis in such circumstances. The only means of obtaining motor unit action potentials in the setting of general anesthesia is to ask the anesthesiologist to "lighten up" the anesthesia, especially for agents with short half-lives such as propofol, in the hopes of eliciting a withdrawal response and some motor unit activity before the patient wakes up completely. If this is attempted, the lightening of anesthesia should only be performed once, and the patient should in the end be permitted to wake up regardless of the quantity and quality of the data obtained (i.e., the patient should not be subjected to multiple rounds of general anesthesia).

In summary, needle examination with assessment of spontaneous activity and voluntary motor unit activity may be performed with a high degree of accuracy and utility in most children. Given the limitations of data collection, especially in infants and younger children, a skilled neurophysiologist is essential to the proper collection and interpretation of these data.

References

1. Stalberg E. Invited review: electrodiagnostic assessment and monitoring of motor unit changes in disease. Muscle Nerve. 1991;14(4):293–303.
2. Daube JR, Rubin DI. Needle electromyography. Muscle Nerve. 2009;39(2):244–70.
3. Gertken JT, Hunt CH, Chinea NI, Morris JM, Sorenson EJ, Boon AJ. Risk of hematoma following needle electromyography of the paraspinal muscles. Muscle Nerve. 2011;44(3):439–40.
4. Shah DU, Darras BT, Markowitz JA, Jones HR Jr, Kang PB. The spectrum of myotonic and myopathic disorders in a pediatric electromyography laboratory over 12 years. Pediatr Neurol. 2012;47(2):97–100.
5. Hanisch F, Kronenberger C, Zierz S, Kornhuber M. The significance of pathological spontaneous activity in various myopathies. Clin Neurophysiol. 2014;125(7):1485–90.

Chapter 10
The Use of Stimulated EMG in the Diagnosis of Neuromuscular Junction Abnormality

Matthew Pitt

Introduction

Despite the increasing availability of gene panels, an accessible and cost-effective genetic screen for children with myasthenic conditions remains elusive for many clinicians. The number of genes associated with the condition increases yearly [1–13]. The clinical manifestations are so protean that it is very likely that without some direction by neurophysiological testing a large number of children will be screened unnecessarily. Of the different tests available repetitive nerve stimulation will be discussed in another chapter and has its proponents. However, it is not always sensitive, especially for certain diagnoses such as ocular myasthenia gravis, and when performed to its greatest extent uncomfortable for many children [14]. Performing it under general anaesthesia is a considerable undertaking and usually not necessary. Single fibre EMG (SFEMG) is a technique developed by Erik Stålberg in the 1970s that detects excessive variations in neuromuscular transmission, termed "jitter", among single muscle fibers. This test modality has higher sensitivity than repetitive stimulation for disorders of the neuromuscular junction, but has less specificity as increased jitter may be seen in other neuromuscular disorders. In its purest form, namely with volition activating the potentials, SFEMG is really technically impossible in children under 8 years of age consistently. It is true that on occasion experts in the technique will be able to achieve it in a particularly cooperative younger child but this is not a basis for universal application particularly if one is hoping to develop a neurophysiological screening test for myasthenia. It is therefore necessary to talk about the use of stimulated techniques for producing potentials that can be analysed. In most centres this would be called stimulated single-fibre EMG (stimSFEMG) [15, 16] but this name is most probably a misnomer because

M. Pitt, M.D., F.R.C.P.
Department of Clinical Neurophysiology, Great Ormond Street Hospital for Children NHS Foundation Trust, London, WC1N 3JH, UK
e-mail: matthew.pitt@gosh.nhs.uk

© Springer International Publishing AG 2017
H.J. McMillan, P.B. Kang (eds.), *Pediatric Electromyography*,
DOI 10.1007/978-3-319-61361-1_10

even when studying a normal neuromuscular junction it is very difficult to be sure that one is recording from single fibre potentials as opposed to small compound motor potentials representing a few fibers. As the test becomes more abnormal, reflecting abnormality of the neuromuscular junction, this becomes increasingly impossible. The technique evolved in our department from the work of Dr. Payan [17] using the "blanket technique" to reveal the components of a motor unit potential and by these means identify any instability that might be present. It was never intended to be a single fibre assessment and was unequivocally distanced from classic single fibre methodology by the author. In its original form it was used qualitatively and was a very useful adjunct to pediatric EMG allowing identification of likely abnormalities not only of the neuromuscular junction, but also other conditions affecting the peripheral nervous system such as neurogenic disorders. The technique lends itself very easily to quantification using peak detection algorithms used for the single fibre recording, particularly around the normal range of responses.

To avoid any possible confusion with single fibre methodology and also to remove it from the legitimate criticisms of proponents of traditional single fibre methodology, our group calls the test "SPACE", which is an acronym for ***S***timulated ***P***otential ***A***nalysis with ***C***oncentric needle ***E***lectrodes. Because it does not include single fibre within its definition, SPACE is a neutral term and will be the focus of the remainder of this chapter. Concentric needle electrodes (CNE) enter into the definition of SPACE because the neurophysiological world has been obliged to turn to single use needles as a result of the discovery of prion disease, which cannot be eliminated by autoclaving. Reusable needles can no longer be used, one example of which is the single fibre electrode (SFE). Official SFE are quite costly, hence the previous practice of autoclaving and reusing them. In contrast concentric needles are significantly cheaper and are thus disposable. Until the price drops for single-use single fibre EMG needles it is likely that the situation of using a CNE, usually the facial needle with the smallest diameter, will continue for some time into the future.

Methods

The technique of SPACE is well recognisable in the descriptions of stimSFEMG and the important elements ensuring success of the technique will be summarised here. One of the most important is how you prepare the parents and the child, if old enough. It is very important that parents realise the importance of the condition that we are attempting to identify. While it may be vanishingly rare with only 10 per million of population affected [18], it is a condition that is treatable and should not be missed as it is associated with significant morbidity and in some cases mortality. If the parents understand the importance of the test and the reason you are doing it, even if in all honesty it is unlikely to show an abnormality in nearly 90% of the studies, they are complicit in what follows. It is also very important to stress to the parents that the technique when using local anaesthetic produces a minimal amount of discomfort, and therefore any distress that is displayed by the child is more likely to be a reaction to the unfamiliar settings and people as discomfort. Ametop (active ingredient tetracaine 4%) is the anaesthetic used in some centers in preference to EMLA (active ingredients lidocaine 2.5%, prilocaine 2.5%) as the former is approved for use in children down to the age of 1 month and has a more rapid onset of action, reaching its maximum anaesthetic level at around 30 minutes. After application over the orbicularis oculi (taking care not to expose the eye itself) and covering of the anaesthetic with an occlusive dressing the parents and child are sent away for that period. On their return it is very important to wash the dressing off the face as otherwise you may inadvertently pull the hair which may set the child on edge and make future investigation difficult.

The studies are performed using any modern EMG machine, in our department this is a KeyPoint. The filter settings for the recording are 3–10 kHz. The low-frequency filter setting derives from the work of Dr. Payan, already mentioned, which was the forerunner of the development of SPACE in our department. There have been criticisms of using such a high low-frequency filter with recommendations that it should not exceed 1 kHz mainly because of the phenomenon of ringing when potentials appear that are not real. In a study of normal subjects we were unable to demonstrate this phenomenon and also identified the peak detection algorithm showed no difference in the jitter measurements according to the low-frequency filter setting [19]. The stimulus duration is set at 0.04 ms. Surface electrodes are placed on the forehead as the earth (known as the ground in North America) and just below the tragus as the indifferent (known as the reference in North America). A monopolar stimulating electrode of 15 mm length and 30G diameter (SpesMedicaS.r.l, Genoa, Italy) is inserted just above the midpoint of the upper margin of the zygomatic arch (Fig. 10.1). The operator will press with the digit of his/her non-dominant hand on the zygomatic arch and while the pressure is being exerted place the needle just above it with the dominant hand. The Ametop removes the sting from the insertion but not the pressure and disguising the insertion with the pressure on the zygomatic arch is very effective. The needle is secured with tape to avoid accidental injuries to delicate structures, and then stimulation applied while slowly increasing the threshold to 1 mA. Looking for a twitch in the orbicularis oculi, it is anticipated that this should be seen before the 1 mA stimulation threshold is reached. If it is not the stimulating needle is repositioned and if this is still ineffective the needle is removed and placed in a different point. It is crucial to have the stimulation threshold below 1 mA as it means that the child does not experience any discomfort, and equally important the operator can be certain that the needle is placed close to the nerve and can expect an "all or nothing response" to increasing levels of stimulation. If any abnormality occurs this is then more likely to be pathological than technical. Even saying this most of us when seeing abnormal jitter or blocking will increase the stimulus further to be sure this is not a technical effect. Usually the response, if your insertion technique has been good, is that the abnormality remains in the potentials you identified but other potentials are recruited, sometimes with normal jitter. Next the recording electrode, a concentric needle electrode of the facial type (French gauge 30G) (Ambu A/S DK-2750

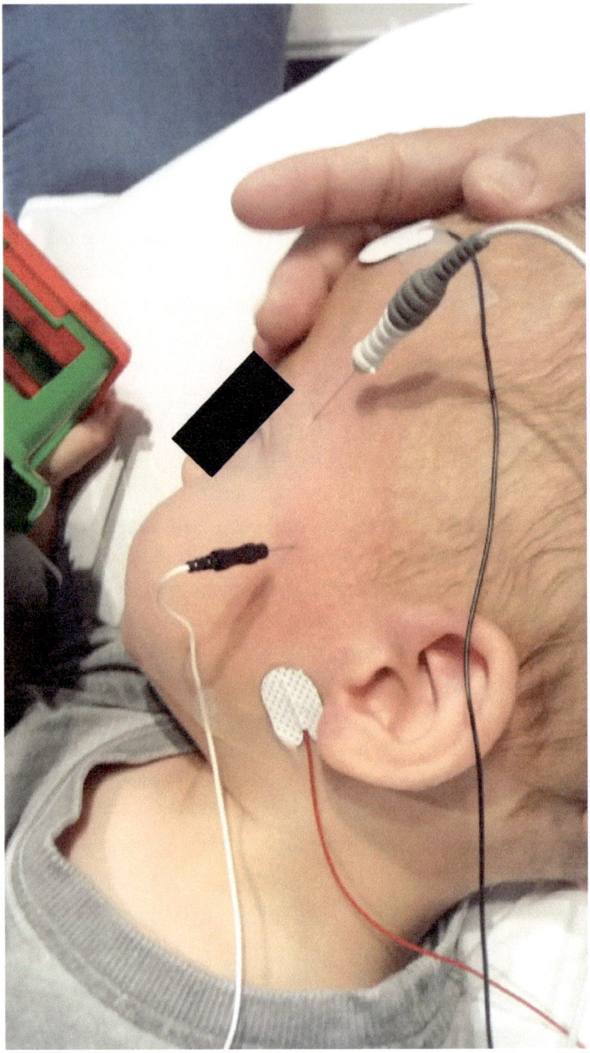

Fig. 10.1 Position of the stimulating and recording electrodes when assessing jitter in the *left orbicularis oculi*

Ballerup) with a recording surface of 0.019 mm^2 is placed at the outer margin of the eyebrow aiming at the ipsilateral hip and protecting the eye by placing the thumb of the non-EMG hand into the corner of the orbit, lying gently over the eyeball.

The stimulation is given individually by single shocks gradually increasing the intensity until waveforms are seen. The threshold is returned to 0 and the rate increased to 10 Hz. Continuous low frequency repetitive stimulation is given until the waveforms appear and continue until a screen full of potentials is recorded which approximates to around 25 repetitions. The process is repeated with single shocks being given with the needle moved slightly in order to obtain a different population of potentials. When seen the process is repeated. The aim is to collect at least 25 different potentials. The technique itself if everything goes smoothly will take less than 10 minutes although sometimes if there is difficulty identifying the potentials it may take longer.

If no abnormality is found on SPACE, the study is followed by a routine nerve and EMG study. Whatever the finding on the examination of the jitter it is important to leave the needle in orbicularis oculi and get the children to contract the muscle to see the interference pattern in the muscle. If the traces are abnormal this examination of the interference pattern in orbicularis oculi allows the determination of whether there is neurogenic change, which is an important cause for abnormalities of jitter and is associated with a bulbar palsy. If there is any doubt of the normality of the interference pattern in orbicularis oculi, particularly if the jitter is abnormal, it is obligatory to study the genioglossus, easily approached from the submental route. Whatever the findings in all of the initial investigations, nerve conduction studies and sampling of a peripheral muscle must be performed, the latter is particularly important if a bulbar palsy is identified as it may demonstrate that the neurogenic changes are part of a widespread motor neuronopathy.

SPACE of orbicularis oculi may miss some of the limb girdle myasthenias and particularly some of the more recently described disorders of N-glycosylation such as *GMPPB* and *DPAGT* [20–23]. Reports so far have demonstrated significant abnormalities on repetitive nerve stimulation of a peripheral muscle and if the jitter is normal and this is the suspected diagnosis it is necessary to perform repetitive nerve stimulation (RNS). RNS of the accessory nerve recording trapezius is very well tolerated by many children and can be reliably performed.

Interpretation of Results

Our software package uses a peak detection algorithm. The work on filter settings was performed using that algorithm and therefore what follows in the description here may not apply to programs using an algorithm which is triggered by the slope of the potential as this may be affected by the low-frequency filter settings. There is good deal of debate as to what the potentials produced by stimulation of the nerve or muscle represent [24–26]. It is for this reason that we have tried to distance ourselves from strict single fibre methodology because the requirements for single-fibre potentials to be accurately identified are necessarily extremely stringent and very rarely met by the technique of SPACE. The number of potentials that can safely be considered to be from a single fibre are very few indeed in most examinations. Using the alternative term apparent single fibre action potentials (ASFAP) [24] to cover this in many ways does not go far enough. Our technique is to use the peak detection algorithm to identify the potentials by the algorithm set by the software. If the study is normal and the peaks do not show much variation clearly the peak detection algorithm will have little difficulty in identifying jitter. However, sometimes several potentials may be seen with varying confidence as to their origin. Such a situation is shown in Fig. 10.2 where five potentials are seen none of which would fulfil criteria for a single fibre potential but the measurement, albeit

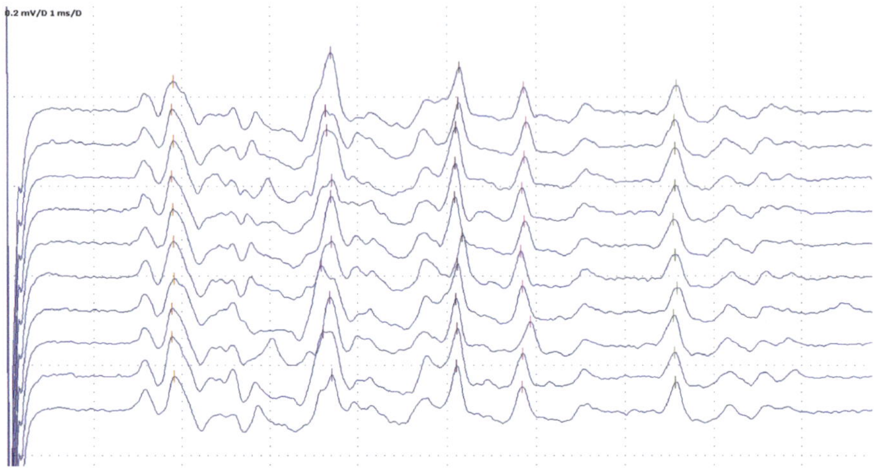

Fig. 10.2 Five potentials identified by the peak algorithm, none of which completely fulfill criteria for single fiber potentials, all showing slight variations in shape or amplitude

inaccurate, does give you some indication of the degree of abnormality when compared with normative data obtained from similar technique. Once the abnormality becomes pronounced the abnormality on peak detection increases exponentially and any linear relationship between degree of abnormality of the neuromuscular junction and abnormality on jitter measurement can be discounted (Fig. 10.3).

When analysing the data as we increase the intensity from zero until the threshold for individual potentials is reached there is a need to remove those first potentials particularly as they may show some minor jitter until supramaximal stimulation is achieved. Once this is done it is normally acceptable to use the measurements provided by the peak detection algorithm. The only time this is contested is if the program is clearly picking up alternating peaks from a potential with two peaks. This is shown in Fig. 10.4. It is possible to go through and identify those waveforms which only focus on one peak, or more easily, discount that potential from your examination.

Normative Data

Early on in our departmental experience with the technique we formed the impression that the neuromuscular junction was extraordinarily mature with samples of seemingly unaltered potentials appearing in children as young as 6 weeks of age which were indistinguishable to the blinded observer from a child in their teenage years. For this reason we used for a while the normative data obtained in stimulated single fibre EMG or volition SFEMG with the correction factor applied (×0.8) [27] in normal adults [24, 28–34] . With E-norm methodology, which extracts the normative data from laboratory attendances we have been able to confirm the jitter

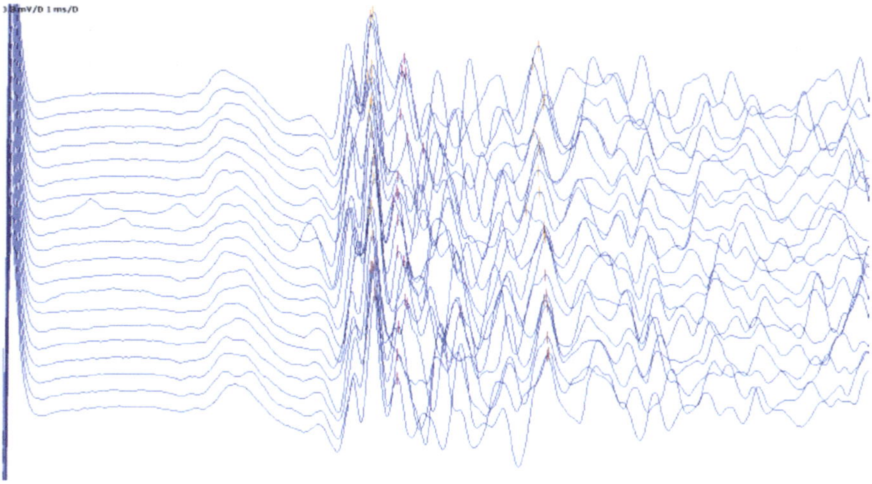

Fig. 10.3 A severely abnormal recording in a 20 month female with proven *COLQ*-associated congenital myasthenic syndrome illustrating that in some cases accurate estimation of jitter, other than having been identified as abnormal, is not always possible

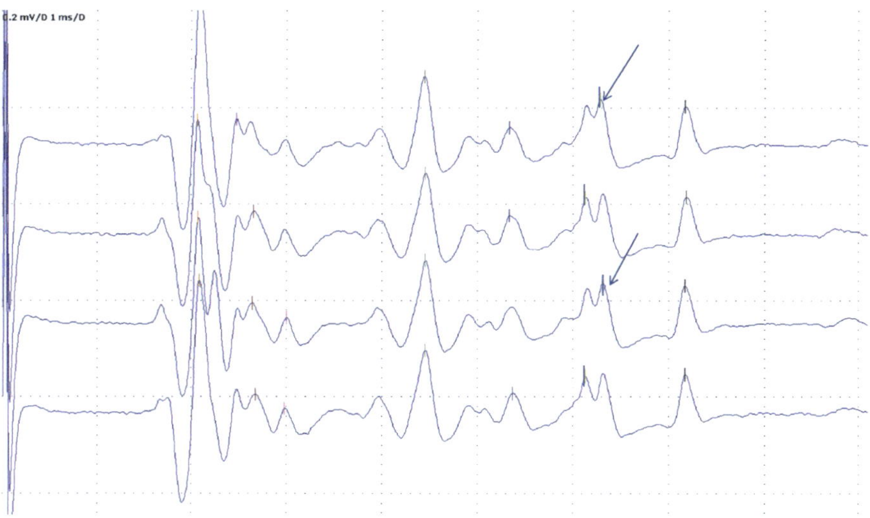

Fig. 10.4 An algorithm induced abnormality with a peak detection algorithm is identifying different peaks from a potential, which has a double peak, with the arrows showing, when the second of the two peaks are chosen

measurements in older children are indeed very similar to adults [35]. From a cohort of 600 cases, we derived an upper limit of normal of 26 μs for the mean jitter for children 2 years of age and older. More detailed analysis of the group under 2 years of age suggested that while some may have extraordinarily mature neuromuscular junctions this state is by no means the rule and we therefore found that under 1 year an upper limit of the mean jitter was 45 μs decreasing in the next year to 33 μs with the adult level being reached at 2 years of age [36]. Our results are calculated as the mean consecutive difference index or MCD-I which is calculated as the value obtained divided by the upper limit of normal.

Results

There are few if any centres that have much experience of the use of this technique in children, which is inexplicable, and whilst there have been a few papers [37, 38] reporting results in limited numbers of subjects our experience is unique. For a period of time certainly from around 1997–2007 our attempts to perform the technique were often greeted by failure and the numbers done per year were very few (Fig. 10.5). Sometimes a maximum of only ten would come through our department in a year. However, after that time possibly related to changes in technique such as

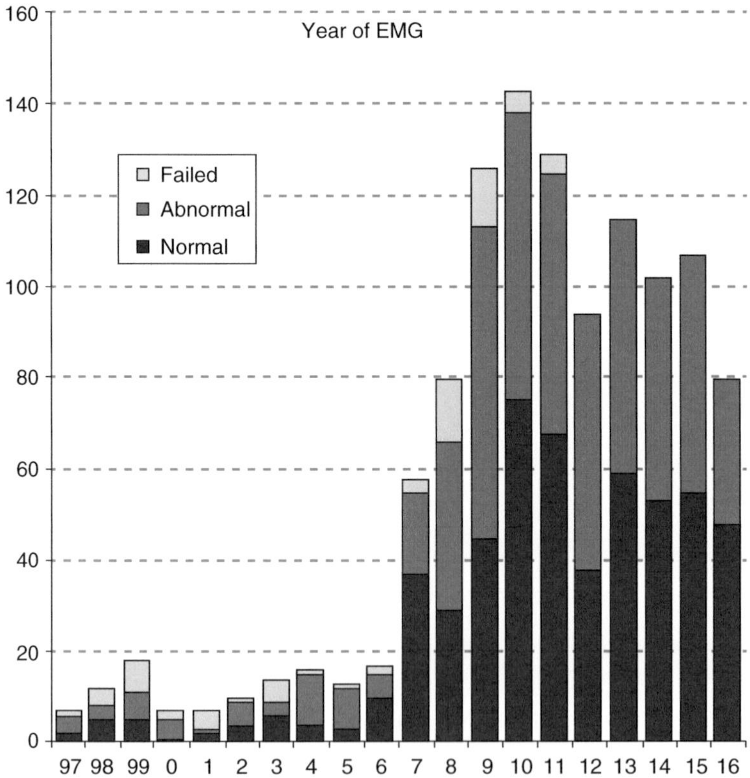

Fig. 10.5 Figures of the number of SPACE examinations since 1997. The open squares are those cases in which the study failed, the light grey those in which the test was abnormal and the *dark grey* those in which the test was normal

using shorter stimulating electrodes, which did not need to be held in position and also the more frequent application of local anaesthetic we saw an exponential increase in the number of cases, which are now at around 120 per year. A recent audit of our experience from 7 July 2007 to 8 February 2016 identified a total of 878 investigations, 501 boys and 377 girls [39]. The mean age was just over 5 years (66 months) but was skewed towards the younger age group with the median 46.5 months. Our hospital is a tertiary referral centre and because of this 114 cases were lost to follow-up. Many of these were from overseas often attending for one visit only. In this group 23 had an abnormal MCD-I ranging between 101 and 294% with 10% of them having MCD-I significantly elevated, defined as greater than 125%. A further group of 104 patients had not completed their investigations and were excluded from the analysis. Thirty six of these had a raised MCD-I, 25 of which were greater than 125%. The remaining cohort was 660 children in whom a diagnosis had been made or neuromuscular abnormality had been ruled out by a neuromuscular specialist.

Diagnoses

The diagnosis of myasthenia was considered definite if an associated genetic abnormality was identified or antibodies against the acetylcholine receptor or the MuSK protein had been identified. A further category of probable myasthenia was included in which the diagnosis of myasthenia was felt to be highly likely based on examination by a neuromuscular specialist with additional support from response to pyridostigmine. Ninty four patients had a diagnosis of myasthenia and these are shown in Table 10.1 along with other causes of NMJ abnormality such as botulism, when persistence of neuromuscular blocking agents (NMBA), bringing the total to 106.

Table 10.1 Primary disorders of the NMJ with number having normal MCD

Diagnosis	Number	Number having normal MCD
AIMG (anti-MuSK n = 2)	23	2
DOK 7	15	0
COLQ	9	1
CHRNE	4	0
Rapsyn	3	0
CHRNG	3	1
Slow channel syndrome	2	0
GFPT1	2	0
GMPPB	7	5
Agrin	1	0
Probable myasthenia gravis or congenital myasthenic syndrome	25	6
Botulism	9	2
NMBA	3	0
	106	17

Table 10.2 Non-primary NMJ disorders with number having abnormal MCD and the range of abnormal MCD-I

Diagnostic grouping	Number	Number having abnormal MCD	Abnormal MCD range as MCD-I
Neurogenic disorders			
Bulbar palsy	84	34	102.4–248.5
Cranial neuropathy	22	9	120.5–349.2
Generalised motor neuronopathy	70	18	105.8–264.4
Neuropathy	8	5	115.0–240.7
Myopathic disorders			
Specified myopathy	75	24	101.9–364.4
Non-specified myopathy	111	28	101.2–290.8
Mitochondrial disease	13	4	104.2–166.9
Unspecified, likely musculoskeletal			
Chromsomal defect	11	7	117.7–212.3
Chronic fatigue	4	0	
Congenital ptosis	10	0	
Ligamentous laxity	28	3	111.9–136.2
Others			
Central (including functional)	16	0	
Miscellaneous	30	5	110.4–138.1
No neuromuscular abnormality	60	17	103.1–140.8
Prader-Willi	6	4	114.7–161.8
Syndromic	6	0	
Totals	554	158	

In 554 alternative diagnoses were made (Table 10.2). The diagnoses were made with combination of clinical assessment, genetic, histopathological and other ancillary investigations. The diagnosis of a neurogenic abnormality was felt to be secure on neurophysiological grounds only. A proportion of these other cases had abnormalities of jitter and the range of that abnormality as an MCD-I is also shown.

Analysis of Test Parameters

Analysis showed sensitivity 84%, specificity 71%, negative predictive value 96%, and finally positive predictive value 36%. Certain subgroups within this cohort are worthy of additional comment. The sensitivity for the diagnosis of myasthenia was a little reduced, when compared to other studies [31, 40–42] but this was influenced by such cases as the five patients with *GMPPB* mutations, who are known not to have abnormalities of jitter when testing orbicularis oculi [21]. When looking at figures for sensitivity for the diagnosis of myasthenia gravis our figures (91%

sensitivity) are comparable with other studies. The two cases of autoimmune myasthenia gravis (AIMG) where autoantibodies had been demonstrated but no jitter abnormality was present included one patient in whom the abnormality appeared to be restricted to the ocular muscles. Amongst those patients with alternative diagnoses to myasthenia but abnormalities of jitter, the most important are those with neurogenic abnormalities and these were either isolated bulbar palsies or generalised motor neuronopathies. In the age group of under 2 years of age an isolated bulbar palsy as a reason for the apparent jitter abnormality was more common than myasthenia. If these cases, that is the generalised and bulbar motor neuronopathies, are removed from the analysis of test parameters the specificity is improved to 74% and the positive predictive value to 46%, with no alteration to sensitivity. The final group of interest are those are patients with myopathies either specified or non-specified in whom a proportion have been shown to have jitter abnormalities. What is emerging is that there are certain myopathies that do seem to have an associated neuromuscular transmission disorder and determining whether the condition is one of these or whether the myopathic changes are from the severity of the myasthenic syndrome can be a very difficult in practice [43–45] . As a rough guideline most myasthenics, with the exception of *DOK7* mutations, which may show patchy change, usually show severe abnormalities of jitter.

Discussion

SPACE is an imprecise and rather inelegant technique, which must be clearly delineated from the volitional single fibre EMG, which must be considered the gold standard for the diagnosis of neuromuscular junction abnormalities. However, whatever the criticisms that can be levelled at the former, it is highly practical and applicable in children and it is better to have an imperfect technique that you can do rather than a perfect technique that you cannot. While the author could additionally be criticised in calling this anything other than stimulated single fibre EMG, there is a strong feeling that the identification with single fibre methodology has led to the technique being resisted in its more widespread application in children. It evolved not only from single fibre methodology in particular use of peak detection algorithms but also from the "blanket technique" as a very useful technique for analysing the components of the motor unit potential [17]. The discoverer of the "blanket technique" was adamant when he described it that this was not single fibre methodology and our group would certainly agree.

With attention to some of the details given here it is possible to perform the technique in most conscious children of any age. Resort to general anaesthetic is very rarely needed and is to be resisted as it prevents the all-important EMG examination of bulbar and limb muscles taking place in the same attendance. The technique itself is quickly performed and we have shown that its results are to be trusted. It has formed an important part of the examination of children with hypotonia in our hospital with clinicians using it freely to examine those difficult cases in which myasthenia has not been excluded. The high negative predictive value is of particular importance in this subgroup. As a rule if the jitter abnormality is highly abnormal and a neurogenic abnormality has been excluded it has been our experience that the most likely cause is a myasthenic syndrome rather than a myopathic process with secondary neuromuscular junction changes. In the cases where the jitter is elevated but perhaps not very significantly, less than 115% [39], most clinicians would still arrange for a muscle biopsy while screening for some of the more common myasthenic conditions.

Further work that is needed in the development of this technique is to determine the normal range in the very youngest babies, under 3 months of age, for example. Most congenital myasthenic conditions are symptomatic from birth and to have a test that can identify these patients early on in the course of their disease, at a time when they are perhaps the most vulnerable from the consequences of serious associated symptoms, such as episodic apnoea, would be very useful. Additionally, but certainly not likely to find a solution in paediatric practice, refinement of this technique such that one could restrict the number of fibres stimulated and thus enable the indisputable identification of single fibre potentials, is awaited eagerly.

References

1. Beeson D. Congenital myasthenic syndromes: recent advances. Curr Opin Neurol. 2016;29:565–71.
2. Ravenscroft G, Davis MR, Lamont P, Forrest A, Laing NG. New era in genetics of early-onset muscle disease: breakthroughs and challenges. Semin Cell Dev Biol. 2017;64:160–70.
3. Shelton GD. Myasthenia gravis and congenital myasthenic syndromes in dogs and cats: a history and mini-review. Neuromuscul Disord. 2016;26:331–4.
4. Engel AG, Shen XM, Selcen D, Sine SM. Congenital myasthenic syndromes: pathogenesis, diagnosis, and treatment. Lancet Neurol. 2015;14:420–34.
5. Eymard B, Hantai D, Fournier E, Nicole S, Sternberg D, Richard P, Fardeau M. Congenital myasthenic syndromes; French experience. Bull Acad Natl Med. 2014;198:257–70.
6. Rodriguez Cruz PM, Palace J, Beeson D. Congenital myasthenic syndromes and the neuromuscular junction. Curr Opin Neurol. 2014;27:566–75.
7. Eymard B, Hantai D, Estournet B. Congenital myasthenic syndromes. Handb Clin Neurol. 2013;113:1469–80.
8. Finlayson S, Beeson D, Palace J. Congenital myasthenic syndromes: an update. Pract Neurol. 2013;13:80–91.
9. Hantai D, Nicole S, Eymard B. Congenital myasthenic syndromes: an update. Curr Opin Neurol. 2013;26:561–8.
10. Engel AG. Current status of the congenital myasthenic syndromes. Neuromuscul Disord. 2012;22:99–111.
11. Lorenzoni PJ, Scola RH, Kay CS, Werneck LC. Congenital myasthenic syndrome: a brief review. Pediatr Neurol. 2012;46:141–8.
12. Nance JR, Dowling JJ, Gibbs EM, Bonnemann CG. Congenital myopathies: an update. Curr Neurol Neurosci Rep. 2012;12:165–74.
13. Barisic N, Chaouch A, Muller JS, Lochmuller H. Genetic heterogeneity and pathophysiological mechanisms in congenital myasthenic syndromes. Eur J Paediatr Neurol. 2011;15:189–96.
14. Pitt M. Neurophysiological strategies for the diagnosis of disorders of the neuromuscular junction in children. Dev Med Child Neurol. 2008;50:328–33.

15. Trontelj JV, Khuraibet A, Mihelin M. The jitter in stimulated orbicularis oculi muscle: technique and normal values. J Neurol Neurosurg Psychiatry. 1988;51:814–9.
16. Trontelj JV. Stimulation SFEMG in myasthenia gravis. Muscle Nerve. 1990;13:458–9.
17. Payan J. The blanket principle: a technical note. Muscle Nerve. 1978;1:423–6.
18. Parr JR, Andrew MJ, Finnis M, Beeson D, Vincent A, Jayawant S. How common is childhood myasthenia? The UK incidence and prevalence of autoimmune and congenital myasthenia. Arch Dis Child. 2014;99:539–42.
19. Patel A, Gosk M, Pitt M. The effect of different low-frequency filters on concentric needle jitter in stimulated orbicularis oculi. Muscle Nerve. 2016;54:317–9.
20. Rodriguez Cruz PM, Belaya K, Basiri K, Sedghi M, Farrugia ME, Holton JL, Liu WW, Maxwell S, Petty R, Walls TJ, Kennett R, Pitt M, Sarkozy A, Parton M, Lochmuller H, Muntoni F, Palace J, Beeson D. Clinical features of the myasthenic syndrome arising from mutations in GMPPB. J Neurol Neurosurg Psychiatry. 2016;87:802–9.
21. Belaya K, Rodriguez Cruz PM, Liu WW, Maxwell S, McGowan S, Farrugia ME, Petty R, Walls TJ, Sedghi M, Basiri K, Yue WW, Sarkozy A, Bertoli M, Pitt M, Kennett R, Schaefer A, Bushby K, Parton M, Lochmuller H, Palace J, Muntoni F, Beeson D. Mutations in GMPPB cause congenital myasthenic syndrome and bridge myasthenic disorders with dystroglycanopathies. Brain. 2015;138:2493–504.
22. Klein A, Robb S, Rushing E, Liu WW, Belaya K, Beeson D. Congenital Myasthenic syndrome caused by mutations in DPAGT. Neuromuscul Disord. 2015;25:253–6.
23. Selcen D, Shen XM, Brengman J, Li Y, Stans AA, Wieben E, Engel AG. DPAGT1 myasthenia and myopathy: genetic, phenotypic, and expression studies. Neurology. 2014;82:1822–30.
24. Ertas M, Baslo MB, Yildiz N, Yazici J, Oge AE. Concentric needle electrode for neuromuscular jitter analysis. Muscle Nerve. 2000;23:715–9.
25. Sanders DB. Measuring jitter with concentric needle electrodes. Muscle Nerve. 2013;47:317–8.
26. Stalberg E. Jitter analysis with concentric needle electrodes. Ann N Y Acad Sci. 2012;1274:77–85.
27. Stalberg EV, Trontelj JV, Sanders DB. Single fibre EMG. Fiskebackskil, Lysekil: Edshagen Publishing House; 2010.
28. Gilchrist JM. Single fiber EMG reference values: a collaborative effort. Ad hoc committee of the AAEM special interest group on single fiber EMG. Muscle Nerve. 1992;15:151–61.
29. Kouyoumdjian JA, Stalberg EV. Reference jitter values for concentric needle electrodes in voluntarily activated extensor digitorum communis and orbicularis oculi muscles. Muscle Nerve. 2008;37:694–9.
30. Kouyoumdjian JA, Stalberg EV. Concentric needle jitter on stimulated orbicularis oculi in 50 healthy subjects. Clin Neurophysiol. 2011;122:617–22.
31. Sarrigiannis PG, Kennett RP, Read S, Farrugia ME. Single-fiber EMG with a concentric needle electrode: validation in myasthenia gravis. Muscle Nerve. 2006;33:61–5.
32. Stalberg E, Trontelj JV. Single fiber electromyography studies in healthy and disease muscle. New York: Raven Press Ltd; 1994.
33. Trontelj JV, Fernandez JM. Single fiber EMG in juvenile idiopathic scoliosis. Muscle Nerve. 1988;11:297–300.
34. Valls-Canals J, Povedano M, Montero J, Pradas J. Stimulated single-fiber EMG of the frontalis and orbicularis oculi muscles in ocular myasthenia gravis. Muscle Nerve. 2003;28:501–3.
35. Jabre JF, Pitt MC, Deeb J, Chui KK. E-norms: a method to extrapolate reference values from a laboratory population. J Clin Neurophysiol. 2015;32:265–70.
36. Pitt MC, Jabre JF. Determining jitter values in the very young by use of the e-norms methodology. Muscle Nerve. 2017;55(1):51–4.
37. Verma S, Lin J. Stimulated jitter analysis for the evaluation of neuromuscular junction disorders in children. Muscle Nerve. 2016;53:471–2.
38. Verma S, Lin J, Barkhaus PE. Stimulated jitter analysis in the early diagnosis of infant botulism. Muscle Nerve. 2015;52:309–10.
39. Pitt MC, McHugh JC, Deeb J, Smith RA. Assessing neuromuscular junction stability from stimulated EMG in children. Clin Neurophysiol. 2017;128:290–6.

40. Lyu RK, Cheng SY, Tang LM. Electrodiagnostic studies in myasthenia gravis. Changgeng Yi Xue Za Zhi. 1993;16:164–9.
41. SJ O, Kim DE, Kuruoglu R, Bradley RJ, Dwyer D. Diagnostic sensitivity of the laboratory tests in myasthenia gravis. Muscle Nerve. 1992;15:720–4.
42. Sanders DB, Howard JF Jr. AAEE minimonograph #25: single-fiber electromyography in myasthenia gravis. Muscle Nerve. 1986;9:809–19.
43. Illingworth MA, Main M, Pitt M, Feng L, Sewry CA, Gunny R, Vorstman E, Beeson D, Manzur A, Muntoni F, Robb SA. RYR1-related congenital myopathy with fatigable weakness, responding to pyridostigimine. Neuromuscul Disord. 2014;24:707–12.
44. Munot P, Lashley D, Jungbluth H, Feng L, Pitt M, Robb SA, Palace J, Jayawant S, Kennet R, Beeson D, Cullup T, Abbs S, Laing N, Sewry C, Muntoni F. Congenital fibre type disproportion associated with mutations in the tropomyosin 3 (TPM3) gene mimicking congenital myasthenia. Neuromuscul Disord. 2010;20:796–800.
45. Robb SA, Sewry CA, Dowling JJ, Feng L, Cullup T, Lillis S, Abbs S, Lees MM, Laporte J, Manzur AY, Knight RK, Mills KR, Pike MG, Kress W, Beeson D, Jungbluth H, Pitt MC, Muntoni F. Impaired neuromuscular transmission and response to acetylcholinesterase inhibitors in centronuclear myopathies. Neuromuscul Disord. 2011;21:379–86.

Part IV
Advanced Electrodiagnosis

Chapter 11
Artifacts

Hugh J. McMillan

Neurophysiologists must be aware of the many physiological, environmental, and/or operational factors that can influence data collection and analysis. These factors are collectively referred to as artifacts as they have the potential to lead to inaccurate or erroneous test results and ultimately to potential misdiagnosis. Erroneous test results, whether due to errors in the collection of data or the interpretation of results, can result in the pursuit of costly diagnostic procedures such as genetic testing and/or the unnecessary pursuit of invasive therapies such as surgical biopsies. Just as it is important for neurophysiologists to possess proper knowledge of the anatomical courses and positions of nerves and muscles, so is it essential to show constant vigilance for common pitfalls that may arise.

Artifacts will be classified into one of three broad categories: (1) patient factors, (2) environmental factors and (3) equipment/operator factors (Table 11.1).

Patient Factors

Age

Age is one of the most commonly encountered variables encountered by neurologists and neurophysiologists who work with children. Clinicians are well aware of the dramatic changes in neurodevelopmental milestones that occur during the first few years of life. The changes in central and peripheral nerve myelination are equally remarkable, though less commonly recognized, over these years. Interpretation of pediatric nerve conduction studies must always include consideration of a child's age. Axon diameter and myelination gradually increase

H.J. McMillan, MD, MSc, FRCPC, FAAN
Division of Neurology, Children's Hospital of Eastern Ontario, University of Ottawa, Ottawa, ON, Canada
e-mail: hmcmillan@cheo.on.ca

© Springer International Publishing AG 2017

H.J. McMillan, P.B. Kang (eds.), *Pediatric Electromyography*,
DOI 10.1007/978-3-319-61361-1_11

Table 11.1 Technical factors influencing nerve conduction studies and electromyography

Patient factors
Age
Height and/or length
Weight
Temperature
Anatomic variability (e.g., Martin-Gruber anastamosis)
Environmental factors
Electrical (60 Hz) interference
Drug administration (pyridostigmine, neuromuscular blockade, botox)
Machine/operator factors
Stimulation malposition
Electrode malposition
Cathode position (erroneous reversal of stimulator polarity)
Submaximal stimulation applied
Stimulus artifact
Adjacent nerve co-stimulation
Filter settings
Measurement errors
Sweep speed and sensitivity errors

from birth until adult values are attained at 4–5 years of age [1]. Not surprisingly, the normal reference ranges for electrodiagnostic tests also change with age, reflecting the progressive myelination that occurs in the first few years of life. Several reports have documented term newborns to show ulnar nerve motor conductions in the range of 20–35 m/s, with adult nerve conduction velocities not consistently observed until 3–5 years of age (Fig. 11.1) [2, 3]. This maturation must be considered when interpreting nerve conduction studies of infants and young children so as to avoid misinterpreting normal physiological differences as a sensorimotor polyneuropathy with demyelinating features. Normal values have been derived from prior published reports and are detailed in Chap. 24.

Temperature

Temperature is another important and common artifact. Practically, there are several reasons why aberrant skin temperatures may be encountered in the EMG laboratory. Patient anxiety or apprehension is not unusual, particularly in children who are about to undergo nerve conduction testing. Physiologically, this anxiety may be associated with the increased circulation of epinephrine. Blood vessel constriction occurs as part of the "fight or flight" response such that blood is shunted to muscle [4]. Circulation to the skin is also reduced to potentially mitigate blood loss in the event of injury. As a result, the hands and feet of anxious individuals tend to be cooler than usual [5]. Sweating may further cool the hands. Cool ambient air

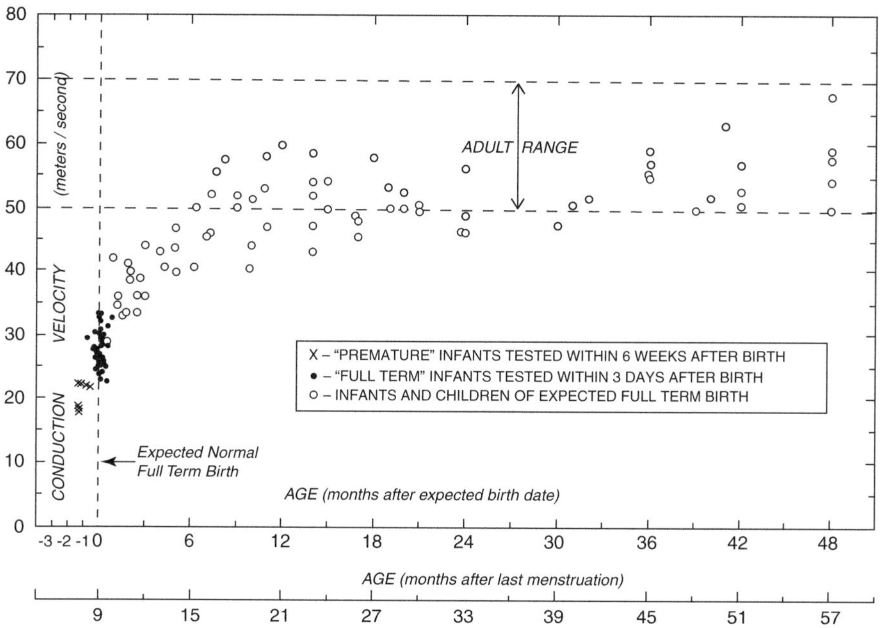

Fig. 11.1 Normal changes in ulnar motor nerve conduction velocity within the first few years of life, reflecting progressive growth and myelination [2]

temperatures including air conditioning in a patient wearing summer attire can further augment this problem. Regardless of the exact cause, temperature artifacts are common and can lead to interpretation error and misdiagnosis.

Temperature can affect peripheral nerve function by influencing ion channel function as well as neuromuscular transmission by altering acetylcholinesterase activity. Cooler temperatures will affect both sensory nerve action potentials (SNAPs) and motor compound muscle action potentials (CMAPs) by: (1) reducing conduction velocities; (2) increasing onset or peak latencies; and (3) increasing SNAP or CMAP amplitudes (Fig. 11.2). This pattern of abnormality can mimic compression neuropathies and potentially give rise to erroneous diagnoses; a common example is carpal tunnel syndrome.

Limb cooling affects both sensory and motor nerves. Action potentials are propagated along a myelinated axon as the voltage-gated sodium channels at each node of Ranvier open and sodium ions move along their electrochemical gradient into the axon. After the initial influx of sodium ions, these channels close. Potassium channels then open, resulting in an efflux of potassium ions, thereby restoring the resting membrane potential. Physiologically, cooling slows the rate at which sodium channels open and, to an even greater extent, the rate at which they close. The slower rate of opening gives rise to the delay in the propagation of action potential along the axons resulting in a slower conduction velocity. This delayed closing results in higher amplitude and longer duration action potentials which are reflected in the higher SNAP and CMAP amplitudes that are observed in patients with cool limbs.

Median Nerve Antidromic Sensory Responses at 25°C and 32°C

Median Nerve Motor Responses at 26°C and 32°C

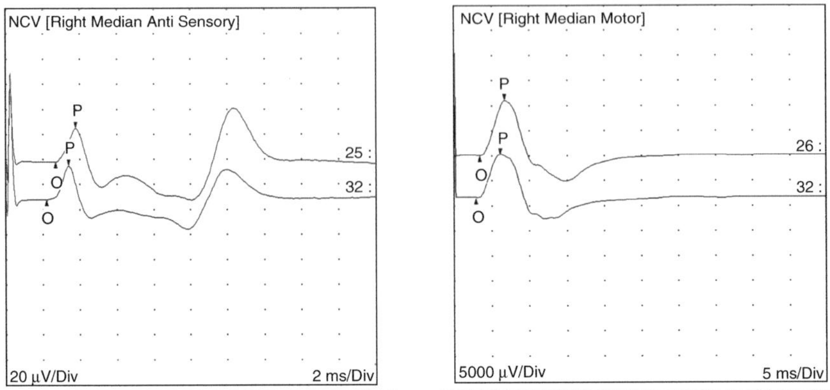

Site	Temp	Onset (ms)	Amp (µV)	Dist (cm)	Vel (m/s)
Right Median Anti Sensory (2nd Digit)					
Wrist	25°C	2.9	28.8	14.0	55
Wrist	32°C	2.0	26.4	14.0	64

Site	Temp	Onset (ms)	Amp (mV)	Dist (cm)	Vel (m/s)
Right Median Motor (Abd Poll Brev)					
Wrist	26°C	3.4	11.0	6.0	43
Wrist	32°C	2.9	8.7	6.0	52

Fig. 11.2 Median nerve sensory and motor responses showing faster conduction velocity and shorter onset latencies at warmer (32 °C) temperature compared to cooler limbs

Studies have shown predictable neurophysiological changes with cooling. Ulnar sensory and motor nerve conduction velocities decrease by 1.6–2.1 m/s for every 1 °C of cooling and distal latencies increase by 0.2 ms for every 1 °C of cooling [6]. Other studies have confirmed a conduction velocity decrease of 1.5–2 m/s for each degree of cooling [7, 8]. As such, limb temperatures should be measured and, if necessary, re-warmed to attain temperatures in the 33–34 °C range [9]. Other sources recommended a range of 34–36 °C for the upper limbs and 31–34 °C for the lower limbs [10]. Caution must be taken when hands are warmed since the superficial tissue will warm more quickly than deeper tissue, which can cause the limbs to cool off more quickly than expected after the study has been restarted [11].

Weight

Adipose tissue will insulate peripheral nerves such that stimulating electrodes may have greater difficulty delivering supramaximal stimulation. This is more problematic at proximal stimulation sites and can be observed in healthy infants as well as children and adults who have limb edema and/or obesity. Practically this is reflected in an amplitude drop at the proximal stimulation site compared to the more distal stimulation site(s) which can mimic axonal injury and/or conduction block. Caution must be taken not to overcall conduction block in such individuals, particularly when studying the tibial nerve motor response. Subcutaneous adipose tissue distributions often makes it difficult to elicit sural sensory responses in infants.

Height

Patients' heights or limb lengths are known to influence late responses (e.g., F-response minimum latency) when completing neurophysiological testing in adults. Correction factors, namely the F-estimate, can be used to calculate the minimum F-responses in patients who are tall and consequently have longer limb lengths [12]. However, several studies have also demonstrated an inverse relationship between sensory nerve conduction velocity and adult patients' height [13–15]. Cadaver studies have established that sensory nerve conduction velocities are slowed by 3.9 m/s for every 10 m of axonal length.

Normal pediatric values exist for pre-pubertal children of various ages. The precise contribution of height versus age-related myelination changes is less well known for this population. As such, greater emphasis is placed upon age rather than height per se when evaluating pediatric studies. Exception may be taken for very tall adolescents who should follow adult rules for correction factors as they apply to late responses.

Anatomic Variability

Children can demonstrate the same patterns of anomalous innervation seen in adults, especially as these anatomical variants are generally congenital. The classic Martin-Gruber anastomosis (MGA) should be considered in any child who demonstrates a higher CMAP amplitude when stimulating the ulnar nerve at its distal stimulation site (wrist) relative to a proximal site (below or above the elbow). MGA has been reported in up to 15–20% of adult patients [16], and presumably a similar proportion of children are affected. MGA results from the cross-over of median-to-ulnar nerve motor fibers supplying the hypothenar muscles. It has been referred to as a "pseudo-conduction block" as it has the potential to mislead inexperienced electromyographers into thinking that it represents evidence for a demyelinating disorder such as chronic inflammatory demyelinating polyradiculoneuropathy (CIDP) or multifocal motor neuropathy. The presence or absence of MGA can be confirmed by stimulating the median nerve proximally (elbow) while leaving the recording electrodes over the hypothenar muscles. The sum of the CMAP amplitudes recorded over the hypothenar muscles while stimulating the proximal median and ulnar sites should equal that seen with stimulation at the distal ulnar site in this condition. Other anomalous innervations include the Marinacci anastomosis (forearm ulnar-to-median communication), Riche-Cannieu anastomosis (palmar median-to-ulnar communication) and Berrettini anastomosis (palmar ulnar-to-median communication).

Anomalous innervation can also occur in the lower limb. Approximately 10–20% of adult patients are reported to have an accessory peroneal nerve [17] that contributes to innervation of the extensor digitorum brevis (EDB). This anomaly is detected when the peroneal motor CMAP amplitude (recorded at the EDB) is higher at the proximal stimulation sites compared to the distal (ankle) site. To differentiate an accessory peroneal nerve from submaximal stimulation at the ankle, the neurophysiologist should stimulate the lateral calf posterior to the lateral malleolus. If a small CMAP amplitude is recorded at the EDB when stimulating at this location, the anomalous innervation is confirmed.

Environmental Factors

Electrical (60 Hz) Interference

Electrodiagnostic testing relies on measuring very small bioelectrical signals that range from microvolts (for sensory studies) to millivolts (for motor studies). Given how sensitive the recording equipment must be, it is not surprising that external, non-biological electrical energy can contaminate or interfere with testing. Electromagnetic interference is widespread and can represent a source of considerable frustration for neurophysiologists. Overhead lighting, medical equipment and/or adjustable beds are common sources of electrical interference, especially in the setting of alternating currents. Intensive care units are particularly problematic due to the frequent presence of continuous infusion pumps and monitoring equipment. Neurophysiologists are often able to reduce electrical interference by taking a systematic approach to identifying its sources and temporarily eliminating any non-essential sources for the duration of the test. It is important, however, to discuss the disconnection of any device with the primary team. Patients themselves may carry hand held electronic devices including smart phones, but our experience has been that these introduce little to no perceptible electrical interference, and such devices may help distract children during EMG testing.

Drug Administration

Medications can have a significant impact upon nerve conduction study results. Neuromuscular blocking agents (NMBA) are commonly administered to patients in an intensive care setting to facilitate ease of ventilation and/or prevent inadvertent extubation. Depolarizing agents such as succinylcholine bind to acetylcholine receptors, causing persistent depolarization. Non-depolarizing agents such as rocuronium or pancuronium are competitive antagonists of nicotinic receptors, effectively blocking the action of acetylcholine. Motor nerve CMAP amplitudes may be absent or dramatically reduced if nerve conduction studies are performed upon a patient who has received such medications. Neurophysiologists must ensure that sufficient time has passed from administration of these medications until the time of testing, particularly in patients who are comatose and/or show flaccid paralysis as well as those who may have hepatic and renal dysfunction which may alter the pharmacokinetics of these drugs.

Botulinum toxin (or BOTOX) is often administered to children with spastic cerebral palsy and/or other forms of acquired injuries to the central nervous system. Since BOTOX impairs the release of acetylcholine from the pre-synaptic membrane it chemically denervates muscle. As such CMAP amplitudes may again be decreased, and active or chronic denervation changes may be apparent upon needle examination.

Machine/Operator Factors

Submaximal Stimulation Applied

Accurate nerve conduction studies rely on the delivery of supramaximal stimulation. This ensures that all axons contained within the nerve are depolarized. If stimulation is submaximal, only a subset of the axons will be depolarized, and the resulting SNAP or CMAP amplitude will be artifactually reduced. This can give the false impression of an axonal sensory and/or motor neuropathy where one does not exist. Often this may occur if a patient, particularly a child, finds the test uncomfortable and the nerve conduction studies are not performed as thoroughly as they should be. In such circumstances the possibility of submaximal stimulation should be documented by the technician and/or neurophysiologist to avoid misinterpretation. When such factors may have important consequences for a child's care, the nerve in question can be retested at a later point in the study, or consideration may be given to performing the study under conscious sedation or general anesthesia.

Adjacent Nerve Co-stimulation

Although it is important to ensure supramaximal stimulation, the application of excessively high currents may have the undesired effect of co-stimulating adjacent nerves. Typically this is seen in patients with neuropathies, where higher than normal stimulation is required. It can also occur in younger children where their smaller limb size places nerves in closer proximity. Common sites of co-stimulation include stimulation of the peroneal nerve above the knee (recording at the EDB) causing inadvertent co-stimulation of the tibial nerve. One clue that should alert the neurophysiologist to this phenomenon is a sudden change in the wave form morphology that is distinct from more distal stimulation sites and/or different from wave forms at lower stimulation intensities. The neurophysiologist may also notice muscles twitching that are not ordinarily innervated by the stimulated nerve. This artifact may be corrected by ensuring that the site of stimulation is directly over the desired nerve and that the intensity of stimulation is reduced if the aforementioned changes are noted in the waveform.

Measurement Errors

The distance between the cathode and the recording electrode must be carefully measured. Errors in measurement can have significant implications on the validity of the results since this can increase or decrease conduction velocity, influence the interpretation of latency measurements, and also give rise to apparent slowing across a possible compression site, mimicking conduction block. Measuring distance for ulnar nerve motor studies for example must ensure the measuring tape follows the normal physiological path of the nerve (i.e., distance is obtained following the course of the ulnar nerve, with the elbow flexed at 90°). If the arm is not maintained in flexion then the measured distance will be shorter than the actual length of the nerve, thereby overestimating the conduction velocity in this segment. It is important for all distance measurements that the technologist or neurophysiologist be aware that this error can only be corrected if it is identified at the time of testing. Although the neurophysiologist reporting a study may later be suspicious values obtained, he or she cannot verify the distance after the patient has left the clinic or laboratory. Children are particularly susceptible to measurement errors, due to the shorter distances involved and the squirming that often occurs during testing.

Stimulation Malposition

Stimulating at the incorrect site can result in no response or, if a response is obtained, decreased SNAP or CMAP amplitudes as the stimulation will be submaximal resulting from distance-related decay in stimulation intensity. Potential co-stimulation of nearby nerves can also occur if stimulation is administered at the incorrect location.

Recording Electrode Malposition

Recording electrodes must be placed immediately over the sensory nerves being studied, or in the case of motor nerves over the center of the muscle belly known as the motor point. If the recording electrode (G1) is incorrectly placed, then the CMAP amplitude will be reduced, giving the impression of axonal loss or a myopathy. A clue to misplacement of the recording electrode is an initial positive (downward) dip in the CMAP waveform, which should not be present in a correct recording. The downward dip can also make it more difficult to determine the precise onset of muscle depolarization, making latency measurements less reliable.

The two recording electrodes (G1 and G2) should be placed 3–4 cm apart, which is the typical distance of most bar recording electrodes. Larger distances can be associated with changes in amplitude and waveform duration due to alternation in the summation of action potentials and waveform cancellation [10]. Incorrect G2 position also has the potential to affect CMAP onset latencies by 0.1–0.5 ms [18].

Cathode Position (Erroneous Reversal of Stimulator Polarity)

Cathode malposition refers to the reversal of the relative positions of the cathode and anode of the stimulator. Typically when the hand-held stimulator is used the depolarization first occurs in the segment of nerve immediately under the cathode. The cathode should always be closer to the recording electrode (G1) than the anode. If the orientation of the stimulator is reversed, then the sensory and motor latencies will be increased since the recording represents the standard distance between the cathode and the recording electrode, plus the distance between the cathode and anode (usually 2–3 cm), yet only the distance between the cathode and the recording electrode is typically measured.

Stimulus Artifact

Stimulation artifact can be particularly problematic when performing sensory studies. When the initial baseline leading to the waveform is shifted it can make it difficult for the examiner to gauge where the onset point (initial deflection of the waveform) is located, which determines the onset latency. Sensory latency is marked either at the initial deflection of the waveform (onset latency) or the highest negative peak (peak latency). Different EMG laboratories favor one versus the other, and normal values have been established for both approaches.

Artifact from muscle can also impede the measurement of sensory responses. This is particularly problematic for young children due to the smaller sizes of their limbs and thus the closer proximity of nerves and muscles. A large motor CMAP can potentially obscure or even obliterate the SNAP in some instances during antidromic stimulation of a sensory nerve. One way of overcoming this problem is to reduce the stimulating current in an attempt to reduce or remove the artifactual CMAP. Another is to attempt orthodromic sensory nerve testing rather than antidromic testing. This is particularly easy to perform for the median, ulnar, medial plantar and lateral plantar sensory responses in children. Orthodromic stimulation involves distal stimulation of sensory fibers such that the signal travels in the same direction it would normally travel when a physiological response is carried along sensory nerve. Recording electrodes are placed more proximally. Since this technique selectively stimulates sensory fibers, it avoids the potential problem of muscle artifact near the recording site that occurs when a mixed nerve is stimulated in an antidromic manner. Antidromic stimulation, as the name suggests, sends a signal in the opposite direction than a sensory response would normally travel. Antidromic stimulation is often easier to perform than orthodromic stimulation, but when the former is used for a mixed nerve, distal muscles innervated by that nerve may be stimulated, leading to the generation of artifactual CMAPs. Since SNAP amplitudes are in the microvolt range, compared to CMAP amplitudes in the millivolt range, it is understandable why an aberrant motor response could be problematic.

For sensory and motor testing, care should be taken to avoid the excessive application of cream or gel at the stimulation site as this can created a bridge between the cathode and anode, causing cancellation of stimulation. This is especially important in children who may move their limbs more than adults tend to do during testing which can cause cream or gel to spread.

Filter Settings

High and low frequency filters have the benefit of screening out various artifacts, including electrical artifact. However, alterations to these filters can also have an adverse effect upon neurophysiologic test results. Increasing the low-frequency filter setting will reduce some electrical artifact but can also reduce SNAP or CMAP amplitudes. As such, caution must be taken when adjusting the filters away from standard settings.

Sweep Speed and Sensitivity Errors

Most machines will use standard settings for sensitivity and sweep speed. Sensitivity settings (also known as the gain) typically range from 10–20 μV per division for sensory studies and approximately 5 mV per division for motor studies. Sweep speed settings typically range from 2 to 5 msec per division. Latencies are longer for motor studies since they must account not only for the speed of conduction along a segment of motor nerve, but also neuromuscular transmission and muscle action potential propagation before the CMAP is generated.

Sensitivity and sweep speed should remain constant within any given study to ensure comparison of nerves (especially median and ulnar) is accurate and not influenced by this potential artifact. Additionally settings should not be permitted to deviate too far from standard ranges to ensure the validity of test results. However, in certain circumstances these settings may need to be adjusted at least temporarily. For example, when a CMAP is difficult to obtain and is suspected of having a profoundly low amplitude, the sensitivity setting may need to be adjusted to help detect a small CMAP. Similarly, in some demyelinating neuropathies the conduction velocities are so slow that the action potentials do not appear on the screen with standard sweep speeds, and thus the sweep speed may need to be adjusted to bring the action potential onto the screen.

Summary

Neurophysiologists must be vigilant to potential artifacts and ensure that technologists assisting with these studies are also aware of these factors. Several of the artifacts described, particularly temperature and operator factors can only be identified and rectified if they are discovered at the time of testing. Attention to these potential sources of error can prevent misdiagnosis and the negative consequences that may ensue.

References

1. Schroeder JM. Introduction. In: Schroder JM, editor. Pathology of peripheral nerves: an atlas of structural and molecular pathological changes. 1st ed. Berlin: Springer; 2001. p. 1–14.
2. Thomas JE, Lambert EH. Ulnar nerve conduction velocity and H-reflex in infants and children. J Appl Physiol. 1960;15:1–9.
3. Wagner AL, Buchthal F. Motor and sensory conduction in infancy and childhood: reappraisal. Dev Med Child Neurol. 1972;14(2):189–216.
4. Blair DA, Glover WE, Greenfield ADM. Excitation of cholinergic vasodilator nerves to human skeletal muscle during emotional stress I. Physiology. 1959;148:633.
5. Crawford DG, Friesen DD, Tomlinson-Keasey C. Effects of cognitively induced anxiety on hand temperature. Biofeedback Self Regul. 1977;2(2):139–46.
6. Halar EM, DeLisa JA, Soine TL. Nerve conduction studies in upper extremities: skin temperature corrections. Arch Phys Med Rehabil. 1983;61:412–6.
7. Edelwejn Z. Trials of evaluation of conduction velocity in motor fibers of different size under conditions of local hyperthermia. Acta Physiol Pol. 1964;15:503–11.
8. Halar EM, DeLisa JA, Brozovich FV. Peroneal motor conduction velocity: the importance of temperature correction. Arch Phys Med Rehabil. 1981;62:439–43.
9. Preston DC, Shapiro BE. Artifacts and technical factors. In: Shapiro DC, Shapiro BE, editors. Electromyography and neuromuscular disorders. 2nd ed. Philadelphia: Elsevier; 2005. p. 87–106.
10. Gooch CL, Weimer LH. The electrodiagnosis of neuropathy: basic principles and common pitfalls. Neurol Clin. 2007;25:1–28.
11. Halar EM, DeLisa JA, Brozovich FV. Nerve conduction velocity: relationship of skin, subcutaneous and intramuscular temperatures. Arch Phys Med Rehabil. 1980;61(5):199–203.
12. Panayiotopoulos CP, Scarpalezos P. Nastas 1: F-wave studies on the deep peroneal nerve. Part I Control Subjects J Neurol Sci. 1977;31:319–29.
13. Rivner MH, Swift TR, Malik K. Influence of age and height on nerve conduction. Muscle Nerve. 2001;24:1134–41.
14. Wu PB, Neff J, Kingerly WS, Date ES. Sensory nerve conduction velocity is inversely related to axonal length. Electromyogr Clin Neurophysiol. 1999;39(1):61–3.

15. Robinson LR, Rubner DE, Wahl PW, Fujimoto WY, Stolov WC. Influences of height and gender on normal nerve conduction studies. Arch Phys Med Rehabil. 1993 Nov;74(11):1134–8.
16. Roy J, Henry BM, Pekala PA, Vikse J, Saganiak K, Walocha JA, Tomaszewski KA. Median and ulnar nerve anastomoses in the upper limb: a meta-analysis. Muscle Nerve. 2016;54(1):36–47.
17. Tzikaa M, Paraskevasa GK, Kitsoulis P. The accessory deep peroneal nerve: a review of the literature. Foot. 2012;22:232–4.
18. Phongsamart G, Wertsch JJ, Ferdjallah M, King JC, Foster DT. Effect of reference electrode position on the compound action potential (CMAP) onset latency. Muscle Nerve. 2002;25(6):816–21.

Chapter 12
Motor Unit Number Estimation

Peter B. Kang

Due to the anatomic location of motor neurons, it is has not been possible to directly quantify motor neuron loss in anterior horn cell disease. Motor neurons are located in the anterior spinal cord, one of the areas within the nervous system that are not amenable to biopsy and histological analysis in living patients. The spinal cord has a high density of eloquent fiber tracts. Biopsy-induced injury to these tracts would result in significant weakness, paraesthesiae and/or sphincter dysfunction. As a result, estimating the degree of actual motor neuron loss has remained elusive for motor neuron diseases such as amyotrophic lateral sclerosis (ALS) and spinal muscular atrophy (SMA). ALS is primarily an adult-onset disease, while SMA is typically identified in infancy or early childhood.

Given the limitations described above, an electrophysiologic test has been designed to act as a surrogate measure of motor neuron integrity. This method, known as motor unit number estimation (MUNE), provides a reliable estimate of the number of functional motor units present. MUNE was first described in 1971 [1] in patients with amyotrophic lateral sclerosis. Since then, it has also been applied to patients with other neuromuscular diseases such as Duchenne muscular dystrophy [2] and poliomyelitis [3]. More recently, it has been shown to be a reliable and useful electrophysiologic outcome measure for spinal muscular atrophy [4, 5].

There has been some discussion in the literature about the relative merits of two different electrophysiologic measures to quantify motor unit loss: the compound muscle action potential (CMAP), which is a standard measurement in nerve conduction studies, versus the MUNE, which requires specialized nerve conduction studies that are not routinely performed in clinical settings. The CMAP is easier to obtain and provides a more global assessment of the motor unit for a selected muscle [6, 7]. It is also widely used in routine clinical practice and is thus easy for a

P.B. Kang, M.D., F.A.A.N., F.A.A.P.
Division of Pediatric Neurology, Shands Children's Hospital, University of Florida College of Medicine, Gainesville, FL, USA
e-mail: pbkang@ufl.edu

© Springer International Publishing AG 2017

H.J. McMillan, P.B. Kang (eds.), *Pediatric Electromyography*,
DOI10.1007/978-3-319-61361-1_12

neurophysiologist to obtain for research purposes without substantial additional training. However, determination of the MUNE is a more complex calculation that has the potential to yield more in depth analysis, especially as the component variables are the CMAP and the mean single motor unit action potential (SMUP), which in theory represents a single motor unit [8]. The MUNE calculation is as follows:

$$\text{MUNE} = \text{CMAP (converted to } \mu\text{V)/mean SMUP (recorded in } \mu\text{V)}$$

Several methods have been developed for obtaining the data needed for MUNE calculations, primarily focusing on various approaches to obtaining an accurate mean SMUP calculation. Among these, the multipoint stimulation method has been used in children [5, 8], but other methods such as spike-triggered averaging, F wave methods, and statistical methods are also used, primarily in adults [9–12]. More recently, a new method that combines features of the multipoint and incremental approaches has been developed that provides sufficient reliability to be especially useful in human clinical trials [13].

Obtaining the data needed to calculate MUNE accurately in children is feasible, requires a minimum degree of cooperation, and does not involve substantial discomfort. The only equipment needed is a standard electrodiagnostic (NCS/EMG) machine. Either before or after the MUNE data are obtained, an accurate CMAP should be recorded at the muscle by administering a supramaximal current to the motor nerve, usually at the standard distal stimulation point, as the CMAP amplitude is included in the MUNE calculation. Ideally the EMG machine would include software settings for performing MUNE, but if not, a protocol can easily be programmed into the settings. Filter settings are generally 10 Hz (low) and 10 kHz (high). As the action potentials to be obtained represent single motor units, the amplitude of the voltages recorded are mostly less than 500 μV, and are often less than 100 μV, though sometimes larger motor units are seen in patients with motor neuron disease and significant denervation. The software settings should be adjusted accordingly (i.e., the standard sensitivity settings for a motor nerve conduction study are not sensitive enough to detect these action potentials, the ranges are more aligned with what is seen with sensory nerve action potentials). For research protocols, a specific nerve and muscle pair are typically specified for study, for example the right ulnar nerve recording the abductor digiti minimi. The currents administered to the child should be small and raised slowly, as the goal is to stimulate conduction in a single motor unit only, either in isolation or as an incremental increase over a previous stimulation.

The two MUNE approaches that have been used most extensively in children are the traditional multipoint stimulation approach and the combined multipoint incremental approach which will be described in further detail.

Traditional Multipoint Stimulation Approach

In a traditional multipoint stimulation approach, the recording electrodes are maintained in the same location throughout the study, while the investigator moves the stimulator from site to site over the course of the nerve, seeking distinct single motor unit action potentials. The first motor unit obtained at any given stimulation point is recorded; the presence of only one motor unit in the potential obtained should be confirmed by observing an "all or none" response when the stimulation is reduced a bit below the level needed to generate that potential, and then increased again past the threshold. Stimulation points can be selected along the length of the nerve under study, within the limits set by the research protocol. Certain locations may yield motor units more readily than others. For example, along the ulnar nerve, the sites just proximal to the wrist and around the elbow are especially fruitful for this purpose, whereas sites between these two along the forearm may be more difficult. Only one motor unit action potential is recorded for each stimulation site. The current needed to stimulate a single motor unit action potential is usually less than 10 mA, and almost always less than 20 mA. One potential pitfall of this approach is the possibility of recording the same motor unit action potential at multiple stimulation points, which may affect the accuracy of the final calculations. Thus, it is important to observe the amplitude and morphology of each single motor unit action potential obtained, and to eliminate those that are redundant. After the required number of single motor unit action potentials at various stimulation sites are measured, these may be averaged for the MUNE calculation. Figure 12.1 provides an example of this approach.

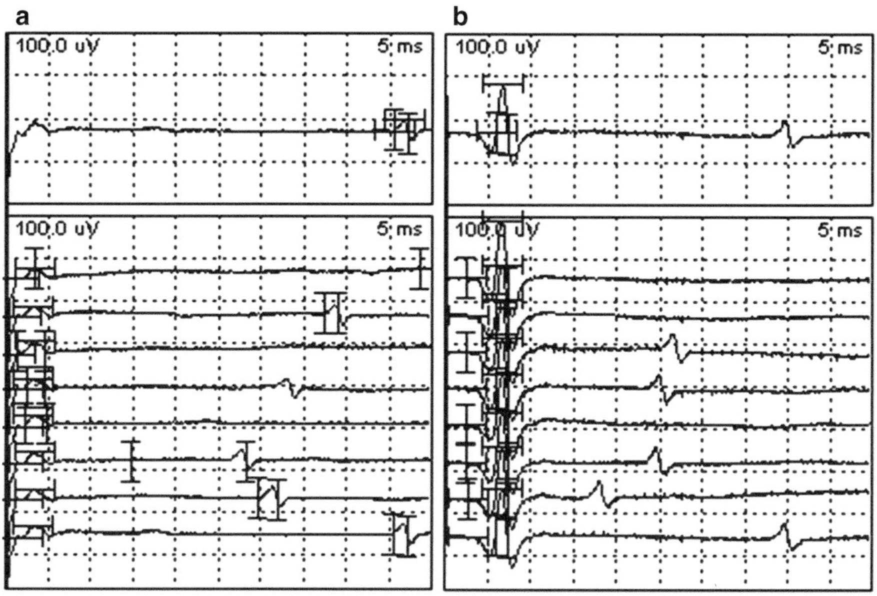

Fig. 12.1 Representative examples of single motor unit potentials (SMUPs) stimulating the right ulnar nerve and recording abductor digiti minimi using the multipoint approach. One set of SMUPs had amplitudes ranging from 23–30 μV (**a**), while the other had amplitudes ranging from 112–128 μV (**b**). Note the similar morphology of the waveforms in each set of tracings. The full examination identified 8 distinct sets of SMUPs that averaged 116.68 μV. With a CMAP amplitude recorded to be 1.9 mV at the same site, the MUNE was calculated to be 16.285

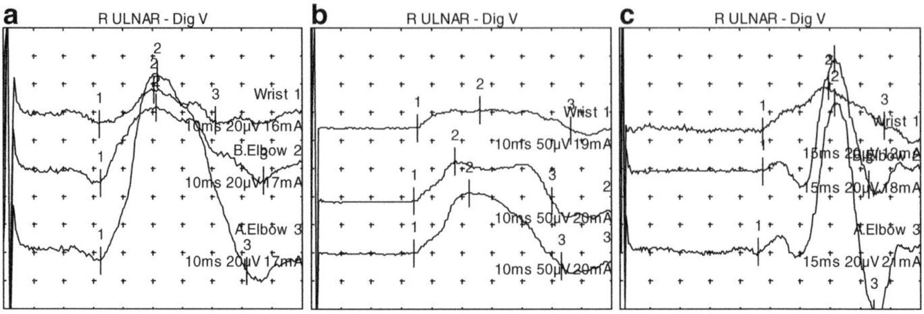

Fig. 12.2 Images of SMUPs stimulating the right ulnar nerve and recording abductor digiti minimi using the incremental approach. Three increments are recorded at each of three different sites: 2 cm proximal to the wrist crease (**a**), 6 cm proximal to the wrist crease (**b**), and 1 cm proximal to the ulnar groove at the elbow (**c**). The average increment, representing the SMUP, for the nine stimulations is 38.9 μV. With a CMAP recorded at 9.5 mV, the MUNE is then calculated to be 244.2

Combined Multipoint Incremental Method

The combined multipoint incremental method involves the use of a single recording site for a nerve/muscle pair, and a defined set of stimulation points, typically three [13]. At each stimulation site, the nerve is stimulated at low currents that are increased slowly, as in the multipoint approach. However, once the first motor unit action potential is obtained and recorded, the current should continue to be increased slowly until a second incremental ("all or none") jump in the action potential amplitude occurs. Once the second is recorded, then the stimulation is again increased slowly until a third incremental jump occurs. This protocol is repeated at each of the three stimulation sites, yielding a total of 9 measurements. At each site, the first motor unit amplitude is equivalent to the first action potential obtained, while the second is calculated by subtracting the first from the second, while the third is calculated by subtracting the second from the third. These nine motor unit amplitudes are then averaged and used for the standard MUNE calculation (Fig. 12.2). Redundant motor unit action potentials are tolerated in this protocol, as opposed to the multipoint stimulation technique.

MUNE is increasingly used as an outcome measure for clinical trials in spinal muscular atrophy [7, 14, 15], and has yielded interesting information about the disease, including natural history data [16, 17] and evidence suggesting that new motor development may be occurring as a compensatory mechanism in spinal muscular atrophy [8]. Thus far, it does not appear to have obvious diagnostic applications in routine clinical settings, as it is not clear that it would detect signs of motor unit dysfunction that would not be seen by other means, such as CMAP amplitudes and signs of denervation/reinnervation on needle examination. However, as more data accumulate regarding the correlation of MUNE values with disease progression, such applications may be proposed in the future.

References

1. McComas AJ, Fawcett PR, Campbell MJ, Sica RE. Electrophysiological estimation of the number of motor units within a human muscle. J Neurol Neurosurg Psychiatry. 1971;34(2):121–31.
2. McComas AJ, Sica RE, Brandstater ME. Further motor unit studies in Duchenne muscular dystrophy. J Neurol Neurosurg Psychiatry. 1977;40(12):1147–51.
3. Sorenson EJ, Daube JR, Windebank AJ. Motor unit number estimates correlate with strength in polio survivors. Muscle Nerve. 2006;34(5):608–13.
4. Galea V, Fehlings D, Kirsch S, McComas A. Depletion and sizes of motor units in spinal muscular atrophy. Muscle Nerve. 2001;24(9):1168–72.
5. Bromberg MB, Swoboda KJ. Motor unit number estimation in infants and children with spinal muscular atrophy. Muscle Nerve. 2002;25(3):445–7.
6. Lewelt A, Krosschell KJ, Scott C, Sakonju A, Kissel JT, Crawford TO, et al. Compound muscle action potential and motor function in children with spinal muscular atrophy. Muscle Nerve. 2010;42(5):703–8.
7. Swoboda KJ, Prior TW, Scott CB, McNaught TP, Wride MC, Reyna SP, et al. Natural history of denervation in SMA: relation to age, SMN2 copy number, and function. Ann Neurol. 2005;57(5):704–12.
8. Kang PB, Gooch CL, McDermott MP, Darras BT, Finkel RS, Yang ML, et al. The motor neuron response to SMN1 deficiency in spinal muscular atrophy. Muscle Nerve. 2014;49(5):636–44.
9. Shefner JM. Motor unit number estimation in human neurological diseases and animal models. Clin Neurophysiol. 2001;112(6):955–64.
10. Daube JR. Motor unit number estimates—from A to Z. J Neurol Sci. 2006;242(1–2):23–35.
11. Bromberg MB. Updating motor unit number estimation (MUNE). Clin Neurophysiol. 2007;118(1):1–8.
12. Gooch CL, Doherty TJ, Chan KM, Bromberg MB, Lewis RA, Stashuk DW, et al. Motor unit number estimation: a technology and literature review. Muscle Nerve. 2014;50(6):884–93.
13. Shefner JM, Watson ML, Simionescu L, Caress JB, Burns TM, Maragakis NJ, et al. Multipoint incremental motor unit number estimation as an outcome measure in ALS. Neurology. 2011;77(3):235–41.
14. Swoboda KJ, Scott CB, Reyna SP, Prior TW, LaSalle B, Sorenson SL, et al. Phase II open label study of valproic acid in spinal muscular atrophy. PLoS One. 2009;4(5):e5268.
15. Swoboda KJ, Scott CB, Crawford TO, Simard LR, Reyna SP, Krosschell KJ, et al. SMA CARNI-VAL trial part I: double-blind, randomized, placebo-controlled trial of L-carnitine and valproic acid in spinal muscular atrophy. PLoS One. 2010;5(8):e12140.
16. Kaufmann P, McDermott MP, Darras BT, Finkel R, Kang P, Oskoui M, et al. Observational study of spinal muscular atrophy type 2 and 3: functional outcomes over 1 year. Arch Neurol. 2011;68(6):779–86.
17. Finkel RS, McDermott MP, Kaufmann P, Darras BT, Chung WK, Sproule DM, et al. Observational study of spinal muscular atrophy type I and implications for clinical trials. Neurology. 2014;83(9):810–7.

Chapter 13
Concentric Macro EMG

Joe F. Jabre

Introduction

Needle electromyography (EMG) can be grouped into one of three classifications for use by neurophysiologists in clinical practice. Listing them by "size" from small to large (Table 13.1 and Fig. 13.1), the first is single fiber EMG (SFEMG) that can be considered a "micro EMG" technique. SFEMG records activity of one or two single muscle fibers of a motor unit at a given time and is used in the evaluation of fiber density and neuromuscular transmission disorders. The second technique that is the most familiar to neurophysiologists and widely used in routine clinical practice is that using a concentric or monopolar needle electrode to record from 10 to 20 muscle fibers of a motor unit at a time. This second technique is what is usually meant when the term "needle examination" or "needle EMG" is used. The last technique, macro EMG, records from the majority of muscle fibers in a motor unit at any given time. This technique uses an electrode's cannula referenced to a nearby surface electrode. Each of these techniques provides the neurophysiologist with a different set of tools to measure and analyze the motor unit waveform.

The difference in these recording techniques is dependent largely upon the recording surface area of each needle. Single fibre EMG needles are characterized by a very small side-port that is 25 μm [1] in size and serves as the recording surface. This gives rise to a very small recording radius enabling potentials to be recorded from only 1–2 muscle fibers at a time. Conventional EMG utilizes needles with a larger recording surface area that may be either concentric or monopolar. Concentric needles are characterized by their beveled tips that contain a side port with a recording area of 150 × 580 μm [1]. Monopolar needles are characterized by their pointed tip with a recording surface area of 640 μm [1]. Of note, when concentric needles

J.F. Jabre, M.D.
Department of Neurology, David Geffen School of Medicine, UCLA, Los Angeles, CA, USA
e-mail: jjabre@mednet.ucla.edu; jjabre@teleemg.com

© Springer International Publishing AG 2017

H.J. McMillan, P.B. Kang (eds.), *Pediatric Electromyography*,
DOI 10.1007/978-3-319-61361-1_13

Table 13.1 Needle characteristics and utility for various needle EMG techniques

Technique	Recording surface	Recording area (mm^2)	Number fibers in one motor unit studied (fibers)	Utility
Single fiber EMG	Small; 25 μm at side-port	0.0005	1–2	Analysis of neuromuscular transmission
Concentric EMG	Medium; 150 × 580 μm of beveled tip	0.07	10–20	Analysis of individual MUAPs
Monopolar EMG	Medium; 640 μm at tip	0.12–0.34	10–20	Analysis of individual MUAPs
MacroEMG	Large; un-insulated distal 15 mm of needle	Large	300–2000	Analysis of entire motor unit

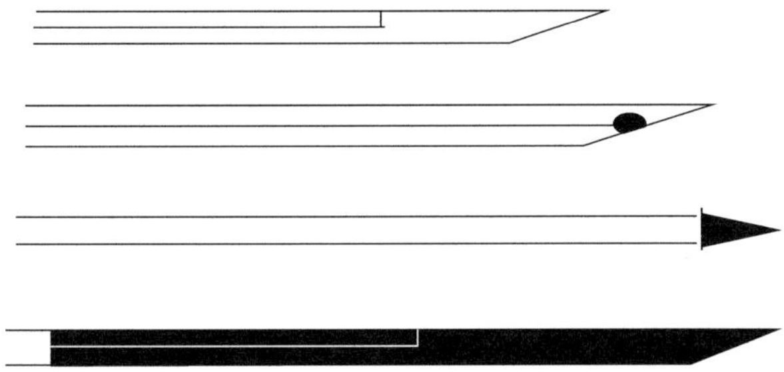

Fig. 13.1 Comparison of needles used for various types of electromyography studies. Line drawings illustrate, from *top* to *bottom*: single fiber, concentric, monopolar and macroEMG needles. The dark area corresponds to the recording area for each needle

are used, a single ground surface electrode is required, while the use of a monopolar needle requires both ground and reference surface electrodes. MacroEMG needles are unique since they possess a recording surface area that is many times larger than these other needles. Although the needle contains a side-port similar to single fiber EMG, the distal 15 mm of the macroEMG needle is un-insulated, which gives rise to the larger recording surface area allowing it to perform analysis of all muscle fibers belonging to an individual motor unit (Table 13.1 [1, 2]).

Some of the traditional motor unit action potential (MUAP) measurement and analysis techniques described by Buchtal in the 1950s [3, 4] are time-consuming and pose significant challenges even in cooperative adult patients. Pediatric neurophysiologists are frequently called upon to differentiate normal versus abnormal neuromuscular pathology without the luxury of time and patient cooperation. In infants and younger children, the term "burst" EMG analysis is sometimes used to describe the sampling that occurs with a patient who is not able to follow commands consistently, in contrast to the traditional motor unit analysis technique used in older children, adolescents, and adults. Though experienced pediatric neurophysiologists are usually able to obtain accurate and valuable data from these smaller samplings, there are circumstances in which the amount of data collected is not optimal.

Compounding this difficult undertaking is that concentric needle electrodes record from about 10–20 muscle fibers of a motor unit at a time. While in adults one can overcome this limitation by moving the needle electrode inside the corridor of a motor unit's territory to explore other areas, in children, especially infants and toddlers, this luxury of needle motor unit territory exploration is not always consistently attainable. Figure 13.2 shows a schematic representation of a concentric needle electrode inside the muscle, and the contribution of the nearby muscle fibers belonging to the same motor unit to the MUAP.

Macro EMG as described by Stålberg [5] is a well-accepted technique for estimating the electrical size of a motor unit. It makes use of a large recording surface that makes it possible to sample the majority of muscle fibers of a motor unit, in contrast to the 10–20 muscle fibers sampled by the tip of a concentric needle electrode. As useful as the Stålberg technique is, a practical limitation is that it uses a single fiber needle electrode to record the cannula potential and does not afford a concomitant view of the concentric MUAP from which the Macro potential is derived. Another practical limitation is the significant cost associated with the purchase of macroEMG needles. To overcome these limitations, a technique known as concentric macro EMG or ConMac was developed by Jabre [6] that uses the cannula of a standard concentric needle electrode to record the concentric electrode's cannula potential, referenced to a nearby surface electrode, allowing for a simultaneous view of the concentric MUAP and its corresponding macro potential [7]. To clearly

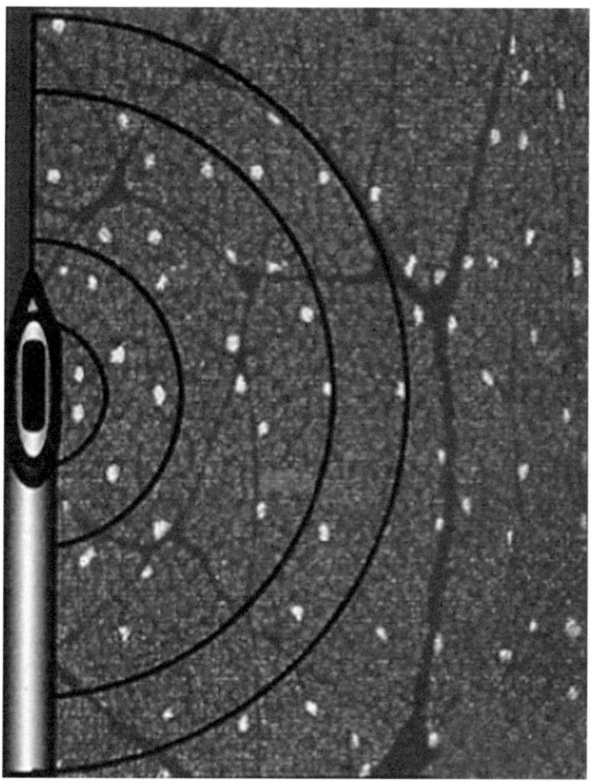

Fig. 13.2 Schematic representation of a concentric needle electrode inside a normal muscle, showing the contribution to the MUAP of the nearby muscle fibers (simulated as white dots) belonging to a single motor unit. The semi circles (from closest to furthest from the needle electrode) approximate the muscle fibers that contribute to the MUAP amplitude, followed by those that contribute to its spike component, area, and lastly to its duration

distinguish between macro potentials derived from these two electrode types, we refer to the single fiber electrode cannula derived potential as the Macro potential, and to the concentric electrode cannula derived potential as the ConMac potential.

In this chapter, we will describe the ConMac EMG technique and its applicability to quickly and easily distinguish between normal, neurogenic, and myopathic motor unit changes.

In our experience, ConMac EMG is a fairly simple technique to learn and can be performed in under 5 minutes with a conventional concentric needle electrode using an EMG machine that allows for two channel recording.

Technical Description of the ConMac EMG Technique

The ConMac EMG technique requires a two-channel EMG machine, with one channel, typically channel 1, being used to record the concentric MUAP. This potential serves as a trigger to the cannula potential recorded on the other channel, in this case channel 2.

To extract the time-locked cannula potential on channel 2 from interfering MUAPs of nearby units, the channel 2 signal is averaged between 16 and 32 times, or until it remains stable and its amplitude and area can be measured easily. Filters used are 20–8 kHz for the concentric potential, and 8 Hz to 8 kHz for the ConMac potential. The technique and recording principle are shown in Fig. 13.3.

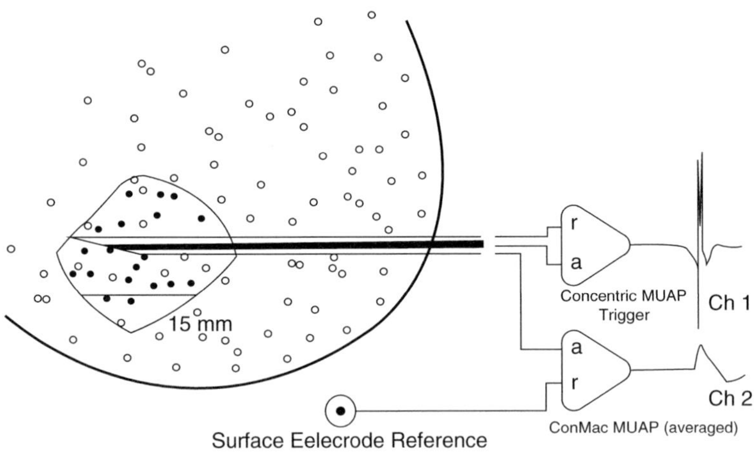

Fig. 13.3 Concentric Macro EMG (ConMac) recording principle using a two-channel EMG machine. In the first channel (Ch 1), a concentric MUAP is recorded from the electrode's active recording tip (**a**), with the cannula used as reference (r). This concentric MUAP is used to trigger a time-locked potential on the second channel (Ch 2), where the needle's cannula is now the active (**a**) recording area, and a surface electrode nearby is used as reference (r). Because of the size and non-selective nature of the electrode's cannula, there is much interference from nearby active motor units on channel 2. Interference can be greatly reduced by averaging this time-locked potential to generate the ConMac MUAP

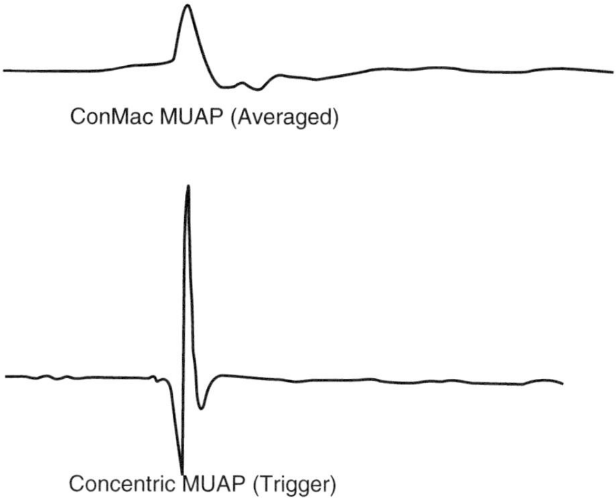

Fig. 13.4 Typical concentric MUAP (bottom) used to trigger and average a ConMac MUAP (*top*) in a normal subject. Sweep speed: 10 ms/division. Sensitivity: Concentric MUAP 300 μV/division; ConMac MUAP 500 μV/division

ConMac action potentials look like a small motor response, very similar to an F-wave as shown in Fig. 13.4.

ConMac EMG in Clinical Use

Our experience with the clinical use of ConMac EMG spans three decades. Several publications have explored the use of this technique in normal adults and in patients with neurogenic and myopathic pathology [8, 9].

These studies have shed some light not only on the motor unit territory and its architecture, but also on the validity of currently available MUAP normal values in the literature [10], and on the relationship between the cannula potential and the motor unit twitch force [11]. ConMac EMG has also been used for the demonstration of the motor unit recruitment size principle [12]. Finally, the shape of the ConMac MUAP remains relatively stable during needle manipulations, as shown by the scanning study in Fig. 13.5.

This property of the ConMac technique makes it especially useful in children who typically do not tolerate the traditional sampling protocol that requires multiple movements of the needle electrode inside the muscle.

Normal Subjects

In normal adult subjects, cannula potentials usually have one or two phases, but occasionally may show more, such as in the tibialis anterior muscle [13]. Since the needle electrode's cannula is non-selective, the ConMac MUAP is derived from the

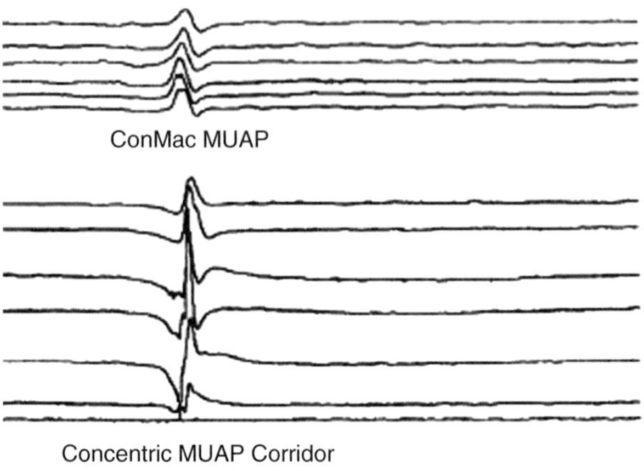

Fig. 13.5 Scanning EMG. The concentric electrode is dragged through a motor unit territory's corridor while recording its MUAP at different positions in the corridor (bottom), and trigger averaging the corresponding ConMac MUAP from these same positions in the corridor (top). Note the changes in the concentric MUAP morphology as the needle is moved through the corridor, and the stability of the corresponding ConMac MUAP's morphology throughout the move. Sweep speed: 10 ms/division. Sensitivity: Concentric MUAP and ConMac MUAP 500 μV/division

temporal and spatial summation of the majority of muscle fibers inside a motor unit [14]. Additionally, the ConMac potential's area and amplitude are related to both the number and size of muscle fibers in the motor unit, a property that makes it especially sensitive to changes in muscle fiber size seen in neurogenic and myopathic pathology.

Normal values for ConMac MUAPs have been developed for the upper and lower extremity muscles of healthy adult volunteers (Table 13.2) at mild, moderate, and full contraction levels [10].

Patients with Nerve and Muscle Disease

Our studies have spanned a spectrum of patients who suffered from various types of neurogenic and myopathic pathology. These included patients with motor neuron disease or amyotrophic lateral sclerosis (ALS), poliomyelitis, syringomyelia, and lumbosacral root lesions with neurogenic pathology; and patients with polymyositis, congenital myopathy, and steroid myopathy with myopathic pathology. While we found ConMac EMG to be useful in all, our experience has shown that its major contribution has been especially striking in the evaluation of patients with early or mild myopathy. We believe that this may be due to the reliance on visual data alone for ConMac EMG interpretation, as opposed to the combination of visual and auditory data used for traditional concentric MUAP

Table 13.2 ConMac amplitudes and areas mean and standard deviation for upper and lower extremity muscles in healthy adult subjects at mild, moderate, and full contraction levels

Muscle	Contractions	ConMac Amp (μV)	ConMac Area (μV ms)
		Mean (SD)	Mean (SD)
FDI	Mild	107.5 (56.3)	409.6 (225.5)
	Moderate	200.6 (92.5)	749.7 (420.9)
	Full	230.9 (54.8)	966.8 (295.1)
BR	Mild	52.0 (21.1)	324.3 (117.1)
	Moderate	98.4 (39.1)	531.7 (135.2)
	Full	159.3 (61.4)	846.6 (403.9)
TRI	Mild	79.6 (19.7)	401.4 (53.6)
	Moderate	133 (23)	582.6 (40.8)
	Full	169.4 (2.3)	853.9 (51.7)
DEL	Mild	68.4 (37)	446.1 (246.9)
	Moderate	114.2 (42.7)	853.1 (283.9)
	Full	169 (72.7)	1068.4 (418.3)
EDB	Mild	146.3 (70.4)	432.0 (210)
	Moderate	191.3 (128.2)	953.9 (282.3)
	Full	313.0 (274.4)	1337.4 (813)
TA	Mild	125.7 (5.7)	885.0 (193.3)
	Moderate	166.9 (81.1)	1154.9 (529.8)
	Full	276.2 (72.2)	2199.7 (916.0)
VL	Mild	61.0 (9)	349.8 (155.7)
	Moderate	122.1 (24.4)	570.9 (85.5)
	Full	246.9 (132.5)	1032.2 (216.1)

FDI first dorsal interosseous, *BR* brachio-radials, *TRI* triceps, *DEL* deltoid, *EDB* extensor digitorum brevis, *TA* tibialis anterior, *VL* vastus lateralis

interpretation, as the latter leads the neurophysiologist to naturally avoid end stage muscle tissue that does not generate as much auditory feedback, and seek areas that generate more sound than others near the electrode's tip to study the MUAP as seen in Fig. 13.6.

In those areas where the healthier muscle fibers of a myopathic muscle can be found, the concentric MUAP may display a near normal amplitude, although its duration may be shorter than normal. A cannula potential recorded from that same area, however, may show that the majority of muscle fibers of that unit are very depressed, both as a result of a drop in the number of muscle fibers, and a decrease in the size of those remaining in the affected areas, resulting in a very low, or nearly flat ConMac MUAP as seen in Fig. 13.7. At later stages of myopathic disease, both test modalities should have reasonable sensitivity for abnormal muscle physiology.

The opposite is true in patients with neurogenic MUAP changes, where in most instances, the neurophysiologists cannot get away from sound-rich areas in the

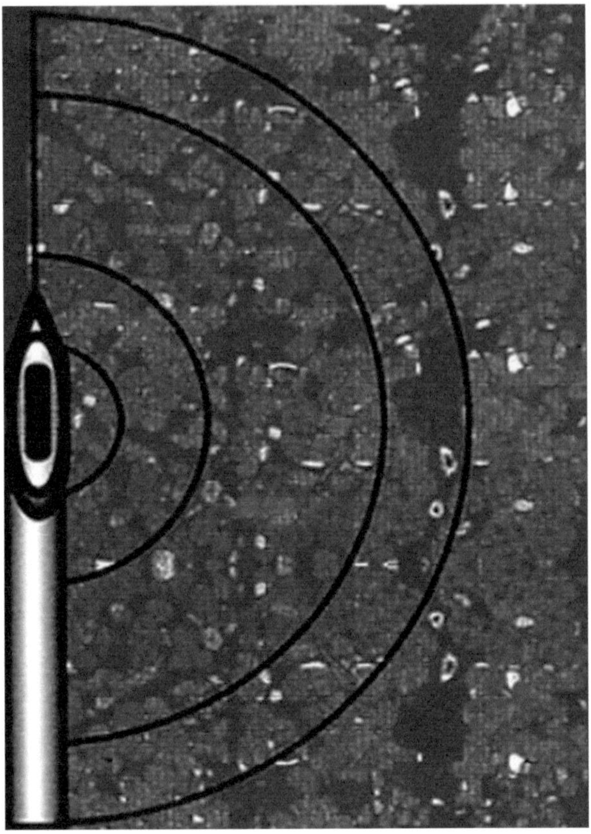

Fig. 13.6 Schematic representation of a concentric needle electrode inside a myopathic muscle, showing the contribution to the MUAP of the nearby muscle fibers (simulated as white dots) belonging to a single motor unit. Note that the two muscle fibers nearest to the electrode tip appear normal and may result in a normal MUAP amplitude, though its duration will be decreased. The semi circles (from closest to furthest from the needle electrode) approximate the muscle fibers that contribute to the MUAP amplitude, followed by those that contribute to its spike component, area, and lastly to its duration

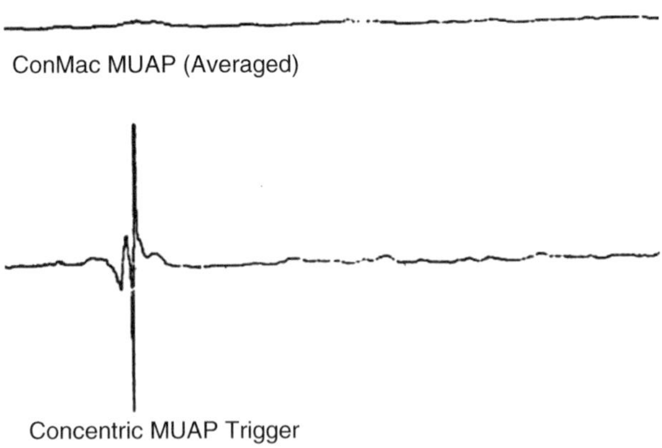

Fig. 13.7 Concentric (*bottom*) and averaged ConMac (*top*) MUAPs in a patient with polymyositis. Note the nearly "normal" concentric MUAP's waveform, and the clearly abnormal, almost flat, ConMac MUAP waveform. Sweep speed: 10 ms/division. Sensitivity: Concentric MUAP 300 μV/division; ConMac MUAP 500 μV/division

unit's territory because of the higher density of muscle fibers in their vicinity due to reinnervation as seen in Fig. 13.8.

Under those circumstances, both the concentric and ConMac MUAPs will easily display high amplitude and polyphasia as seen in Fig. 13.9.

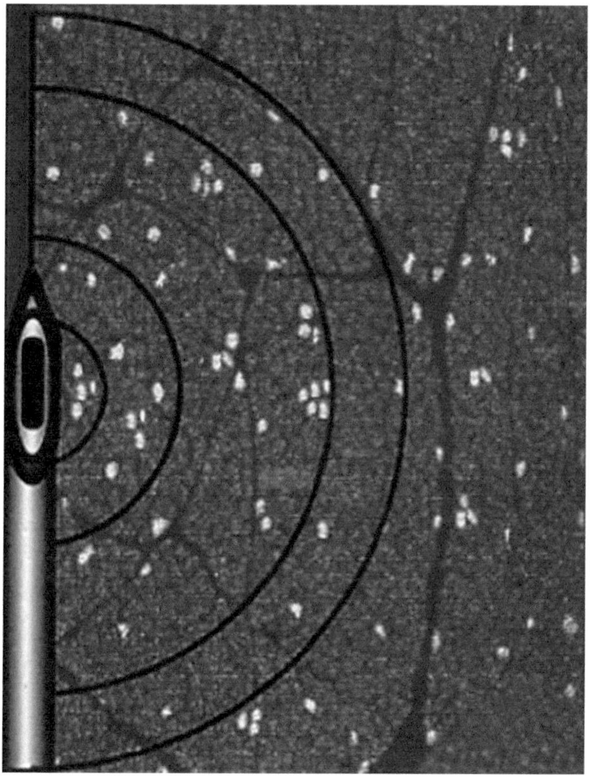

Fig. 13.8 Schematic representation of a concentric needle electrode inside a neurogenic muscle, showing the contribution to the MUAP of the nearby muscle fibers (simulated as white dots) belonging to a single motor unit. Note that the higher fiber density nearest to the electrode tip will result in an increased amplitude and likely polyphasic MUAP. The semi circles (from closest to furthest from the needle electrode) approximate the muscle fibers that contribute to the MUAP amplitude, followed by those that contribute to its spike component, area, and lastly to its duration

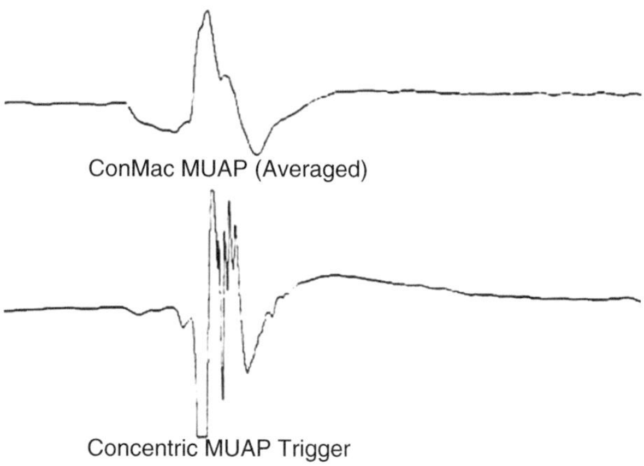

Fig. 13.9 Concentric (*bottom*) and averaged ConMac (*top*) MUAPs in a patient with syringomyelia. Note the clearly abnormal concentric and ConMac MUAP waveforms. Sweep speed: 10 ms/division. Sensitivity: Concentric MUAP 300 μV/division; ConMac MUAP 500 μV/division

To that end, one can summarize the findings detected by the ConMac electrode in nerve and muscle pathology as follows:

- In early or mild myopathic pathology, the concentric MUAP may appear normal, depending on the needle position inside the motor unit territory, while the ConMac MUAP will be very depressed or nearly flat. At later stages of disease, both test modalities should show abnormalities depending on the number and distribution of muscles tested.

- In neurogenic pathology, both the concentric and ConMac MUAPs will show abnormal changes due to the widespread distribution of reinnervation changes throughout affected muscles.

ConMac MUAP Samples in Neurogenic and Myopathic Pathology

ConMac EMG in Myopathy

We show here some typical myopathic MUAP changes seen in a patient with congenital myopathy (Fig. 13.10) and another with polymyositis (Fig. 13.11).

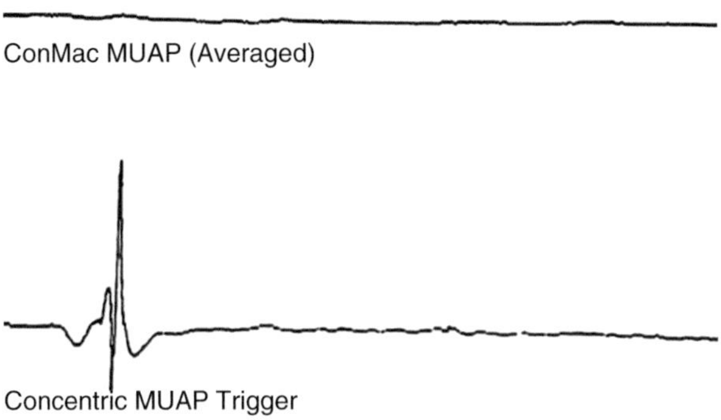

Fig. 13.10 Concentric (*bottom*) and averaged ConMac (*top*) MUAPs in a patient with congenital myopathy. Note the concentric MUAP's waveform, and the clearly abnormal, nearly flat, ConMac MUAP waveform. Sweep speed: 10 ms/division. Sensitivity: Concentric MUAP 100 μV/division; ConMac MUAP 500 μV/division

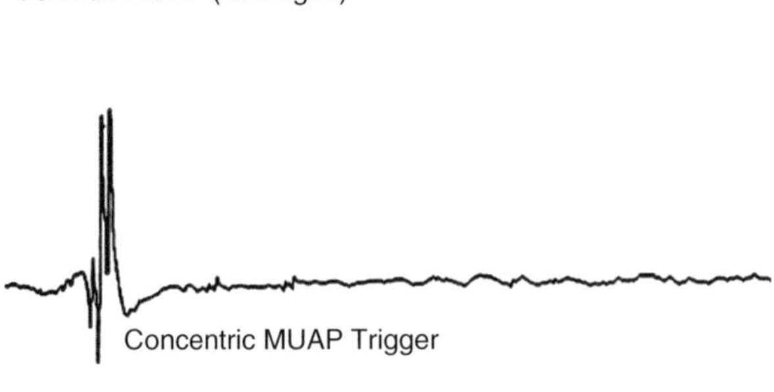

Fig. 13.11 Concentric (*bottom*) and averaged ConMac (*top*) MUAPs in a patient with polymyositis. Note the concentric MUAP's waveform, and the clearly abnormal, nearly flat, ConMac MUAP waveform. Sweep speed: 10 ms/division. Sensitivity: Concentric MUAP 300 μV/division; ConMac MUAP 500 μV/division

ConMac EMG in Neurogenic Reinnervation

We show here some typical neurogenic MUAP changes seen in a patient with old poliomyelitis (Fig. 13.12), and another with ALS (Fig. 13.13).

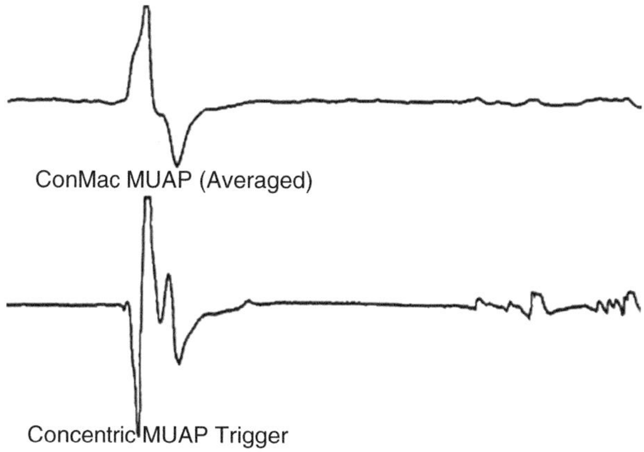

Fig. 13.12 Concentric (*bottom*) and averaged ConMac (*top*) MUAPs in a patient with old poliomyelitis. Note the concentric MUAP's waveform, and the clearly abnormal ConMac MUAP waveform. Contrast the shape and size of the ConMac MUAP with those seen in Figs. 13.9 and 13.10. Sweep speed: 10 ms/division. Sensitivity: Concentric MUAP 300 μV/division; ConMac MUAP 700 μV/division

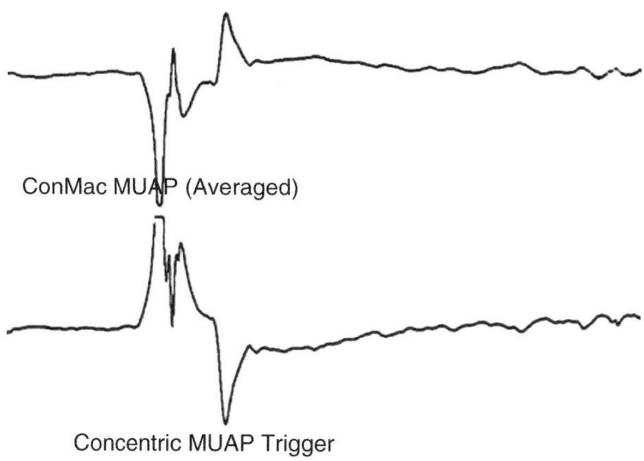

Fig. 13.13 Concentric (*bottom*) and the averaged ConMac (*top*) MUAPs in a patient with ALS. Note the concentric MUAP's waveform, and the clearly abnormal ConMac MUAP waveform. Sweep speed: 10 ms/division. Compare the shape and size of the ConMac MUAP with those seen in Figs. 13.9 and 13.10. Sensitivity: Concentric MUAP 300 μV/division; ConMac MUAP 500 μV/division

Conclusion

The concentric Macro or ConMac EMG technique described above can be a valuable addition to the pediatric neurophysiologist's toolbox when evaluating infants and children with nerve or muscle pathology in situations where diagnostic findings on traditional concentric MUAP analysis may be subtle and equivocal, especially in early and mild cases of myopathic disorders.

ConMac EMG can be performed quickly and effectively using a regular concentric electrode and a two-channel EMG machine with trigger and delay capabilities, modalities that are found in just about every EMG machine on the market today. In our experience, the procedure adds little time to routine EMG studies and does not require much skill to learn by a trained neurophysiologist, and even less so by a pediatric neurophysiologist who faces these daily challenges with much less luxury of time and patient cooperation. Thus, it may be worth implementing in cases when traditional nerve conduction studies and concentric MUAP analysis do not yield definite diagnostic findings, especially when the clinical index of suspicion for a myopathic disorder is high.

References

1. Feinstein B, Lindegard B, Nyman E, Wohlfart G. Morphologic studies of motor units in normal human muscles. Acta Anat (Basel). 1955;23(2):127–42.
2. Kohara N, Kaji R, Kimura J. Comparison of recording characteristics of monopolar and concentric needle electrodes. Electroencephalogr Clin Neurophysiol. 1993;89(4):242–6.
3. Buchthal F, Guld C, Rosenfalck P. Action potential parameters in normal human muscle and their dependence on physical variables. Acta Physiol Scand. 1954;32(2–3):200–18.
4. Buchthal F, Pinell P, Rosenfalck P. Action potential parameters in normal human muscle and their physiological determinants. Acta Physiol Scand. 1954;32(2–3):219–29.
5. Stålberg E. Macro EMG, a new recording technique. J Neurol Neurosurg Psychiatry. 1980;43(6):475–82.
6. Jabre JF. Concentric macro electromyography. Muscle Nerve. 1991;14(9):820–5.
7. Stålberg E. Macro electromyography, an update. Muscle Nerve. 2011;44(2):292–302.
8. Bauermeister W, Jabre JF. The spectrum of concentric macro EMG correlations. Part I. Normal subjects. Muscle Nerve. 1992;15(10):1081–4.
9. Gan R, Jabre JF. The spectrum of concentric macro EMG correlations. Part II. Patients with diseases of muscle and nerve. Muscle Nerve. 1992;15(10):1085–8.
10. Jabre JF, Guan Y, Chui KKH. Motor unit potential change with contraction level: a concentric macro electromyography study. Muscle Nerve. 2013;48(4):551–6.
11. Vogt T, Nix WA. Functional properties of motor units in motor neuron diseases and neuropathies. Electroencephalogr Clin Neurophysiol. 1997;105(4):328–32.
12. Jabre JF, Spellman NT. The demonstration of the size principle in humans using macro electromyography and precision decomposition. Muscle Nerve. 1996;19(3):338–41.
13. Stålberg E, Fawcett PR. Macro EMG in healthy subjects of different ages. J Neurol Neurosurg Psychiatry. 1982;45(10):870–8.
14. Nandedkar S, Stålberg E. Simulation of macro EMG motor unit potentials. Electroencephalogr Clin Neurophysiol. 1983;56(1):52–62.

Chapter 14
Electrical Impedance Myography and Its Application in Pediatric Neuromuscular Disorders

Seward Rutkove

Introduction and Basics of Impedance Techniques and EIM

Electrical impedance myography (EIM) is a relatively new technology for the assessment of neuromuscular disorders. In EIM a high frequency electrical current is passed via surface electrodes through a muscle of interest and the consequent surface voltages are measured by a second set of electrodes [1]. Unlike standard electrophysiological testing, such as electromyography and nerve conduction studies, the technique does not measure the inherent bioelectrical signals produced by the nerve or muscle, but rather evaluates how the tissue transforms the current. In some respects, EIM is analogous to diagnostic ultrasound, but instead of high frequency sound waves being emitted and reflected by the tissue, high frequency electrical current is being transmitted through the tissue. In addition, unlike ultrasound, the main interest is in obtaining quantifiable data rather than in producing images with anatomical details, although the latter could potentially be developed.

Electrical impedance techniques are broadly based on the basic concept that alterations in tissue morphology and composition will impact the measured impedance [2]. Thus, unlike standard electrophysiological testing, the technology is very sensitive to pathological change per se, including alterations in muscle and muscle fiber size, the presence of connective tissue, fat or edema, the number of muscle fibers, loss of the normal columnar structure of the tissue, and alterations in the broader muscle architecture and shape of the muscle.

A major characteristic of impedance measures is their dependence on frequency of the applied current, supported by theoretical work that was first spearheaded and developed by Kenneth Cole in the early-mid twentieth century [3]. The basic under-

S. Rutkove, M.D.
Beth Israel Deaconess Medical Center, Harvard Medical School, Boston, MA, USA
e-mail: srutkove@bidmc.harvard.edu

© Springer International Publishing AG 2017

H.J. McMillan, P.B. Kang (eds.), *Pediatric Electromyography*,
DOI 10.1007/978-3-319-61361-1_14

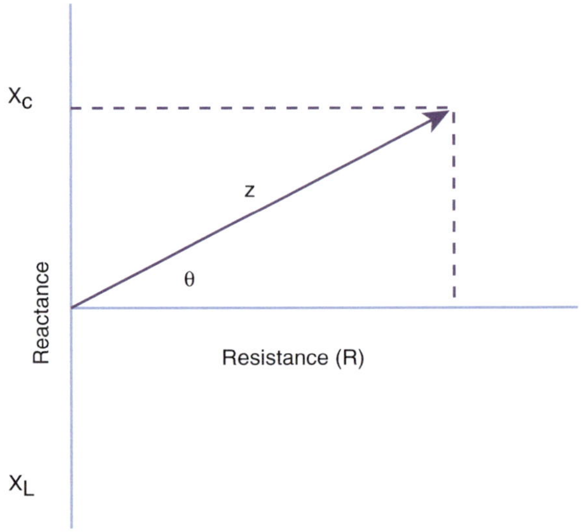

Fig. 14.1 Standard diagram explaining the concept of electrical impedance showing both capacitive and inductive reactance values (X_C and X_L), with signs reversed for convenience, resistance, and the impedance (Z) magnitude. When dealing with direct current, Ohm's law states V = IR, or that the measured voltage is the product of the applied current (I) and the resistance (R) of the tissue measured. However, when dealing with an alternating current, the equation is changed to V = IZ, where Z = R + *i*X, where R is the resistance (also called the "real" component) and X is the reactance (or the "imaginary" component). The "*i*" indicates that this is a complex number ("*i*" is favored by mathematicians for this value; engineers use "*j*" so the term doesn't get confused with the symbol for electrical current). Mathematically, Z can be considered to be a vector made of two components. The phase angle (q) can be derived trigonometrically from the measured X and Z values. In most biomedical impedance applications, R is considerably larger than X_C; so much larger in fact, that Z is not typically utilized since it may approximate the value of R

lying concept is that at low frequencies, electrical current mainly passes through the extracellular space; at very high frequencies the electrical current can pass through the cells since the membranes, which act as capacitors, become completely invisible to the electrical current at high frequency.

Electrical impedance (Z) is usually a complex number (Fig. 14.1). X itself actually consists of two components—X_C and X_L that point in opposite directions, with X_C representing the capacitive reactance (that due to the charge being stored briefly in the tissue and then being released as the alternating current flips direction) and X_L being due to the inductive or magnetic effects of the current passing through the tissues. Fortunately, biological tissues induce no meaningful inductive component, so X_L is generally dropped from the equation and X_C remains the only value being measured. Whereas X_C is a negative value (i.e., $X = X_L - X_C$), for convenience in most bioimpedance work, the sign is flipped to positive.

Technological Approaches and Electrode Arrays

As with most basic bioimpedance technologies, 4 electrodes are generally positioned in a linear array, with either a transverse or linear orientation—the two outer ones supplying the electrical current and the two inner ones measuring the generated voltages [1]. There are two major reasons for using a 4-electrode system rather than a 2-electrode system, which can also be utilized to measure impedance. First, the two-electrode approach is adversely affected by electrode polarization at the electrode-skin interface, adding an additional component to the measured impedance values that has no relevance to tissue condition. The second reason is that the two inner electrodes are measuring the voltages across tissue at a distance from the current electrodes, allowing the electrical current to substantially penetrate the subcutaneous fat into the muscle at the point of measurement. The use of 4 electrodes thus captures more data representing muscle than subcutaneous fat.

Outside of the restriction of using 4 electrodes in a specific order (Current-1, Voltage-1, Voltage-2, and Current-2), EIM can applied to the body using a variety of approaches. For example, in early EIM work, the current emitting electrodes: silver (Ag)—silver chloride (AgCl) adhesive electrodes, were placed at a distance from the voltage measuring electrodes, usually on the feet or hands and the voltage electrodes were placed over a muscle or muscle group of interest (e.g., over the quadriceps or biceps) [4]. An advantage of this approach is that it ensures that most of the electrical current flows through deeper tissues and thus is less affected by fat. In addition, large current-emitting electrodes can be used to ensure a relatively broad application of current throughout the limb. Disadvantages include the clumsiness of the approach (with multiple long cables attaching to the patient), the potential for even small changes in joint angle to have a significant impact on the data (a joint acting as a lens distorting the current flow as it passes through it), and the potential of substantial variations due to hydration status, associated with the current's flowing through deep veins and arteries.

For these reasons a simple and more convenient approach is taken in which all 4 electrodes are placed within several centimeters of one another [1]. This has obviated many of the problems associated with the initial approach, although it has the disadvantage of a requirement that the patient not move the limb during measurement (since changes in the shape of the muscle will affect the data) and a significant contribution of subcutaneous fat to the measured impedances (although there are approaches for disentangling these effects as described below). This approach also allows measurement of the muscle's anisotropy, discussed further below, as well as the use of pre-formed electrical arrays, expediting the process of data acquisition. Finally, this approach appears to be much less impacted by hydration status since the current does not readily penetrate deep blood vessels [5].

Using this "near" electrode description still leaves open many aspects of the possible configuration including the best size and shape of the electrodes for a given muscle and the ideal inter-electrode distances [6]. Ongoing work continues to model and improve these electrode configurations attempting to develop arrays that are effective at achieving excellent penetration of muscle while ensuring high repeatability and ease of use.

Frequency Dependence

A basic tenet of all impedance work is that by varying frequency one can learn a great deal more about tissues than by applying current at just a single frequency. As noted above, applying electrical current at multiple frequencies allows one to investigate the actual structure of the tissue being studied, which is not possible with single frequency approaches. Figure 14.2 gives an example of the frequency spectra for reactance, resistance, and phase of a healthy child, and one with Duchenne muscular dystrophy. As can be seen the entire spectrum for all three measures alters in complex ways, although lower reactance and phase values are perhaps the most prominent feature. Moreover, if multiple frequencies are not utilized (e.g., data from only a single frequency is obtained), it is impossible to tell if there is an artifact present in the data. Such distortions are readily identifiable when performing a multifrequency analysis.

A challenge of obtaining multifrequency data, or impedance spectroscopy, is that it is necessary to condense or collapse all the values into a single output value of interest. One approach is by applying simple mathematical operations that attempt to capture this change, such as the determination of linear fits of the data over certain

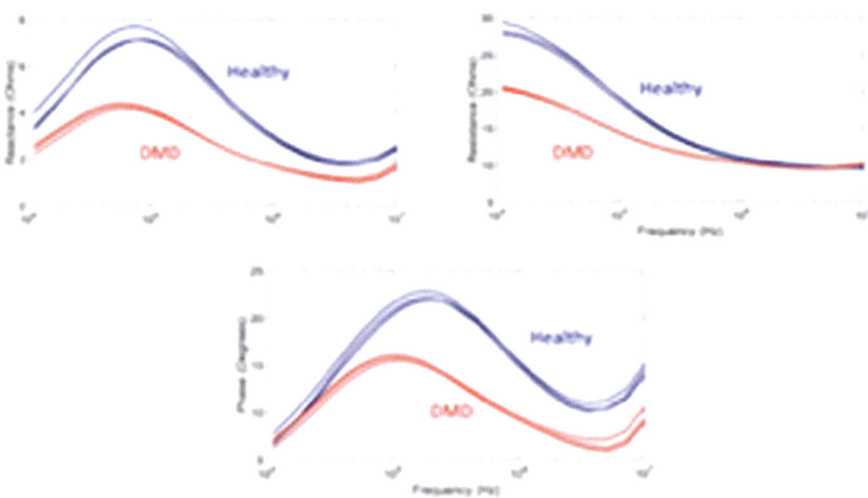

Fig. 14.2 Examples of multifrequency EIM data obtained from a healthy 10-year old boy and a 10-year old boy with DMD. Although the overall impedance characteristics of both children share similarities, the boy with DMD boy has considerably lower reactance and phase values with broadening out of the impedance curves

frequency ranges [7] or calculating simple ratios of data from individual frequencies [8]. Another is by using "Cole parameters" which are based on a basic simple impedance circuit model [2]. These parameters include: f_c, the center or characteristic frequency, corresponding to the highest reactance value, and an indirect measure of muscle cell size; α, an index of variation of muscle fiber size (one being perfectly homogeneous); and R_0 and R_{inf}, corresponding to the resistance at 0 kHz and infinite kHz respectively, providing measures of cell density.

Anisotropy

Another aspect of muscle is a property termed anisotropy, or directional dependence of electrical current flow [9]. Since muscle fibers are essentially long cylinders arranged in compact bundles (fascicles), applied electrical current will flow more easily along the fibers than across them [10]. The anisotropic nature of muscle, however, may be disturbed in situations in which there is alteration or destruction of muscle fibers or interposition of other materials into the muscle such as fat and connective tissue. Thus, myopathic diseases, including muscular dystrophies, will manifest a reduction in the normal anisotropic features of muscle [11]. In addition, a given direction of applied current flow may provide a better measure of disease status than another direction.

Which Impedance Feature Is Best for Assessing Neuromuscular Disease?

One challenge of performing impedance measurements is identifying which impedance characteristic is most informative of a specific muscle disease. Given the range of frequencies, the anisotropy issues, and varying electrode designs, it is challenging to know which values are best for assessing disease status. Much early work looked at single frequency measures, such as the 50 kHz phase [4, 12, 13]. While this value appeared repeatable and sensitive to progression in amyotrophic lateral sclerosis, it has proven less useful in other disorders. The reason for choosing this value initially was simply convenience: it was readily obtainable with relatively inexpensive impedance measuring equipment. Since then, other outcomes have been assessed including some of the multifrequency phase parameters we have discussed above, such as slopes, ratios, and Cole parameters. Moreover, in some conditions, rather than focusing on the phase value, the single or multiple frequency reactance or resistance values appear useful [14]. Moreover, of the three parameters, reactance appears to be least correlated with subcutaneous fat thickness [15], but at the same time is the most variable of the three parameters. Thus, for the most part, the question as to the "best" impedance parameter remains unsettled. In choosing any given parameter or set of parameters to use as a biomarker, it will be important that such measures be tested in separate populations and can survive verification by other investigators to ensure that it is truly robust and meaningful. Moreover, for such a parameter to be useful longitudinally, it not only should track disease status and demonstrate outstanding reproducibility, but should also be sensitive to the beneficial impact of an effective drug or other therapy.

Overview of EIM in the Pediatric Population

Although initial uses of EIM focused on adults with neuromuscular disorders including amyotrophic lateral sclerosis, it became clear early on that since the technique was entirely painless and could be applied at the bedside or in clinic, it could have special value in the pediatric population. A list of the potential advantages and disadvantages to using EIM in children is shown in Table 14.1. To date, the technique has been mainly studied in children with spinal muscular atrophy (SMA) and Duchenne muscular dystrophy (DMD) [7, 16, 17]. However, it was also recognized that in order to assess longitudinal changes in pediatric disease, it would also be necessary to evaluate changes in healthy children with growth. Given the sensitivity of impedance technologies to muscle histology, our a priori anticipation was that we might observe the effect of increasing muscle fiber size with age. Thus, in nearly all our human studies to date, both a healthy cohort of children has been included along with those affected by disease processes.

As for EIM's potential application in pediatric disease, the focus is currently more on tracking disease status over time and not for providing an initial diagnosis, although the latter application remains a possibility for future development. Thus, it may ultimately be used in clinical care settings to assess the effects of treatment or to evaluate the progression of a disease rather than for the more typical diagnostic applications of most electrodiagnostic technologies such electromyography and nerve conduction studies.

Table 14.1 Advantages and limitation of using EIM in a pediatric population

Advantages	Disadvantages
Very fast to apply	Data impacted by subcutaneous fat and edema
Painless; does not produce any sensation	Alterations may be challenging to interpret; the best parameters remain uncertain
Possible to use in children of all ages, including newborns	Normal growth causes changes in the impedance values, so comparison to control population needed
Can be used flexibly at the bedside or in clinic to evaluate a variety of muscles	Has uncertain diagnostic value; greatest use will be in tracking diseases over time and response to therapy
Can evaluate trunk muscles	
No image analysis required	
Electrode arrangements can be modified to fit any muscle of child	

EIM in Healthy Children

EIM has been performed in healthy children of all ages during several clinical studies [17, 18] (*and the NeuroNEXT SMA biomarker study*). Marked alterations in the impedance values with growth are observed, including increasing phase values, and alterations in the frequency spectrum, including reductions in peak frequency with growth. These changes may be multifactorial and may relate to increasing muscle fiber size per se and also increasing muscle volume over time. EIM values for healthy older children are fairly similar to those of adults. This relationship to muscle fiber size has also been studied in rats [19] and healthy immature mice, the data showing a strong inverse relationship between muscle fiber size and peak frequency (*personal communication*).

EIM in SMA

The first study of EIM in SMA evaluated a group of children with mainly Type II and Type III spinal muscular atrophy (SMA) and compared them to age-matched control subjects [7, 17]. Data were obtained at baseline as well as over an approximately 18-month follow-up period. Baseline EIM values, including single- and multi-frequency parameters, correlated with functional measures that included strength. Over time, differences were observed between the healthy and SMA children with increasing EIM values in the healthy children and relatively stable, unchanging values in the children with SMA, suggesting that SMA types II and III tend to be non-progressive over periods of time up to 18 months. The technique was also shown to have relatively high reproducibility.

More recently, EIM has been included in the NeuroNEXT SMA biomarker study which specifically sought to evaluate children with Type 0 or I SMA, and thus only enrolled children aged 0–6 months [20] (*personal communication*). This study also included a group of healthy age-matched children. All children were followed for up to 2 years from the time of enrollment. A number of potential outcomes for disease assessment were evaluated beyond EIM, including CMAP and functional measures. While single frequency EIM parameters did not show a clear difference between the affected and control groups at baseline, several multifrequency parameters did, including those identified in the earlier SMA study. One of these, the multifrequency reactance slope, also identified a difference in trajectories comparing the two groups, suggesting that the technique was sensitive to differences in muscle health and maturation.

These data in humans have been supported by a limited amount of work in SMA mouse models. One study identified differences in EIM values between wild type (WT) mice and those with a mild form of SMA [21]. More interestingly, another study showed that EIM could capture the effects of disease progression in the severe SMAΔ7 mouse and the impact of early interventional therapies with antisense oligonucleotides [22]. Such data, in conjunction with the human data described above, indicates that the technique may have value as an SMA biomarker. In particular, EIM has potential for the assessment of muscle health in SMA, since there is increasing evidence that SMA may have a substantial primary myopathic component [23].

EIM in DMD

DMD is the other pediatric disorder in which EIM has been studied extensively. This work has included one major study of about 36 DMD boys ranging in age from 2 to 14 years followed for up to 2 years [18]. Baseline cross-sectional data showed substantial differences in single frequency (50 kHz) EIM data between healthy and DMD boys as well as high reproducibility of the data between visits [16]. This measure also correlated well ($R = 0.65$, $P = 0.022$) with standard functional measures such as the 6 minute walk test. Longitudinal analysis also confirmed that the differences between DMD and healthy boys persisted over time, the latter showing the anticipated changes in multifrequency measures, including a phase ratio measure and a multifrequency phase-slope measure first used in the SMA population [20]. Interestingly, changes over time correlated with functional changes over time in both the 6 minute walk test and a timed test of getting up from the floor to a standing position.

As with SMA, mouse investigations have also been performed using EIM. As expected, substantial differences between healthy and *mdx* mice were identified with those changes being more substantial in older (2-year-old) as compared to younger (6-month-old) mice [24]. Importantly, both cell size and connective tissue deposition correlated with EIM values. A second mouse study showed a correlation of EIM values to T2 values on muscle MRI [25].

EIM in Other Pediatric Conditions

Investigators have pursued or currently are pursuing EIM applications for a number of other inherited muscle diseases, including congenital muscular dystrophy, facioscapulohumeral muscular dystrophy, and myotonic dystrophy, as well as acquired neuromuscular conditions such as obstetric brachial plexopathy and critical illness myopathy. Along with these efforts, EIM could have broader applicability in various conditions associated with muscle atrophy including orthopedic injury, prolonged hospitalization, cachexia, and even potentially malnutrition.

Ongoing Work and Future Developments

EIM is a technology that is still in the process of being developed and refined, though the volume of rigorous research on it is rising rapidly. While commercial systems are available, much of the work has been performed with off-the-shelf impedance devices with customized handheld arrays or with adhesive electrodes. EIM values are very sensitive to electrode configuration and a great deal remains unknown about the "best" configuration designs. Limitations are related to the fact that subcutaneous fat may play a substantial role in the acquired data, depending on the thickness of the fat layer [6] as well as anisotropic effects of the muscle itself. In addition to these electrode challenges, identifying which set of multifrequency parameters for use is best for a given disease remains an open question at this time. Evaluating the multifrequency alterations in disease may not only be dependent on the specific disease, but also on the electrode design as well.

Outside of these technical factors, other EIM-related work is underway, including additional studies in animal models, with correlations to pathology. Indeed, one potential use of EIM is as a "virtual muscle biopsy" in which the EIM data could provide information non-invasively on histological characteristics of the myofiber, including cell size, the presence of abnormal mitochondrial, glycogen deposition, or internalized nuclei, as well increased interstitial fat and connective tissue. These studies are ongoing.

Another major benefit of EIM is its ease of use, with people requiring relatively little training in order to employ the technology successfully. This has led to the development of a commercial fitness product for self-measurement, but this also raises the distinct possibility of encouraging EIM data to be collected at home by older children on themselves or by parents or caregivers for ongoing evaluation of muscle status during a specific therapy or during a treatment trial. By obtaining frequent measurements there is improved sensitivity to subtle changes in muscle that may not readily achievable when measurements are performed just occasionally (e.g., once every several months) as is standard in most clinical trials. Frequent measurements could lead to a substantial reduction in noise and thus improved sensitivity to the effects of therapy on muscle condition. This concept has served as the basis of a new clinical study in amyotrophic lateral sclerosis (ALS-at-home) but could also be readily expanded to pediatric conditions as well.

The next decade will likely see increased use of EIM as a tool for the assessment of pediatric neuromuscular disorders as clinicians and researchers gradually become more familiar with the technology, its related terminology, its challenges, and its potential promises.

References

1. Rutkove SB. Electrical impedance Myography: background, current state, and future directions. Muscle Nerve. 2009;40:936–46.
2. Martinsen OG, Grimnes S. Bioimpedance and Bioelectricity Basics. 2nd ed. Cambridge: Academic Press; 2008.
3. Cole KS, Cole RH. Dispersion and absorption in dielectrics. I. Alternating current characteristics. J Chem Phys. 1941;9:341–51.
4. Rutkove SB, Aaron R, Shiffman CA. Localized bioimpedance analysis in the evaluation of neuromuscular disease. Muscle Nerve. 2002;25:390–7.
5. Li J, Sanchez B, Rutkove SB. The effect of profound dehydration on electrical impedance of mouse skeletal muscle. Conf Proc IEEE Eng Med Biol Soc. 2014;2014:514–7.

6. Jafarpoor M, Li J, White JK, Rutkove SB. Optimizing electrode configuration for electrical impedance measurements of muscle via the finite element method. IEEE Trans Biomed Eng. 2013;60:1446–52.
7. Rutkove SB, Shefner JM, Gregas M, Butler H, Caracciolo J, Lin C, et al. Characterizing spinal muscular atrophy with electrical impedance myography. Muscle Nerve. 2010;42:915–21.
8. Schwartz S, Geisbush TR, Mijailovic A, Pasternak A, Darras BT, Rutkove SB. Optimizing electrical impedance myography measurements by using a multifrequency ratio: a study in Duchenne muscular dystrophy. Clin. Neurophysiol: Elsevier; 2014.
9. Aaron R, Huang M, Shiffman CA. Anisotropy of human muscle via non-invasive impedance measurements. Phys Med Biol. 1997;42:1245–62.
10. Epstein BR, Foster KR. Anisotropy in the dielectric properties of skeletal muscle. Med Biol Eng Comput. 1983;21:51–5.
11. Garmirian LP, Chin AB, Rutkove SB. Discriminating neurogenic from myopathic disease via measurement of muscle anisotropy. Muscle Nerve. 2009;39:16–24.
12. Rutkove SB, Zhang H, Schoenfeld DA, Raynor EM, Shefner JM, Cudkowicz ME, et al. Electrical impedance myography to assess outcome in amyotrophic lateral sclerosis clinical trials. Clin Neurophysiol. 2007;118:2413–8.
13. Tarulli A, Esper GJ, Lee KS, Aaron R, Shiffman CA, Rutkove SB. Electrical impedance myography in the bedside assessment of inflammatory myopathy. Neurology. 2005;65:451–2.
14. Statland JM, Heatwole C, Eichinger K, Dilek N, Martens WB, Tawil R. Electrical impedance myography in facioscapulohumeral muscular dystrophy. Muscle Nerve. 2016;54(4):696–701.
15. Sung M, Spieker AJ, Narayanaswami P, Rutkove SB. The effect of subcutaneous fat on electrical impedance myography when using a handheld electrode array: the case for measuring reactance. Clin Neurophysiol. 2013;124:400–4.
16. Rutkove SB, Geisbush TR, Mijailovic A, Shklyar I, Pasternak A, Visyak N, et al. Cross-sectional evaluation of electrical impedance Myography and quantitative ultrasound for the assessment of Duchenne muscular dystrophy in a clinical trial setting. Pediatr Neurol. 2014;51:88–92.
17. Rutkove SB, Gregas MC, Darras BT. Electrical impedance myography in spinal muscular atrophy: a longitudinal study. Muscle Nerve. 2012;45:642–7.
18. Rutkove SB, Kapur K, Zaidman C, JS W, Pasternak A, Madabusi L, et al. Electrical impedance myography for assessment of Duchenne muscular dystrophy. Ann Neurol. 2017;81(5):622–32.
19. Ahad M, Rutkove SB. Electrical impedance myography at 50 kHz in the rat: technique, reproducibility, and the effects of sciatic injury and recovery. Clinical Neurophysiology Clin Neurophys. 2009;120(8):1534.
20. Kolb SJ, Coffey CS, Yankey JW, Krosschell K, Arnold WD, Rutkove SB, et al. Baseline results of the NeuroNEXT spinal muscular atrophy infant biomarker study. Ann Clin Transl Neurol. 2016;3:132–45.
21. Li J, Geisbush TR, Arnold WD, Rosen GD, Zaworski PG, Rutkove SB. A comparison of three electrophysiological methods for the assessment of disease status in a mild spinal muscular atrophy mouse model. PLoS One. 2014;9:e111428.
22. Arnold WD, McGovern VL, Sanchez B, Li J, Corlett KM, Kolb SJ, et al. The neuromuscular impact of symptomatic SMN restoration in a mouse model of spinal muscular atrophy. Neurobiol Dis. 2016;87:116–23.
23. Bottai D, Adami R. Spinal muscular atrophy: new findings for an old pathology. Brain Pathol. 2013;23(6):613–22.
24. Li J, Geisbush TR, Rosen GD, Lachey J, Mulivor A, Rutkove SB. Electrical impedance myography for the in vivo and ex vivo assessment of muscular dystrophy (mdx) mouse muscle. Muscle Nerve. 2014;49:829–35.
25. Wu JS, Li J, Greenman RL, Bennett D, Geisbush T, Rutkove SB. Assessment OF aged mdx mice by electrical impedance myography and magnetic resonance imaging. Muscle Nerve. 2015;52:598–604.

Part V
Clinical Applications

Chapter 15
Pediatric Cranial Neuropathies

Francis Renault

Electrodiagnostic examination of orofacial muscles is used to assess dysfunction of the brainstem and paired cranial nerves in newborns, infants, and older children presenting with facial weakness, orofacial malformations, and bulbar weakness.

Cranial Nerves V and VII Electrodiagnostic Studies

Congenital facial weakness or asymmetry may result from obstetrical trauma or reveal a recognizable malformation syndrome, or congenital neuromuscular disorder. A combination of neurophysiologic tests and neuroimaging provides an opportunity for early diagnosis, management, and prognostication.

Correlative Anatomy and Neurophysiology

The motor nucleus of cranial nerve VII originates in the caudal pons. Interneuronal and synaptic V to VII connections in the brainstem provide the basis for neurophysiologic studies exploring blink reflexes (BRs) [1].The close anatomic proximity of cranial nerves V, VI, VII, and VIII in the brainstem and cerebellopontine angle explains the involvement of multiple nerves in malformations, ischemic or compressive disorders. The twin sensory and motor roots of the facial nerve emerge from the brainstem at the level of the bulbopontine sulcus, between the sixth and eighth cranial nerves, at the cerebellopontine angle, then enter the pars petrosal

F. Renault, M.D., A.I.H.P., A.C.C.A.
Neurophysiology Unit, Armand-Trousseau University Hospital, Paris, France
e-mail: docteur.frenault@wanadoo.fr

© Springer International Publishing AG 2017

H.J. McMillan, P.B. Kang (eds.), *Pediatric Electromyography*,
DOI 10.1007/978-3-319-61361-1_15

ossis temporalis via the internal acoustic meatus and follow a common path in the first part of the facial canal. The primary motor bundle of the facial nerve traverses the second and third parts of the facial canal alone. Nerve entrapment is most likely to occur at the narrowest intraosseous segment, the meatal foramen, where it is not protected by epineurium and perineurium [2]. The facial motor nerve emerges from the skull at the stylomastoid foramen, gives off the posterior auricular branch, and then divides into two main terminal branches in the parotid gland. The inferior cervicofacial branch passes down along the mandible to supply the muscles in the lower part of the face, giving off a buccal branch to the risorius, the buccinator, and the orbicularis oris muscles; a mental branch to the depressor anguli oris, the depressor labii inferioris, and the mentalis muscles; and a cervical branch to platysma. The superior temporofacial branch runs horizontally forward, giving off frontal branches to the frontalis and orbicularis oculi muscles; suborbital branches to the levator labii superioris, zygomaticus, levator anguli oris, and dilatator naris muscles; and buccal branches to the buccinator and orbicularis oris muscles. Although there is considerable diversity in its trajectory and divisions, cranial nerve VII innervates all muscles of facial expression except the levator palpebrae superioris.

Facial Nerve Conduction Studies and Electroneuronography

For facial nerve conduction studies (NCSs), surface electrodes are placed over the orbicularis oris muscle to record the compound muscle action potential (CMAP) elicited by an electrical stimulus (0.2 ms, 10–40 mA) that is applied to the nerve, first at a point anterior to the tragus, and then at a point along the horizontal portion of the mandible. During growth, motor latencies show little changes (Table 15.1), while facial nerve conduction velocity (NCV) increases markedly, particularly within the first year of life (Table 15.2) [3].

Electroneuronography (ENOG) uses surface electrodes placed along the nasolabial fold to record a global facial CMAP elicited by a brief supramaximal electrical stimulus applied to the facial nerve at the stylomastoid foramen. The peak-to-peak amplitude of the CMAP is measured bilaterally; an asymmetry greater than 30% is considered abnormal [4]. ENOG is used to evaluate the severity of a lesion to the cranial nerve VII, and has shown prognostic value in complete acute non-traumatic unilateral facial paralysis in childhood [5].

Table 15.1 Normal motor latencies (milliseconds (ms) ± 2 sd) stimulating CN VII and recording at the orbicularis oculi and orbicularis oris muscles from birth to 15 years

Age (years)	Number of subjects	Orbicularis oculi	Orbicularis oris
0–1	120	3.1 ± 0.8	5.3 ± 1.7
1–3	91	3.3 ± 0.5	5.4 ± 1.6
3–9	89	3.5 ± 1.0	5.6 ± 1.5
9–15	44	3.5 ± 0.9	5.6 ± 1.7

Table 15.2 Normal facial nerve conduction velocity (meters per second (m/s) ± 2 sd) stimulating CN VII first at a point anterior to the tragus and then at a point along the horizontal portion of the mandible from birth to 15 years

Age	Number of subjects	Cervicofacial branch NCV
0–30 day	18	19.0 ± 2.5
1–2 months	14	21.4 ± 3.4
2–4 months	12	24.5 ± 3.9
4–6 months	24	26.3 ± 2.8
6–8 months	23	29.1 ± 3.3
8–10 months	15	31.7 ± 3.7
10–12 months	14	33.3 ± 3.3
12–18 months	30	36.1 ± 3.0
18 m–2 years	27	37.5 ± 4.7
2–3 years	34	39.5 ± 2.7
3–4 years	16	41.9 ± 4.5
4–5 years	21	43.4 ± 3.3
5–6 years	12	45.5 ± 4.8
6–7 years	12	45.8 ± 5.3
7–8 years	13	46.5 ± 4.1
8–9 years	15	48.1 ± 3.8
9–11 years	17	48.3 ± 2.8
11–13 years	12	48.7 ± 5.6
13–15 years	15	48.5 ± 2.8

NCV nerve conduction velocity
Distances (mm) between stimulation points are 34.6 ± 6.6 up to 12 months, 48.7 ± 9.7 from 1 to 5 years, and 56.1 ± 6 from 5 to 15 years

Needle Electromyography of Facial Muscles

Conventional needle EMG contributes to the determination of the characteristics and severity of a lesion to the cranial nerve VII, and gives clues regarding pathogenesis and outcome. Needle EMG examination is performed at rest, and with voluntary contraction or after stimulation. EMG is recorded by a concentric needle electrode in at least one muscle innervated by the temporofacial branch (orbicularis oculi or frontalis), and in another innervated by the cervicofacial branch (orbicularis oris or depressor anguli oris). When tolerated, fasting an infant for up to 4 h before the test may facilitate the recording of bursts of activity arising from the facial muscles while the baby is crying or sucking a pacifier. In older children, voluntary contraction can be recorded after asking the child to imitate the examiner by closing the eyes, smiling, and whistling.

The maximum amplitude of a motor unit potential (MUP) is measured from the highest negative peak to the lowest positive peak of the largest EMG burst. Traces are classified as: (1) normal interference pattern; (2) neurogenic (i.e., single or reduced, high-amplitude MUPs units) or; (3) myogenic (i.e., low-amplitude where the maximum amplitude decreased by at least 30%) (Fig. 15.1). The normal maximum MUP amplitude of the interference pattern is 850 μV (range: 400 μV–1.2 mV) with normal MUP duration from 1 to 2.8 ms. The proportion of polyphasic potentials present in a normal muscle may exceed 30% (Table 15.3) [6].

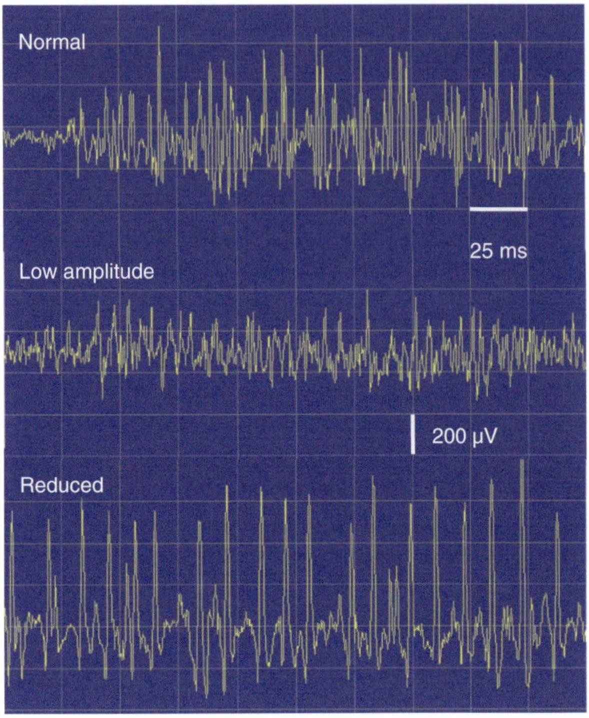

Fig. 15.1 Needle EMG of facial muscles, exemplary recordings: normal pattern (*upper trace*); low-amplitude pattern, reflecting muscle hypoplasia (*middle*); neurogenic reduced recruitment (*lower trace*)

Table 15.3 Needle EMG of muscles of the face, the tongue and soft palate: normal pattern in subjects from 4 days to 3 years old

Muscles	EMG interference pattern		
	Maximal amplitude (range, mV)	MUPs duration (range, ms)	Proportion of polyphasic MUPs (%)
Orbicularis oculi, Orbicularis oris	0.40–1.2	1–2.8	> 30
Genioglossus	0.38–1.5	1–3.9	> 50
Levator veli palatini, Pharyngoglossus, Palatoglossus.	0.42–1.8	1–3.2	> 50

MUPs motor unit potentials

Blink Responses

This technique explores both facial and trigeminal nerve functions, as well as the pathways between their respective cranial nuclei within the brainstem. The blink reflex results from the contraction of the orbicularis oculi muscle provoked by stimulation of the supraorbital branch of the trigeminal nerve [7]. A single electric shock is applied to the supraorbital foramen to elicit BRs recorded from the orbicularis oculi muscle on both sides. Stimulation of the ipsilateral supraorbital trigeminal nerve provokes a direct response with two components: R1, which is immediate and brief, and R2, which is delayed and longer lasting. Stimulation of the contralateral nerve V provokes a crossed R2 response.

The maturation from birth of the electrically elicited BRs has been studied [8]. The R1 response is always present and its latency achieves normal adult values (range: 9–13 ms) at 44 weeks postmenstrual age. The ipsilateral R2 response can be evoked in most newborns at term birth (latency range: 34–43 ms), but the contralateral R2 response is not always obtained before the age of 8 months. The R1 component corresponds to an oligosynaptic reflex arc involving at least two and no more than three synapses in the pons between the main sensory nucleus of cranial nerve V and the motor nucleus of the ipsilateral cranial nerve VII. The R2 component follows polysynaptic medullary pathways, which are more caudal and closer to the bulbar formations. The spinal trigeminal nucleus has projections to the adjacent paramedian reticular formation and the motor nuclei of both seventh nerves. Injury in the trigeminal pathway leads to delayed or absent ipsilateral R1 and R2 responses, and contralateral R2 response, while a lesion in the facial pathway shows delayed ipsilateral R1 and R2, but normal contralateral R2. Lesions at the pons show ipsilateral abnormal R1 response, while contralateral stimulus has normal R1. Lateral medullary lesions show abnormal R2 response on the affected side, stimulating either the non-affected or the affected side [9].

Neurophysiological Assessment of the Trigeminal Nerve

Methods for studying trigeminal afferents have several limitations. The specific clinical assessment of the ophthalmic, maxillary, and mandibular nerves is not reliable in the young child. Supraorbital sensory nerve action potential has been reported only in normal adults so far [10]. Somatosensory evoked potentials are misleading because electrical stimuli to the orofacial area generate muscle potentials and trigeminal reflexes that contaminate the scalp signal [11]. Trigeminal motor function is clinically assessed by palpating the masseter-temporalis muscles at rest and on voluntary contraction after asking the child to bite down. Transcranial motor evoked potentials are not routinely available in an ambulatory setting, and normal values during growth are not available. Surface electrodes placed over masseter and temporalis muscles enable the analysis of the timing and the envelope of EMG bursts, taking into account that bursts are contaminated with signals generated by facial muscles. Conventional needle EMG of the masseter and temporalis muscles remains the way to study trigeminal motor function and to detect neurogenic abnormalities.

Cranial Nerves IX–X and XII Electrodiagnostic Studies

With the aim to explore bulbar dysfunction and evaluate congenital dysphagia, EMG techniques provide information on brainstem structures involved in oral sensorimotor functions. This includes EMG of muscles of the tongue and soft palate and EMG during bottle-feeding, which investigates the electrophysiology of sucking and swallowing.

The Genioglossus Muscle and the Hypoglossal Nerve

The hypoglossal nerve is purely a motor nerve. Its nucleus consists of a column which extends for nearly the full length of the medulla oblongata. Emerging from the skull by the anterior condylar canal, cranial nerve XII crosses the pharyngomaxillary space and curves anteriorly in the carotid groove. In the sublingual area it sends terminal branches to the ipsilateral muscles of the tongue. The genioglossus is a paired paramedian muscle of the tongue; it can be recorded by the endo-oral route. After local anesthesia by swabbing this area with a small amount of lidocaine (the swab should not contain enough lidocaine for the infant to swallow any drops, as that would entail a risk of side effects from inadvertent ingestion), the needle electrode is inserted in the ventral surface of the tongue, slightly lateral to the midline (Fig. 15.2). The interference pattern is recorded when the infant is crying and also when sucking a nipple. The normal maximal amplitude of the interference pattern is from 380 μV to 1.5 mV (Table 15.3).

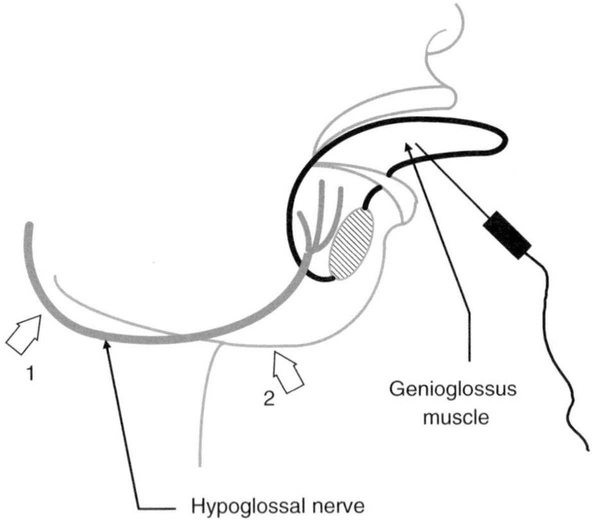

Fig. 15.2 Motor nerve conduction of the hypoglossal nerve stimulus is applied proximally behind the mandible (*large arrow* #1) and then more distally under the chin (*large arrow* #2). EMG needle is inserted into the ventral surface of the genioglossus muscle (tongue), just lateral of the midline

Table 15.4 Normal motor latency (ms ± 2 sd) of the genioglossus muscle when stimulation is applied to cranial nerve XII behind the mandible from birth to 15 years

Age (years)	Number of subjects	Genioglossus motor latency
0–1	120	3.8 ± 1.0
1–3	91	3.5 ± 1.1
3–9	89	3.3 ± 0.9
9–15	44	3.4 ± 0.6

Table 15.5 Normal hypoglossal nerve conduction velocity (m/s ± 2 sd) stimulating CN XII behind the mandible and then at distal submental point under the chin from birth to 15 years

Age	Number of subjects	Hypoglossal NCV
0–30d	18	23.5 ± 2.2
1–2 months	14	24.1 ± 2.2
2–4 months	12	26.6 ± 2.7
4–6 months	24	28.9 ± 2.9
6–8 months	23	31.8 ± 3.4
8–10 months	15	34.3 ± 2.9
10–12 months	14	35.7 ± 3.0
12–18 months	30	37.5 ± 2.1
18 months–2 years	27	40.6 ± 2.6
2–3 years	34	42.1 ± 3.0
3–4 years	16	43.5 ± 3.4
4–5 years	21	46.1 ± 2.5
5–6 years	12	46.5 ± 4.9
6–7 years	12	47.3 ± 2.1
7–8 years	13	48.1 ± 6.9
8–9 years	15	49.0 ± 2.6
9–11 years	17	50.2 ± 7.1
11–13 years	12	50.9 ± 6.4
13–15 years	15	50.7 ± 5.4

NCV nerve conduction velocity

Distances between stimulation points (mm) are: 32.5 ± 9.3 up to 12 months, 36.1 ± 6.5 from 1 to 5 years, and 38.2 ± 9.7 from 5 to 15 years

For hypoglossal NCSs, electrical stimuli (0.2 ms, 10–40 mA) are applied proximally behind the mandible and then more distally under the chin. The motor response has a polyphasic morphology, a mean duration from 6 to 10 ms, and amplitude from 0.8 to 1 mV. Latencies induced by stimulation under the angle of the mandible do not show a significant change between birth and 15 years, ranging from 2.4 to 4.8 ms (Table 15.4). The hypoglossal NCV increases more than 30% in the first year (Table 15.5).

Muscles of the Soft Palate and The Pharyngeal Plexus

The motor fibers of cranial nerves IX and X supplying the muscles of the pharynx arise from the upper part of the nucleus ambiguus. The pharyngeal branches of nerve X merge with the fibers of nerve IX to constitute the pharyngeal plexus, which innervates muscles of the soft palate. The levator veli palatini muscle spreads into the large paramedian section of the soft palate. After local anesthesia by swabbing the mucosa with a small amount of lidocaine, a needle electrode is inserted 1–1.5 cm from the median line. Also, palatoglossus and pharyngoglossus muscles can be easily reached by inserting the needle electrode in the palatoglossal and palatopharyngeal arches respectively. The normal maximal amplitude of the interference pattern in these soft palate muscles is 1.3 mV (Table 15.3).

EMG During Bottle Feeding

This method consists of a two-channel EMG recording while the infant is drinking sugar-water from a bottle (Fig. 15.3). For the oral phase the genioglossus is recorded via a transcutaneous submental route. For the pharyngeal phase, the thyrohyoid is reached on the lateral face of the thyroid cartilage. The recording enables analysis of the activity of each of the muscles and observation of the chronology of their action and the coordination of the two phases of swallowing. A normal pattern features rhythmic spindle-shaped bursts of activity separated by a quiescent period; the two muscles alternate regularly (Fig. 15.4). Initial frequency of sucking ranges from 0.6 to 2 Hz (mean: 1.4). Mean duration of genioglossal bursts, calculated for the first twenty sucks, ranges from 180 to 460 ms depending on the infant, without any correlation with age. The duration of the bursts and quiescent periods between sucks increases progressively (from 35 to 100%) during the course of the feed. This probably reflects both fatigue and decreasing appetite. The EMG activity of the thyrohyoid muscle is also organized into bursts with the same fusiform shape; the mean duration of bursts calculated for the first twenty sucks is 210 to 520 ms. The onset of thyrohyoid activity ranges from 100 ms before to 220 ms after the end of lingual activity, depending on the infant and is unrelated to age. The timing of the two muscle contractions varies from one child to another but varies a little from one swallow to another during feeding in the same child.

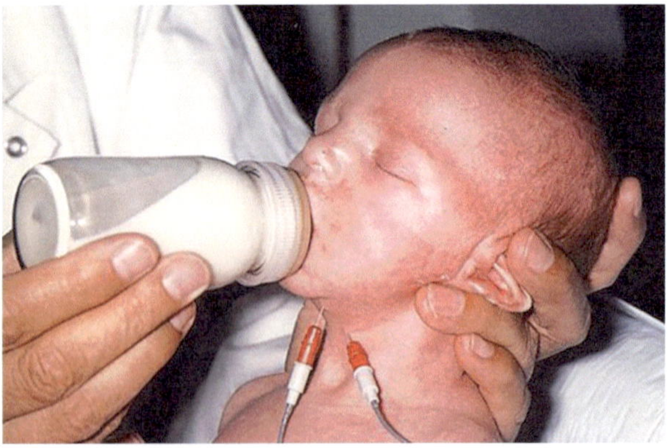

Fig. 15.3 Electromyography during bottle feeding: two-channel needle EMG recording of a muscle reflecting sucking (genioglossus) and another reflecting swallowing (thyrohyoid) while the infant intakes formula milk or sugar water

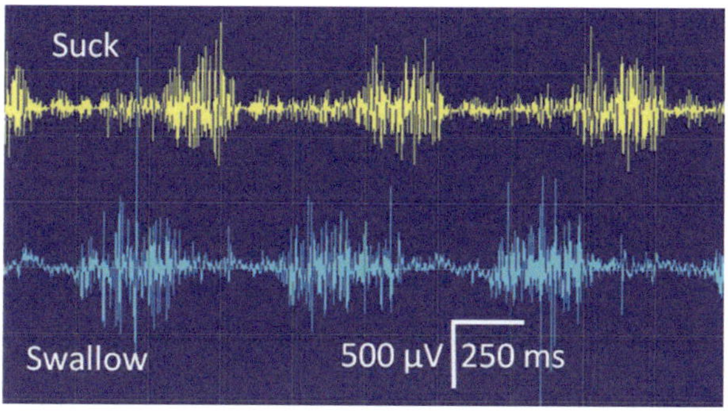

Fig. 15.4 Electromyography during bottle feeding: normal alternating pattern of genioglossus (upper trace) and thyrohyoid muscles in a full-term newborn on day 10

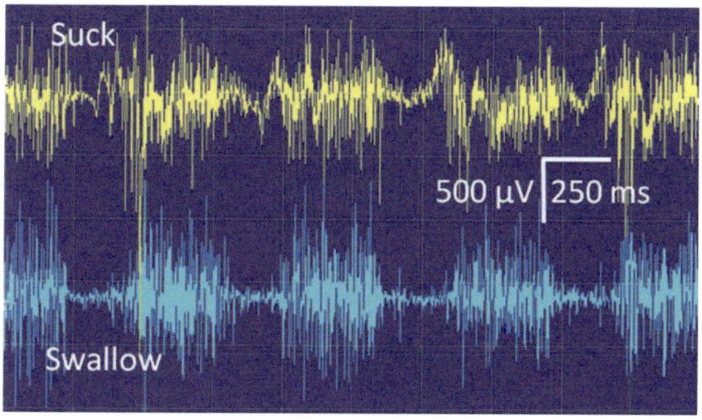

Fig. 15.5 Electromyography during bottle feeding: abnormal result, synchronous oral and pharyngeal phases in a full-term newborn with isolated Pierre Robin sequence

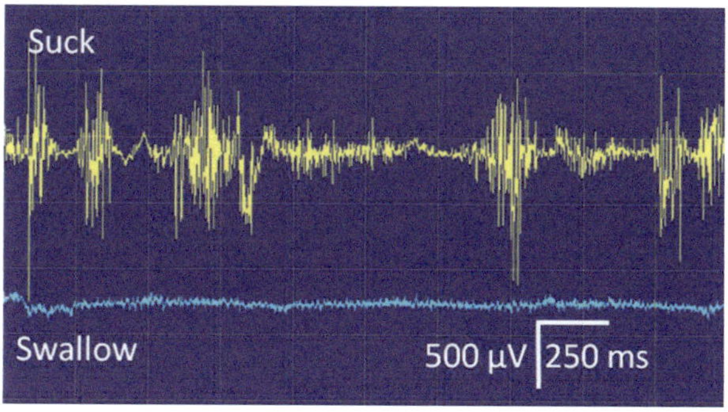

Fig. 15.6 Electromyography during bottle feeding: severely abnormal result, no rhythmic sucking and inactive pharyngeal phase

Abnormal patterns define oropharyngeal incoordination as mild, where sucking is present but the alternation between sucking and swallowing is irregular; moderate, where sucking is present but the pharyngeal phase is either synchronous or random (Fig. 15.5); or severe, where the tongue does not perform rhythmic sucking activity, and the pharyngeal phase is either inactive or tonic (Fig. 15.6). Results are classified as: (1) normal oropharyngeal coordination or mild anomalies; or (2) moderate or severe oropharyngeal incoordination.

Investigating Facial and Bulbar Weakness

Orofacial sensorimotor functions are not easy to assess clinically and involve small-sized brain stem structures that rarely show neuroimaging abnormalities. Neurophysiological techniques help to diagnose neurological dysfunctions as well as to elucidate their pathogenesis, assist therapeutic decisions, and predict outcome.

Congenital Facial Asymmetries and Diplegia

Facial paralysis in a newborn may be due to prenatal or obstetric stress to the nerve. Congenital facial weakness or asymmetry may also reveal a recognizable malformation syndrome or congenital neuromuscular disorder.

Perinatal Facial Nerve Injuries

Alterations in facial NCV and BRs, as well as needle EMG of facial muscles, precisely define the extent and severity of the facial nerve lesion. Moderate forms show only partial denervation and either affect the territories of the two main branches equally, or predominantly involve the cervicofacial branch. Severe forms show absent facial CMAPs and BRs, and very reduced or single EMG recruitment patterns. Clinical and EMG monitoring of congenital facial palsies demonstrates that facial nerve regeneration and muscle reinnervation usually proceed slowly, over several months. Serial facial NCSs and ENOGs help distinguish developmental defects from recovering traumatic insults. The percentage values of facial function over time provided by serial ENOGs correlate with prognosis [5].When the palsy seems to be complete based on clinical presentation, EMG may indicate a more favorable outcome by showing nascent MUPs with the reappearance of a low-amplitude increased-latency motor response. Improvement in facial motor activity and EMG parameters may continue as long as 2 years after nerve injury. In contrast, one must not fail to recognize a definitive facial nerve lesion related to an area of focal compression. Even if CT scan and MRI fail to define a focal VII nerve lesion, consideration of surgical exploration is warranted if there are no signs of clinical or EMG improvement within a reasonable timeframe. Surgical exploration is indicated when two or three successive EMGs demonstrate either the persistence of a major lesion of the two major facial nerve branches without any sign of recovery, or partial recovery of the cervicofacial-branch with persistence of complete paralysis of the temporofacial branch [12].

Asymmetric Crying Facies

Congenital facial asymmetry obvious only when the child is crying, and involving only the lower lip, has several potential causes. Unilateral hypoplasia of the depressor anguli oris muscle (DAOM) is the most frequent condition [13].Typical EMG findings are a low amplitude interference pattern on crying, and normal facial NCV. An EMG diagnosis of hypoplasia of the DAOM should lead to a search for associated visceral malformation and 22q11 deletion [14]. Less often, EMG signs of partial denervation of the DAOM, depressor labii inferioris, and mentalis muscles are indicative of a distal partial facial palsy. The selective topography of these nerve lesions corresponds to the territory of the mental branch of the facial nerve. This branch, arising from the cervicofacial branch, has a course that in the fetus and newborn closely follows the horizontal part of the mandible and is thus easily compressed [15].

Hemifacial Malformation Syndromes

Hemifacial malformations involving the derivatives of the first and second branchial arches can result in lesions of cranial nerves V and VII. Facial paralysis is present in most infants with Goldenhar syndrome [MIM#164210], CHARGE association (Colobomata, Heart disease, Atresia of the choanae, Retarded growth and development, Genital hypoplasia, and Ear anomalies) due to *CHD7* mutations [MIM#214800], and hemifacial microsomia [16]. Facial weakness may be diffuse or localized to one side of the face. EMG activity detected in facial muscles is variably normal, neurogenic, or low amplitude. Neurogenic EMG signs in facial muscles may be associated with multiple cranial neuropathies or malformation of the central nervous system, in particular of the posterior fossa [17].

Moebius Syndrome

Moebius syndrome is characterized by bilateral facial and abducens palsies. Facial diplegia usually involves the upper half of the face, and can be asymmetrical. Facial EMG is an important diagnostic tool contributing to the differential diagnosis and elucidation of the pathogenesis of Moebius syndrome. Most published EMG studies point towards a neurogenic origin, describing sparse motor units, increased latencies, slowing of facial nerve conduction, and sometimes altered BRs [18]. Should facial EMG be difficult to interpret secondary to muscle atrophy, the study of lingual and palatal muscles can be useful in identifying a concomitant neurogenic process (Table 15.6). Myopathic low amplitude EMG patterns may also be detected, but do not necessarily reveal a myopathic disease, but indicate developmental muscular hypoplasia. In the neonatal period, EMG of the limbs distinguishes Moebius syndrome from congenital myotonic dystrophy or other myopathies.

Table 15.6 Needle EMG patterns in orofacial muscles in 61 patients with Moebius syndrome

		EMG pattern			
Muscle	Number	No activity n (%)	Neurogenic n (%)	Myopathic n (%)	Normal n (%)
Temporalis	24	2 (8)	9 (37)	3 (12)	10 (42)
Orbicularis oculi	118	77 (65)	34 (29)	6 (5)	1 (0.1)
Orbicularis oris/DAOM	123	15 (12)	81 (66)	18 (15)	9 (7)
LVP	90	0	21 (23)	17 (19)	52 (58)
Genioglossus	69	0	46 (67)	4 (0.6)	19 (28)

For patients with Moebius syndrome, EMG also elicits useful information before determined whether a child should undergo a temporalis muscle lengthening myoplasty, aiming to improve tightening of the lips and rehabilitate the smile. Electromyographic study of the temporalis can detect muscle denervation or atrophy differentiating this from dyspraxia and help guide decisions regarding myoplasty, as well as to modify rehabilitation programs. Patients and their families must be aware of the modest outcome that myoplasty may offer [19]. Congenital facial diplegia may present as an isolated VIIth nerve involvement in pedigrees with *HOXB1* mutation [20]. EMG studies showed facial denervation, possibly with a progressive course [21].

Neuromuscular Disorders with Congenital Facial Diplegia

Facial weakness is an important clinical sign in several neuromuscular disorders, including congenital myasthenic syndromes, congenital myotonic dystrophy, congenital myopathies, infantile facioscapulohumeral muscular dystrophy, and some metabolic myopathies. Other conditions such as Prader-Willi syndrome and transient neonatal myasthenia gravis should also be considered. Electrodiagnostic studies show normal or myopathic EMG patterns in facial muscles associated with normal facial NCV and BRs. EMG study of proximal and distal muscles of upper and lower limbs may show myopathic abnormalities. Electrical stimulation may provoke repetitive discharges, though clinical myotonia is generally not apparent during infancy [22, 23]. Myopathic EMG changes are frequently associated with neuropathy in patients with congenital muscular dystrophy, especially of the merosin-deficient variety [23]. Stimulated single-fiber EMG may be used, even in the very young, to detect neuromuscular junction disorders [24].

Acquired Facial Palsies

At any age, EMG is particularly useful during the second and third weeks after onset of the facial palsy, once Wallerian degeneration has occurred. Later on in the course of recovery, changing EMG patterns demonstrate nerve regeneration and muscle reinnervation.

Unilateral Facial Palsy

Bell's palsy, local infection, and traumatic injuries account for more than 80% of acquired facial palsies in children, along with Lyme disease in endemic regions. Because more severe conditions may initially resemble an isolated unilateral Bell's palsy, a close follow-up of the patient is required [12]. Bell's idiopathic palsy may occur in the first months of life, but is most frequently seen after age 8 years. Complete spontaneous recovery is the rule, with percentages in different series ranging around 90%; this percentage may be lower if needle EMG is performed to detect residual subclinical nerve injury [25]. Normal CMAP latency and preserved BRs within the first weeks after onset are predictive of complete recovery. Inexcitability of the facial nerve, a marked decrease in CMAP amplitude or absent BR after several weeks, is associated with a poor outcome or delayed recovery [26]. ENOG performed from 8 to 12 days after onset may be used to predict outcome. In idiopathic Bell's palsy, amplitudes reach their nadir 7–14 days after the onset of weakness. A loss of CMAP amplitude of less than 90% compared to the contralateral normal side is usually followed by a complete recovery in 7 or 8 weeks. When the loss is between 90 and 98%, recovery will be slower but usually complete. However, a loss of CMAP of more than 98%, especially later than the third week after onset, carries a worse prognosis. When the paralysis remains clinically complete after the sixth week, improvement in ENOG at successive examinations is a useful predictor of a favorable outcome [27]. Facial palsy may be the presenting sign of Lyme disease, and is its most common neurologic complication in children. Electrodiagnostic studies indicate demyelination in most cases; axonal loss is associated with a worse prognosis. Facial paralysis may occur as a result of temporal bone fractures, penetrating wounds, or iatrogenic injuries. Many cases resolve spontaneously, but surgical exploration is indicated when ENOG shows greater than 98% neural degeneration and no voluntary MUPs are recorded on needle EMG [12].

Acquired Facial Diplegia

The more common causes of bilateral facial weakness in children are idiopathic Bell's palsy, Lyme disease, Guillain-Barré and Miller-Fisher syndromes, multiple idiopathic cranial neuropathy, and brainstem encephalitis. Trauma, tumors of the posterior fossa or meningeal leukemia and neuromuscular disorders such as facioscapulohumeral dystrophy, structural myopathies, and congenital myasthenic syndromes are other possible causes of facial diplegia. [28] Electrodiagnostic studies of the cranial nerves and of the muscles and nerves of the limbs may contribute significantly to the diagnostic evaluation of bilateral facial palsy, by distinguishing neurogenic from myopathic causes, and by differentiating axonal loss from demyelination. Repetitive nerve stimulation facilitates the diagnosis of myasthenia gravis, but in children this technique may present challenges due to movement artifacts. Stimulated single fiber techniques have shown to be very sensitive for detecting abnormalities of neuromuscular transmission [29]. Facial involvement may be the presenting signs of acute polyradiculoneuritis or cranial polyneuritis with sparing of the extremities. Electrodiagnostic studies help to investigate the process, showing prolonged latencies and temporal dispersion of CMAPs and BRs, and EMG signs of denervation of the facial muscles [30]. Patients with Miller-Fisher syndrome may show reduced amplitudes of sensory nerve action potentials (SNAPs) in the extremities and low-amplitude, normal latency facial CMAPs. BRs may be normal or altered, in parallel with the decreased amplitude of the facial CMAPs and denervation of the facial muscles [31, 32].

Neurogenic Dysphagia

An electrodiagnostic protocol including needle EMG of the facial, lingual, and velopharyngeal muscles and EMG during bottle feeding targets the disturbed motor organization, assesses its severity, and shows whether it is isolated or associated with a lesion of the bulbar motor nuclei.

Congenital Neurogenic Dysphagia

EMG highlights multiple cranial neuropathies that can be clinically silent in infants with orofacial dysfunctions [17]. By showing facial, pharyngeal and hypoglossal neuropathies, early orofacial EMG examination contributes to a better understanding of the neurologic origin of congenital facial weakness and dysphagia, and emphasizes the importance of malformation syndromes and neonatal encephalopathies as underlying etiologies (Table 15.7). In patients with Pierre Robin Sequence (PRS), the absence of neurogenic EMG signs in orofacial muscles characterize isolated PRS. At the opposite end of the spectrum, cranial

Table 15.7 Diagnoses of 90 patients with multiple congenital cranial neuropathies

Developmental disorders	*59*
Genetic anomalies	14
Moebius syndrome	8
CHARGE association	7
Other recognizable syndromes	15
Unidentified malformation patterns	15
Encephalopathies	*29*
Preterm (25–34 weeks) with vascular brain injury	7
Localized brainstem ischemia	6
Birth asphyxia at full term	7
Fetal exposure to toxic agents	4
Progressive encephalopathy	5
No apparent underlying disorder	*2*

CHARGE association colobomata, heart disease, atresia of the choanae, retarded growth and development, genital hypoplasia, and ear anomalies or deafness neuropathies were frequently found in patients with associated or syndromic PRS [33]. Moreover, EMG during bottle feeding has contributed to assessing the severity and potential duration of dysphagia [34]. In patients with other facial malformation syndromes showing various anatomic defects, neurogenic EMG signs in orofacial muscles revealed the neurological origin of dysphagia, even in the absence of neurological signs or abnormalities in brain images. Also, neurogenic EMG signs and the severity of oral-pharyngeal incoordination on EMG during bottle feeding correlated with respiratory complications and long-lasting enteral feeding [35].

Newborn infants with congenital bulbar weakness present with facial, lingual, laryngeal, or pharyngeal dysfunction, alone or in combination; all of which have significant developmental and functional consequences. Various etiologies include neuromuscular disorders involving the motor neuron, neuromuscular transmission, or muscle, and cerebral palsies. The evaluation of a child with congenital bulbar weakness requires that major emphasis be placed on an etiological definition and a reliable prognostic assessment because outcomes depend on both the severity of orofacial dysfunction and the nature of the underlying disorder in the peripheral or central nervous system [36]. In a large series of children with congenital bulbar weakness, neurogenic EMG signs were detected in half of the patients. The frequency and duration of respiratory assistance and enteral feeding were not statistically different in patients with or without cranial nerve involvement but BRs abnormalities were significantly associated with high frequencies of respiratory assistance, gastrostomy, and death. Moreover, EMG during bottle feeding identified patients with moderate or severe oropharyngeal incoordination, who showed more need for respiratory assistance, long-lasting enteral feeding, and gastrostomy than patients with normal coordination or mild abnormalities [37]. Thus, orofacial electrodiagnostic studies provide the pediatrician with supplementary information to help anticipate the outcome of bulbar weakness, even in the absence of a clearly defined etiology.

Acquired Bulbar Weakness

Aspiration is most often a complication of a known central nervous system disorder including coma, cerebral lesion, ischemic stroke, acute encephalitis, and degenerative disorders with bulbar or suprabulbar involvement. Aspiration may also complicate peripheral nervous system disorders such as Guillain-Barré syndrome, myasthenia gravis, congenital myopathies, metabolic myopathies, and muscular dystrophies, as well as severe forms of dermatomyositis or polymyositis. The occurrence of a swallowing disorder in these settings suggests a progressive clinical course associated with imminent respiratory failure. Electrodiagnostic studies of the cranial nerves, and also of the upper and lower limbs, contribute to those diagnoses.

Infantile botulism may provoke paralysis of cranial nerves. Motor NCSs reveal markedly reduced CMAP amplitudes. High-frequency repetitive motor nerve stimulation provokes an incremental response. Stimulated single-fiber EMG is another useful way to demonstrate the presynaptic neuromuscular junctional transmission disorder. Needle EMG may show low-amplitude and short-duration spontaneous fibrillation potentials and reduced recruitment pattern with low-amplitude and polyphasic short-duration MUPs. Sensory NCSs are normal.

Swallowing difficulties mark the onset of diphtheric neuropathy. A polyneuropathic feature mimicking GBS may appear during the subsequent weeks.

Isolated temporary pharyngeal paralysis is characterized by acute unilateral velopharyngeal paralysis provoking swallowing difficulty with nasal reflux; needle EMG of the levator veli palatini muscle can detect neurogenic signs [38].

In the same way, neurogenic EMG signs in the soft palate muscle are a means to confirm a velopharyngeal paralysis that may be the presenting sign of an expanding mass in the posterior cranial fossa or a Chiari malformation.

Progressive bulbar paralysis of childhood (Fazio-Londe disease) is a very rare hereditary condition. The EMG findings of reduced interference pattern with enlarged MUPs in bulbar muscles are an important diagnostic sign of the disease.

Salivary stasis and dysphagia associated with trismus and neck stiffness are often the first clinical manifestations of tetanus. Standard motor and sensory NCSs are normal; H waves are easily elicited in distal muscles; F wave amplitudes are high; and EMG may show spontaneous high-frequency discharges.

To conclude, EMG of orofacial muscles and cranial nerves is an important diagnostic tool in congenital facial and bulbar weakness. By contributing to an early diagnosis, this orients the search for associated pathologies. Also, by assessing oral and facial sensorimotor dysfunctions, electrodiagnostic studies help define a therapeutic approach and anticipate outcome.

References

1. Willer JC, Boulu B, Bratzkavski M. Electrophysiologic evidence for crossed oligosynaptic trigemino-facial connections in normal man. J Neurol Neurosurg Psychiatry. 1984;47: 87–90.
2. Eicher SA, Cocker NJ, Alford BR, Igarashi M, Smith RJ. A comparative study of the fallopian canal at the meatal foramen and labyrinthine segment in young children and adults. Arch Otolaryngol Head Neck Surg. 1990;116:1030–5.
3. Raimbault J. Les Conductions Nerveuses Chez L'enfant Normal. Paris: Expansion Scientifique Française; 1988.
4. Esslen E. Electrodiagnosis in facial palsy. In: Miehlke A, editor. Surgery of the Facial Nerve. Philadelphia: WB Saunders; 1973. p. 45–51.
5. Shapiro NL, Cunningham MJ, Parikh SR, Eavey RD, Cheney ML. Congenital unilateral facial paralysis. Pediatrics. 1996;97:261–4.
6. Renault F, Raimbault J. Electromyographie faciale, linguale et pharyngée chez l'enfant: une méthode d'étude des troubles de succion-déglutition et de leur physiopathologie. Neurophysiol Clin. 1992;22:249–60.
7. Kugelberg E. Facial reflexes. Brain. 1952;75:385–96.

8. Vecchierini-Blineau MF, Guiheneuc P. Maturation of the blink reflex in infant. Eur Neurol. 1984;23:449–58.
9. Cruccu G, Deuschl G. The clinical use of brainstem reflexes and hand-muscle reflexes. Clin Neurophysiol. 2000;111:371–87.
10. Therimadasamy A, Wilder-Smith EP, Lim AY, Yap YL, Yeo M, Naidu S, Lee SJ. Supraorbital nerve conduction study in normal subjects. Muscle Nerve. 2012;45:603–4.
11. Cruccu G, Aminoff MJ, Curio G, Guerit JM, Kakigi R, Mauguiere F, Rossini PM, Treede RD, Garcia-Larrea L. Recommendations for the clinical use of somatosensory-evoked potentials. Clin Neurophysiol. 2008;119:1705–19.
12. Renault F, Quijano-Roy S. Congenital and acquired facial palsies. In: Darras BT, Jones HR, Ryan MM, De Vivo DC, editors. Neuromuscular disorders of Infancy, Childhood, and Adolescence. A clinician's approach. Philadelphia: Academic Press/Elsevier; 2014. p. 225–42.
13. Nelson KB, Eng GD. Congenital hypoplasia of the depressor anguli oris muscle: Differentiation from congenital facial palsy. J Pediatr. 1972;81:16–20.
14. Giannotti A, Digilio MC, Marino B, Mingarelli R, Dallapiccola B. Cayler cardiofacial syndrome and del 22q11: Part of the CATCH22 phenotype. Am J Med Genet. 1994;53:303–4.
15. Sammarco J, Ryan RF, Longenecker CG. Anatomy of the facial nerve in fetuses and stillborn infants. J Plast Reconst Surg. 1966;37:556–74.
16. Zentner GE, Layman WS, Martin DM, Scacheri PC. Molecular and phenotypic aspects of CHD7 mutation in CHARGE syndrome. Am J Med Genet. 2010;152A:674–86.
17. Renault F, Flores-Guevara R, Baudon JJ, Vazquez MP. Congenital multiple cranial neuropathies: Relevance of orofacial electromyography in infants. Muscle Nerve. 2015;52:754–8.
18. Cattaneo L, Chierici E, Bianchi B, Sesenna E, Pavesi G. The localization of facial motor impairment in sporadic Möbius syndrome. Neurology. 2006;66:1907–12.
19. Renault F, Sergent B, Charpillet V, Gitiaux C, Vazquez MP. Electromyographic assessment of the temporalis muscle prior to a lengthening myoplasty in patients with Moebius syndrome. Ann Chir Plast Esthet. 2016;62(2):156–62. doi:10.1016/j.anplas.2016.04.007.
20. Vogel M, Velleuer E, Schmidt-Jiménez LF, Mayatepek E, Borkhardt A, Alawi M, Kutsche K, Kortüm F. Homozygous HOXB1 loss-of-function mutation in a large family with hereditary congenital facial paresis. Am J Med Genet A. 2016;170(7):1813–9. doi: 10.1002/ajmg.a.37682.
21. Lehky T, Mills R,Van Ryzin C, Gropman A, Cho H, Jabs EW, Engle E, Toro C, Manoli I. Electrodiagnostic studies in Moebius syndrome and other congenital facial weakness disorders. Muscle Nerve. 2016;54:554.
22. Renault F, Fedida A. Les signes électromyographiques précoces de la dystrophie myotonique congénitale. Neurophysiol Clin. 1991;21:201–11.
23. Quijano-Roy S, Renault F, Guicheney P, Estournet B, Romero N, Fardeau M. EMG and nerve conduction studies in children with congenital muscular dystrophy. Muscle Nerve. 2004;29:292–9.
24. Pitt MC, Jabre JF. Determining jitter values in the very young by use of the e-norms methodology. Muscle Nerve. 2017;55(1):51–4. doi:10.1002/mus.25191.
25. Katusic SK, Beard CM, Wiederholt WC, Bergstralh EJ, Kurland LT. Incidence, clinical features, and prognosis in Bell's palsy, Rochester, Minnesota, 1968–1982. Ann Neurol. 1986;20:622–7.
26. Aminoff MJ. Facial neuropathies. In: Aminoff MJ, editor. Electromyography in clinical practice: clinical and electrodiagnostic aspects of neuromuscular disease. New York: Churchill Livingstone; 1998. p. 513–23.
27. Eavey RD, Herrmann BS, Joseph JM, Thornton AR. Clinical experience with electroneuronography in the pediatric patients. Arch Otolaryngol Head Neck Surg. 1989;115:600–7.
28. Keane JR. Bilateral seventh nerve palsy: Analysis of 43 cases and review of the literature. Neurology. 1994;44:1198–202.
29. Tidswell T, Pitt MC. A new analytical method to diagnose congenital myasthenia with stimulated single-fiber electromyography. Muscle Nerve. 2007;35:107–10.

30. Najim Al-Din AS, Anderson M, Eeg-Olofsson O. Neuro-ophthalmic manifestations of the syndrome of ophthalmoplegia, ataxia and areflexia. Observations on 20 patients. Acta Neurol Scand. 1994;89:87–94.
31. Sauron B, Bouche P, Cathala HP, Chain F, Castaigne P. Miller-Fisher syndrome: clinical and electrophysiological evidence of peripheral origin in 10 cases. Neurology. 1984;34:953–6.
32. Fross RD, Daube JR. Neuropathy in the Miller-Fisher syndrome: clinical and neurophysiological findings. Neurology. 1987;37:1493–8.
33. Renault F, Baudon JJ, Galliani E, Flores-Guevara R, Marlin S, Garabedian EN, Vazquez MP. Facial, lingual, and pharyngeal electromyography in infants with Pierre Robin sequence. Muscle Nerve. 2011;43:866–71.
34. Baudon JJ, Renault F, Goutet JM, Flores-Guevara R, Soupre V, Gold F, Vazquez MP. Motor dysfunction of the upper digestive tract in Pierre Robin sequence as assessed by sucking-swallowing electromyography and esophageal manometry. J Pediatr. 2002;140:719–23.
35. Baudon JJ, Renault F, Goutet JM, Biran-Mucignat V, Morgant G, Garabedian EN, Vazquez MP. Assessment of dysphagia in infants with facial malformations. Eur J Pediatr. 2009;168:187–93.
36. Roig-Quilis M. Oromotor dysfunction in neuromuscular disorders: evaluation and treatment. In: Darras BT, Jones HR, Ryan MM, De Vivo DC, editors. Neuromuscular disorders of infancy, childhood, and adolescence. A clinician's approach. 2nd ed. Amsterdam: Elsevier; 2015. p. 958–75.
37. Baudon JJ, Renault F, Flores-Guevara R, Vazquez MP. Outcomes of neonatal bulbar weakness. Pediatrics. 2016;137(1) doi:10.1542/peds.2015-3004.
38. Roberton DM, Mellor DH. Asymmetrical palatal paresis in childhood: A transient cranial mononeuropathy? Dev Med Child Neurol. 1982;24:842–9.

Chapter 16
Motor Neuron Disease

Bhaskar Roy and Basil T. Darras

Introduction

Spinal muscular atrophies (SMAs) are a group of genetic disorders characterized by progressive muscle weakness and atrophy associated with degeneration of spinal and, in the most severely affected patients, lower bulbar motor neurons. Classic proximal SMA is the most common form of SMA and the leading genetic cause of infant mortality [1, 2]. The incidence of SMA has been estimated to be about 1 per 10,000 live births [3, 4]. Reports from Werdnig of the University of Graz, Austria, and Johann Hoffmann of Heidelberg, Germany, provided the first complete description of the neuromuscular phenotype of the disease and the associated loss of anterior horn cells in the spinal cord, hence the older and now less commonly used eponym, Werdnig-Hoffman disease [5, 6]. Since then, a range of phenotypic variability has been described in autosomal recessive proximal SMA or 5qSMA and also in non-5q SMAs, a heterogeneous group of motor neuron diseases with various genetic mutations and clinical phenotypes [2, 7].

5q Proximal SMA

Classic SMA or 5q SMA results from homozygous deletions or other mutations involving the "survival (of) motor neuron 1" *(SMN1)* gene. Patients with 5q proximal SMA harbor homozygous deletions or mutations involving exon seven of

B. Roy, M.B.B.S., M.M.S.T.
Beth Israel Deaconess Medical Center, Harvard Medical School, Boston, MA, USA

B.T. Darras, M.D. (✉)
Division of Clinical Neurology, Neuromuscular Center, Boston Children's Hospital, Harvard Medical School, Boston, MA, USA
e-mail: Basil.Darras@childrens.harvard.edu

© Springer International Publishing AG 2017

H.J. McMillan, P.B. Kang (eds.), *Pediatric Electromyography*,
DOI 10.1007/978-3-319-61361-1_16

SMN1, but maintain at least one copy of the paralogous gene *SMN2*, which helps compensate for *SMN1* deficiency. The range of phenotypic severity of SMA, based on "maximal functional status achieved," can be divided into four broad clinical subtypes. They represent a continuum extending from the very severe, with onset *in utero,* to the very mild, with onset during adulthood. A spectrum of severity is found within each of these subtypes (Table 16.1) [7, 8]. Broadly, Type I patients are "non-sitters," Type II patients are "sitters," Type III patients are "walkers," and Type IV are adult-onset with mild symptoms [9, 10].

Type I SMA

SMA type I (previously known as Werdnig-Hoffmann disease) has been further subdivided into three groups: type IA (or Type 0 in certain reports[11]) with onset *in utero* and presentation at birth, type IB with onset of symptoms between birth and 3 months of age, and type IC with onset between 3 and 6 months of age. Infants with SMA type I have progressive proximal weakness that affects the legs more than the arms. They have poor head control with hypotonia, leading to a severe head lag, frog-leg posture when supine, slip through on vertical suspension, and draping on ventral suspension, along with areflexia. They are never able to sit independently and are thus also known as "non-sitters" (Table 16.1). Intercostal muscle weakness with relative sparing of the diaphragm produces a bell-shaped chest and a paradoxical pattern of abdominal breathing. They exhibit tongue fasciculations and eventually develop dysphagia, risk of aspiration, and failure to thrive. Other cranial nerves are not as affected, although facial weakness does occur at later stages of the disease. Cognition is usually normal [1, 12, 13].

Type II SMA

Patients with type II SMA, also known as intermediate SMA or Dubowitz disease, are able to sit unsupported at some point and are thus also known as sitters, but they are never able to walk independently (Table 16.1). The onset of symptoms is typically between 6 and 18 months of age. They have progressive proximal weakness affecting legs more than arms, along with hypotonia and areflexia. They also develop progressive scoliosis, which in combination with intercostal muscle weakness results in significant restrictive lung disease as they grow older. They develop joint contractures and can have ankylosis of the mandible [13–15]. Cognition is normal and verbal intelligence may be above average [16]. Patients may live into the third decade, but life expectancy is shortened due to the risk of respiratory compromise [2, 14].

Table 16.1 Clinical and EMG features in classic spinal muscular atrophies (SMAs)

SMA Type (incidence as % of total SMA)	Age at onset	Life span	Highest motor milestone achieved	Other features	EMG findings
Type I (60%): Type IA	Prenatal	<6 months	Mostly unable to achieve motor milestones	• Severe weak-ness at birth • Profound hypotonia • Facial diplegia • Areflexia • Early respiratory failure • Joint contractures	• SNAPs and CMAPs can be normal in the early stage • CMAPs usually lowest among all SMAs but SNAPs are normal • Fibrillation potentials and PSWs are common • Fasciculation potentials are rare • Long duration and large amplitude motor unit potentials can be present but not frequently • Spontaneous motor unit firing is common
Type IB, Type IC	Type IB (0–3 months) Type IC (3–6 months)	<2 years without respiratory support	Never sits unsupported	• Weakness • "Frog leg" posture, hypotonia • Tongue fasciculations • Hyporeflexia, areflexia • Suck and swallow difficulties • Respiratory failure	
Type II (27%)	6–18 months	>2 years ~70% alive at 25 years of age	Sits independently but never walks	• Proximal weakness, hypotonia • Postural hand tremor • Hyporeflexia • Average or above average intellectual skills by adolescence • Scoliosis	• CMAPs are lower than in Type III • Spontaneous motor unit firings can be seen in younger patients • Fibrillation potentials are frequent
Type III (12%)	>18 months Type IIIA (prior to 3 years) Type IIIB (after 3 years)	Almost normal	Walks independently	• May have hand tremor • Resembles muscular dystrophy	• CMAPs are of higher amplitude, especially in ambulatory patients • Duration and amplitudes of motor unit potentials are highest • Smaller and poly-phasic, myopathic looking units can be seen • Fibrillation, fasciculations and complex repetitive discharges can be seen
Type IV (1%)	>21 years	Normal	Normal	• Minimal weakness	

Type III SMA

In 1956, Kugelberg and Welander described a much milder form of SMA characterized by prolonged ambulation [17]. Patients with type III SMA, also known as Kugelberg-Welander disease, are able to walk independently at some point and are thus also referred to as "walkers". The onset of symptoms usually occurs after the age of 18 months. This subset has further been subdivided into type IIIA (onset between 18 months and 3 years) and type IIIB (onset after 3 years). Type III patients have progressive proximal weakness affecting legs more than arms and may ultimately need to use a wheelchair, especially the IIIA group, but they generally develop minor or no respiratory muscle weakness or scoliosis. Loss of ambulation increases the risk of these complications. Type III patients may have tremor or polyminimyoclonus of the hands, which can also be seen in type II or even type I patients [14, 18]. Sometimes, the calves of type III patients can be prominent, and hence type III SMA can be confused with Becker muscular dystrophy. Creatine kinase levels are often elevated, usually no more than fivefold, and may lead to an erroneous evaluation for myopathy. Life expectancy is not significantly different compared to the normal population (Table 16.1) [2, 14, 19].

Type IV SMA

A milder, adult-onset SMA, or type IV SMA, has also been described, with onset of symptoms after age 21 years and essentially normal life span [10].

Electrodiagnostic Testing in SMA

Prior to the identification of the genetic loci for SMA, electrodiagnostic studies were the primary diagnostic tools for suspected cases. Genetic testing has largely supplanted EMG for the diagnosis of SMA. However, there are circumstances in which EMG still plays an important role in the diagnostic evaluation. Genetic testing, even when expedited, often takes several days to return results, whereas EMG is often available the same day, with results reportable immediately. For example, an undiagnosed child who is acutely ill in a critical care setting may benefit from EMG testing. EMG can also help point to the correct diagnosis when there are atypical presentations, especially in some cases of SMA type III [20], and when patients have non-5q related SMAs [1, 21].

Motor nerve conduction studies can be completely normal in the early stages of SMA [21, 22]. With the progression of the disease, nerve conduction studies typically show features of chronic motor axonal loss, specifically reduction of compound muscle action potential (CMAP) amplitudes [23, 24]. Conduction velocities are generally preserved, but mild slowing of conduction velocities secondary to loss of faster conducting fibers can be seen. Distal motor latencies and F wave latencies may similarly be slightly prolonged. Sensory nerve action potentials (SNAPs) are usually preserved throughout the course of disease, even in infants with SMA type I [25, 26].

CMAP amplitudes have been shown to correlate with clinical severity, age, functional status and progression of disease. CMAP amplitudes are most often reduced in SMA type I. Accordingly, SMA type II subjects have lower CMAP amplitudes compared to SMA type III and non-ambulatory SMA type III patients usually have lower CMAP amplitudes than ambulatory type III patients [23, 24]. In some reports, CMAP amplitudes have been shown to decline over time, specifically in SMA type II. Initial CMAP amplitude has been suggested to predict functional outcome [23].

Although SMA is primarily a pure motor neuron disorder with preserved SNAPs, sensorimotor involvement has been described in a few cases [26, 27]. In a small number of infants with SMA type I, sensory action potentials can be reduced, preferentially in the sural nerve, secondary to loss of sensory fibers and ganglion cells [22, 27, 28]. Most of the reported cases of sensory involvement in SMAs involve axonal neuropathy, though occasionally demyelinating neuropathy or mixed axonal and demyelinating features can be seen [26, 29, 30].

Motor unit number estimation (MUNE), an electrophysiologic method to estimate the number of lower motor neurons innervating a specific muscle, has shown motor unit loss in SMA patients [31–33]. The number of functional motor units in some patients progressively decreases, though occasionally an increment in the number of motor units has been noted, suggesting a degree of spontaneous recovery [23, 24, 34]. Please refer to Chap. 12 for a more detailed discussion of MUNE.

In addition, repetitive stimulation studies may show a decremental response with correction after post exercise testing [35]. Decremental responses have also been reported in patients with SMA types II and III at 2–3 Hz repetitive stimulation without facilitation at higher frequency stimulation [35, 36]. Similarly, single fiber EMG may show increased jitter and blocking [37]. It is still uncertain whether these changes are related to a defect in neuromuscular transmission or to a secondary effect of chronic denervation and re-innervation. Typically, these features are uncommon in other motor neuron diseases with more rapid denervation and reinnervation, such as amyotrophic lateral sclerosis [1].

Needle EMG in SMA shows motor neuron or motor axon loss in the form of active denervation and chronic reinnervation. Based on the severity and stage of the disease, as well as the rapidity of disease progression, the proportions and patterns of denervation and reinnervation vary, and different electrophysiological patterns can be seen [38, 39].

In infants with SMA type I, needle EMG shows active denervation in the form of fibrillation potentials and positive sharp waves (PSWs), and residual voluntary motor units are mostly of normal size. Collateral reinnervation is usually absent. In these patients, detection of higher amplitude and normal duration MUAPs does not necessarily indicate collateral sprouting. Several factors may result in such high amplitude, normal duration MUAPs; these factors include loss of smaller motor units, muscle fiber hypertrophy, and other anatomical changes such as contraction of motor unit cross-sectional territory with atrophy of intercalated fibers bringing additional motor units closer to the EMG electrode [15, 21, 38, 39].

Collateral sprouting from the adjacent nerve fibers of healthy neurons is the main reinnervation process that leads to type grouping in cases of partial denervation and reinnervation. At the stage of chronic denervation and successful collateral reinnervation, such as in older infants and children with milder forms of SMA, fibrillation potentials and PSWs, which are usually few, may even disappear. MUAPs are reduced in number and are of giant size [15, 21, 39]. In advanced cases with end-stage individual muscles, MUAPs can be of reduced amplitude and duration, lose their clear neurogenic features, and mimic myopathic units [40].

An unusual form of spontaneous motor unit firing (MUF) at 5–15 Hz has been reported. These continuous potentials can be distinguished from fasciculation potentials by their regular pattern of firing, persistence for long periods and occurrence during sleep. The source of these potentials has not been defined. They are more frequent in SMA type I and in younger type II patients [38, 39]. Fasciculation potentials are absent in most cases of SMA, particularly in type I, but can be seen rarely in later stages of the disease in proximal muscles, particularly the quadriceps [39].

Accurate assessment of EMG features can be difficult in children. They may not be able to cooperate fully, and hence the assessment of number, size, and firing rates can be limited. Secondary to slow progression of SMA, occasionally reinnervation can be complete, features of fibrillation and PSWs can be absent, and abnormalities can be found only in the MUAPs with reduced number, higher amplitude, longer duration and polyphasia. Occasionally, satellite potentials can also be seen. Moreover, in milder SMA, such as SMA type III, MUAPs can appear myopathic with low amplitude and many high frequency components [40]. Some forms of SMAs are focal, and EMG of some muscles is normal [21]. In light of the variability of diagnostic findings, several muscles should be tested in multiple extremities (including genioglossus), if tolerated by the child, to maximize the accuracy of the study.

It is noteworthy that in the early stages of SMA, even in the presence of early weakness, EMG may sometimes be normal. The typical electrophysiologic features of SMA in those cases will emerge later [21]. Therefore, a normal EMG study does not entirely rule out the possibility of SMA, depending upon the circumstances including the extent of needle examination. The degree of electrophysiological abnormality may also not accurately reflect the clinical status. Thus, electrophysiological features should be interpreted carefully. Occasionally, electrophysiologic findings in a patient with SMA can mimic those found in other neuromuscular diseases, such as critical illness neuropathy or Guillain-Barré syndrome [29, 30]. Thus it is important to correlate EMG findings with the clinical context.

Other "Spinal Muscular Atrophies"

Non-5q Spinal Muscular Atrophies

Non-5q SMAs are genetically heterogeneous, clinically diverse and rare compared to 5q SMA [41]. Phenotypic classification may be based on distribution of weakness (distal, proximal or bulbar) and mode of inheritance (Table 16.2) [42, 43]. This classification system, however, does not include all non-5q motor axonopathies or neuronopathies, excludes SMA plus syndromes, and in particular excludes conditions with uncertain nosology or those with no gene/locus information [41].

Table 16.2 Clinical features and EMG findings in major non-5q spinal muscular atrophies (SMA)

Gene/locus	Disease/phenotype, selected distinguishing features	EMG findings
Distal spinal muscular atrophy/distal hereditary motor neuropathy or neuronopathy (DSMA/distal HMN)		
Autosomal recessive		
IGHMBP2	**SMA with respiratory distress (SMARD) or diaphragmatic SMA** • Low birth weight, typically presents within 3–6 months of life with diaphragmatic paralysis • Hypotonia, distal > proximal weakness, sensory and autonomic involvement • Ventilator dependence	• Marked reduction or complete absence of CMAPs (prominent in lower extremities) • Similar but milder findings in sensory studies • Initially EMG shows denervation in distal muscles, later diffuse changes
PLEKHG5	**Lower motor neuron syndrome with childhood onset** • Early involvement of foot and hand muscles. • Rapid progression and early loss of ambulation • Cranial nerves are spared	• SNAPs are present but can be of reduced amplitude, motor and sensory conduction velocity can be mildly slow • EMG shows denervation changes
Autosomal dominant		
GARS	**Distal SMA with upper-limb predominance, Type VA Charcot-Marie-Tooth disease 2D** • Predominant upper-limb weakness • Selective atrophy of the thenar and FDI muscles • Peroneal atrophy and weakness • Reduced vibration senses in CMT 2D	• Absent or markedly reduced CMAPs from APB • Preserved CMAPs from ADM • CMAP amplitudes from peroneal < 2 mV • SNAP amplitudes and conduction velocities are usually normal except sural can be affected • Large MUAPs, reduced recruitment in thenar muscles

(continued)

Table 16.2 (continued)

Gene/locus	Disease/phenotype, selected distinguishing features	EMG findings
BSCL2	**Distal SMA with upper-limb predominance, Type VB** **Silver syndrome/SPG17** • Hand muscle weakness and wasting • Stiffness in lower limbs and foot deformities • Gait abnormalities but ambulation usually maintained	• Reduced CMAPs with occasional chrono-dispersion, partial conduction block and slowing of conduction velocity • Ulnar is less affected • Chronic denervation with large MUAPs • Usually no spontaneous activities
Proximal spinal muscular atrophy (+/- distal involvement) ***Autosomal dominant***		
TRPV4	**Congenital Distal SMA** with arthrogryposis, contractures, asymmetric atrophy and non-progressive weakness with lower limb predominance **Scapuloperoneal SMA** with scapular winging, laryngeal distribution of weakness, distal muscle wasting and absent reflexes **Charcot-Marie-Tooth, Type 2C** with vocal cord and phrenic nerve paralysis	• Normal conduction velocities • Reduced CMAPs • Polyphasic or giant MUAPs • Predominantly motor axonal neuropathy
DYNC1H1, BICD2	**SMA with lower extremity predominance (SMA-LED)** • Abnormal cortical development and epilepsy is common in DYNC1H1 mutation. • Wasting and contracture is common in BICD2, especially around ankle	• NCS can be normal • Mild reduction of CMAPs (especially in common peroneal in BICD 2 mutation) • Chronic denervation in both proximal and distal leg muscles (quadriceps are most affected in DYNC1H1 mutation)
Other non-5q spinal and bulbar muscular atrophies, SMA plus types ***Autosomal recessive***		
RFT2 (C20ORF54)	**Brown-Vialetto-van Laere syndrome** **Fazio-Londe disease, bulbar palsy** • Primarily involves lower cranial nerves • Present with ponto-bulbar palsy • Sensorineural deafness in BVVLS • Respiratory failure	• can be normal initially • repeat testing can suggest MND
EXOCS3 (30–40%), *VRK 1, TSEN54, RARS2*	**Pontocerebellar hypoplasia with SMA,** **PHC1** • Progressive microcephaly combined with brainstem and cerebellar hemispheres atrophy • Relative sparing of the cerebellar vermis. • Severe cognitive and motor limitations, seizures. • Anterior horn cell degeneration	• Neurogenic EMG • In most of the patients no neuropathy • In some EXOSC3 negative patients marked reduction or loss of SNAPs and CMAPs with marked slowing of conduction velocity

Table 16.2 (continued)

Gene/locus	Disease/phenotype, selected distinguishing features	EMG findings
GLE1	Lethal arthrogryposis with anterior horn cell disease or lethal congenital contracture syndrome	
X-linked recessive		
Androgen receptor	**Bulbar SMA, Kennedy disease** • Atrophy and weakness of the facial, bulbar and proximal muscles • Bulbar symptoms • Fasciculation • Mild to severe hyper-CK-emia • Gynecomastia • Testicular atrophy and reduced fertility • Weakness often starts in the lower extremities	• CMAPs and SNAPs are usually reduced with milder involvement of conduction velocities. • In CAG repeat (≥47), CMAPs reduced • In CAG repeat (≤ 47), SNAPs reduced • EMG shows chronic denervation and reinnervation with abnormal spontaneous activities
UBA1	**Infantile SMA with arthrogryposis** • White matter abnormalities on MRI • Prominent motor and sensory involvement • Cerebellar involvement	• SNAPs and CMAPs can be absent • EMG shows reinnervation or denervation

Distal SMAs (DSMA)

Distal SMAs present with predominantly distal weakness. They exhibit significant phenotypic overlap with distal hereditary motor neuropathies or neuronopathies (dHMN).

Spinal muscular atrophy with respiratory distress type 1 (SMARD1) is caused by mutations in the gene *IGHMBP2*, which encodes the immunoglobulin μ-binding protein. Most patients with SMARD1 have low birth weight and present within the first 3 to 6 months of life with diaphragmatic paralysis, hypotonia, distal more than proximal weakness, and sensory and autonomic involvement, followed by ventilator dependency [44, 45]. Life expectancy is usually limited primarily due to the severe respiratory weakness [45]. Respiratory failure between 6 weeks and 6 months combined with the presence of diaphragmatic eventration or preterm birth is a good predictor of the presence of *IGHMBP2* mutations [44]. Patients with SMARD1 usually have normal serum CK levels and no primary cardiomyopathy, but severe autonomic dysfunction can lead to secondary cardiovascular collapse [45, 46]. In a series of 141 patients with respiratory distress and diaphragmatic and intercostal weakness, three distinct phenotypes were noted: (1) SMARD-congenital: arthrogryposis multiplex congenita with associated respiratory failure at birth, (2) SMARD1-like: respiratory distress with onset between 6 weeks to 6 months along with hip flexion weakness with minimal or no movements of the distal muscle groups, and (3) SMARD-late: respiratory distress after age 6 months without multiple congenital contractures; however, the phenotype can be more variable [44, 47].

EMG in SMARD1 shows marked reduction of or complete absence of CMAPs and markedly slow conduction velocities, more predominantly in the lower extremities. Similar but milder findings may be seen in sensory studies [48, 49]. Needle EMG initially shows a denervation pattern only in distal muscles, but diffuse changes can be seen later. EMG of the diaphragm, if performed, may show denervation changes [45, 48, 49].

HMN5A and Charcot-Marie-Tooth type 2D (CMT2D) are allelic conditions caused by mutations in *GARS* [50, 51]. The clinical distinction between HMN5A and CMT2D is usually based on whether sensory abnormalities are present [50]. Patients with *GARS* mutations usually present in their twenties with predominantly upper-limb weakness, most notably including selective atrophy of the thenar eminence and first dorsal interosseous (FDI) muscles. The hypothenar eminence is usually spared until later in the course of the disease. Peroneal weakness and atrophy and reduced vibration sensation are usually present in all patients with CMT2D and about half of the patients with HMN5A [52]. EMG shows a motor axonopathy with typical features of absent or markedly reduced CMAPs recording abductor pollicis brevis (APB) and preserved CMAPs recording abductor digiti minimi (ADM). CMAP amplitudes from peroneal muscles are typically below 2 mV and below 1 mV when leg atrophy is clinically evident. SNAP amplitudes and conduction velocities are usually normal, although sural SNAP amplitude can be reduced. Even in presymptomatic mutation-carrying individuals, large long-duration motor unit potentials with reduced recruitment pattern can be seen in the thenar muscles. Similarly, chronic partial denervation can be seen in the ADM and extensor muscles of the legs even in the absence of apparent muscle atrophy [50, 51].

Mutations in *BSCL2* gene result in allelic phenotypes including spastic paraplegia with amyotrophy of hands and feet (Silver syndrome/SPG17), congenital generalized lipodystrophy, type 2, distal SMA with early hand involvement (dHMNV), and dHMN beginning in the legs (dHMNII) [53, 54]. Phenotypes can be variable, but common features include hand muscle weakness and wasting, gait abnormalities, stiffness in the lower limbs, and foot deformities. Ambulation is usually preserved [53]. EMG shows reduced CMAPs, predominantly in the lower extremities, with occasional temporal dispersion and partial conduction block, and slowing of conduction velocity in the demyelinating range, suggesting that demyelination compounds a presentation that is otherwise predominantly axonal. In the upper extremities, median nerve CMAPs and conduction velocities are typically more affected than the ulnar nerve. EMG shows chronic denervation with large motor unit potentials with or without polyphasia, and without any abnormal spontaneous activity [53].

Non-5q SMAs with Proximal or Diffuse Weakness

SMA with lower extremity predominance (SMA-LED) is caused by dominant mutations in the dynein gene (*DYNC1H1*) encoding a microtubule motor protein in the dynein-dynactin complex and mutations in *BICD2*, which encodes a dynein adaptor protein. Features of SMA-LED with *DYNC1H1* mutations include congenital or very early onset, severe weakness in the proximal legs, specifically quadriceps, and a static or minimally progressive course [43, 55]. In *BICD2* mutations, onset may be in utero, at birth, or in early childhood. The typical presentation consists of delayed motor milestones, along with predominantly lower limb non-length-dependent weakness, with a variable amount of wasting and contractures. Contractures are most commonly found in the ankle. Of note, arthrogryposis or contractures are uncommon in *DYNC1H1*mutations. In some patients, scapular winging is present. A subset of patients can have upper motor neuron signs, but all patients usually have stable or only slowly progressive lower motor neuron disease, and most remain ambulatory throughout their lives [56]. In contrast to *DYNC1H1* mutations, abnormal cortical development and epilepsy are not typical features of *BICD2* mutations [56, 57].

Nerve conduction studies in DYNC1H1-associated SMA-LED may be normal. In older patients, mild CMAP amplitude reductions in the lower extremities may occur. EMG usually shows chronic denervation in both proximal and distal leg muscles [43]. Similar findings may be seen in BICD2-associated SMA-LED. CMAP amplitudes are occasionally reduced, especially in the common peroneal nerve. Nerve conduction velocities and SNAPs are usually normal or borderline reduced. Needle examination shows chronic denervation and large motor units with or without polyphasia [56].

TRPV4-related disorders are another example of diverse phenotypes: (1) congenital distal SMA with arthrogryposis and asymmetric atrophy and weakness, in the lower extremities, (2) scapuloperoneal SMA with scapular winging, laryngeal distribution of weakness, distal muscle wasting and weakness with absent deep tendon reflexes, and (3) CMT2C associated with vocal cord and phrenic nerve paralysis. EMG usually shows normal conduction velocities with reduced CMAP amplitudes and some polyphasic or giant motor units with evidence of a predominantly motor axonal neuropathy [58–62].

Bulbar SMA

Brown-Vialetto-van Laere syndrome (BVVLS) and Fazio-Londe disease are clinically overlapping motor neuron diseases involving primarily lower cranial nerves; they present with ponto-bulbar palsy, sensorineural deafness in BVVLS, and respiratory failure. BVVLS and Fazio-Londe disease have been linked to mutations in the *RFT2* (C200RF54) gene with defective riboflavin transport; riboflavin supplementation has been reported to be helpful in some cases [63, 64]. Early in the course, electrophysiological testing may be normal, but repeat examinations at later time points may detect motor neuron disease with greater sensitivity [64–66].

Pontocerebellar hypoplasias (PCH) are rare inherited progressive neurodegenerative disorders with prenatal onset. To date, 7 PCH clinical syndromes have been described (PCH1-7) [67]. All subtypes feature progressive microcephaly combined with atrophy/hypoplasia of brainstem and cerebellar hemispheres with relative sparing of the cerebellar vermis. Patients have severe cognitive and motor limitations, along with seizures; the cerebrum is variably affected. When PCH is combined with anterior horn cell degeneration, the designation PCH1 is applied. PCH1 has been linked to mutations in the *EXOCS3* gene in about 30–40% of patients and rarely has been associated with *VRK1*, *TSEN54* and *RARS2* mutations. EMG typically shows neurogenic changes. In *EXOSC3* positive patients, neuropathy is usually not seen. In PCH1 with no mutation in known genes, marked amplitude reduction or loss of SNAPs and CMAPs can occasionally be seen with marked slowing of conduction velocity [68, 69].

Other non-5q spinal and bulbar SMAs include Kennedy's disease or X-linked spinal and bulbar muscular atrophy (SBMA/SMAX1), related to an expansion of a CAG trinucleotide repeat in the androgen receptor gene [70]. SBMA presents between 15 and 60 years with atrophy and weakness of the facial, bulbar and proximal muscles. It is associated with bulbar symptoms, fasciculations, mild to severe elevations in serum creatine kinase (CK) levels, gynecomastia, testicular atrophy, and reduced fertility [70, 71].Weakness often starts in the lower extremities. It is usually asymmetric and the dominant side can be affected in about 70% of cases [72, 73]. CMAPs and SNAPs usually have reduced amplitudes, with mild slowing of conduction velocities. In patients with longer CAG repeats (≥47), CMAP amplitudes tend to be reduced, while in patients with a shorter CAG repeats (≤47), SNAP amplitudes are reduced. Needle EMG shows active denervation and chronic reinnervation, enlarged or even giant motor unit action potentials with or without polyphasia, satellite potentials, and reduced recruitment patterns at maximal contraction [71, 73, 74]. Needle EMG may be abnormal even in clinically unaffected muscles [75]. Motor unit numbers, measured by MUNE, may be reduced [73].

Infantile SMA with arthrogryposis with or without bone fractures, dysmorphic features, myopathic facies, hypotonia, areflexia, and digital contractures may represent a lethal X-linked form of SMA (SMAX2) and may be confused with SMA type IA. Mutations in the *UBA1* gene have been detected in this group of patients [76]. A patient with *UBA1* mutation-positive SMAX2 has been reported to be accompanied by white matter and cerebellar abnormalities on brain MRI, prominent motor and sensory system involvement, and widespread inflammatory changes on muscle biopsy. SNAPs and CMAPs may be absent; needle EMG usually shows active denervation and/or chronic reinnervation [77].

Juvenile Amyotrophic Lateral Sclerosis (ALS)

Juvenile ALS is defined as any progressive motor neuron disease affecting both upper and lower motor neurons with onset at age or below 25 years (Table 16.3). Most of the juvenile ALS types are rare autosomal recessive, slowly progressive, non-fatal disorders which may affect non-motor systems as well [78]. ALS2 is a rare, autosomal recessive form of juvenile-onset ALS with mutations in the *ALS2* gene encoding alsin. It is a predominantly upper motor neuron (UMN) syndrome, with slowly progressive spasticity beginning in the lower limbs, and gradual extension upwards to involve the upper limbs and bulbar muscles [79]. ALS4, caused by mutations in the *SETX* gene, is a non-fatal, autosomal dominant, juvenile-onset dHMN with limb weakness, muscle wasting, pyramidal tract signs including brisk reflexes and extensor plantar responses. Bulbar and respiratory muscles are usually preserved [80, 81]. ALS5, linked to chromosome 15q15.1-21.1, was originally described in several kindreds from Tunisia and Germany. Patients present with progressive gait disturbance, mixed UMN and LMN features, and dysarthria (beginning after 3–4 years); survival is generally 10–25 years from symptom onset [78, 82, 83]. ALS6, associated with *FUS* (fused in sarcoma) gene mutations, can present with an aggressive rapid onset form of juvenile ALS [84–86]. A slowly progressive variant of juvenile ALS is associated with predominantly upper motor neuron involvement and *Sig-1R* (sigma-1 intracellular receptor) mutations [87, 88]. A form of juvenile ALS with amyotrophy of limb and bulbar muscles and UMN signs has been reported in a family from Utah with linkage to 6p25 and 21q22 loci [89].

Electrodiagnostic findings in juvenile ALS are similar to adult onset ALS. Reduced CMAPs, normal SNAPs, normal conduction velocities along with signs of an active muscle denervation-reinnervation process are usually seen [78, 82–86]. In ALS4 a graded pattern of distal muscle involvement with chronic partial denervation-reinnervation has been reported; reduced CMAPs and SNAPs were reported in the family with juvenile ALS from Utah [80, 81, 89].

Juvenile Muscular Atrophy of Distal Upper Extremity (Hirayama Disease)

Juvenile muscular atrophy of distal upper extremities (JMADUE), also known as Hirayama disease, was first described in Japan in 1959. It is a clinically distinct anterior horn cell disorder confined to the cervical cord (Table 16.3) [90]. The clinical requirements for the diagnosis of Hirayama disease include: (1) gradual onset of predominantly distal weakness and atrophy of the forearm and hand muscles, (2) onset of symptoms between 10 years to the early 20s, (3) typically unilateral or unilaterally dominant signs and symptoms, (4) gradual progression for the first several years followed by stabilization, (5) lack of any significant sensory changes, abnormal muscle stretch reflexes, or Babinski signs, (6) lack of symptoms in the lower extremities, and (7) exclusion of other disorders including spinal cord tumors, juvenile ALS, syringomyelia, multifocal motor neuropathy, and poliomyelitis [91, 92]. There is an overwhelming male predominance (17:1). The intrinsic hand muscles (interossei, thenar and hypothenar muscle groups) as well as the ulnar side of the forearm are predominantly involved. Brachioradialis and biceps brachii muscles are typically spared, leading to the characteristic appearance of "oblique amyotrophy." Rarely (in 15% of cases), slight triceps brachii atrophy may be seen [92]. This condition is predominantly unilateral in approximately 70% of cases, with the remainder displaying bilateral upper extremity involvement. Reflexes are usually preserved, with occasional hyperactive muscle reflexes in the lower extremities.

Table 16.3 Clinical features and EMG findings in Juvenile amyotrophic lateral sclerosis, hirayama and acute flaccid myelitis

Etiology	Disease/phenotype, selected distinguishing features	EMG findings
Juvenile amyotrophic lateral sclerosis		
AR: *ALS2* *SPG11* *Sig-1R* AD: *SETX* *FUS*	• ALS2: UMN syndrome with slowly progressive spasticity beginning in the lower limbs • ALS5: progressive gait disturbance, mixed UMN and LMN features, and dysarthria • Sig-1R associated with slowly progressive prominent UMN involvement • ALS4: limb weakness, muscle wasting, brisk reflexes and extensor plantar responses • FUS: aggressive rapid onset	• Similar to adult onset ALS. • Reduced CMAPS, normal SNAPs, normal conduction velocity. • Active muscle denervation-innervation process is usually seen. • In ALS4 a graded pattern of distal muscle involvement.
Juvenile muscular atrophy of distal upper extremity (Hirayama disease)		
Probable pathogenic mechanism: Flexion myelopathy arising from contact pressure and axial tension during neck flexion	• Gradual onset of predominantly distal weakness and atrophy of the forearm (usually ulnar side) and hand muscles (interossei, thenar and hypothenar muscle groups). • Onset of symptoms between 10-early 20s • Unilaterally dominant signs and symptoms • Gradual progression followed by stabilization • Lack of any significant sensory changes, abnormal muscle stretch reflexes, or Babinski signs • Lack of symptoms in the lower extremities	• Low amplitude CMAPs of the median and ulnar nerves • SNAPs are usually preserved • Ulnar CMAPs more affected than the median nerve • EMG shows fibrillation potentials, PSWs and signs of reinnervation in the distribution of C7-T1 myotomes • Chronic denervation changes most frequently found in the FDI and FCU muscles
Acute Flaccid Myelitis (AFM)		
Polio West nile Entero D68, Entero 71 Echovirus Coxsackievirus Japanese encephalitis	• Usually a prodromal febrile illness • Develops abruptly and progresses rapidly • Uniformly flaccid weakness involving one or more limbs • Areflexia or hyporeflexia	• Sensory responses are usually spared • CMAP amplitudes are consistently low after the initial 3 weeks • Reduced recruitment and fibrillation potentials are seen persistently after the first week

ADM abductor digiti minimi, *APB* abductor pollicis brevis, *CK* creatine Kinase, *CMAPs* compound motor action potentials, *FCU* flexor carpi ulnaris, *FDI* first dorsal interosseous, *MUAPs* motor unit action potentials, *NCS* nerve conduction studies, *PSWs* positive sharp waves, *SNAPs* sensory nerve action potentials

Pyramidal tract signs are absent. Interestingly, hand muscle weakness may be worse at colder temperatures. Although the condition may initially progress fairly rapidly, in most cases progression slows, with stabilization by about 5 years after onset [92].

Flexion myelopathy, arising from contact pressure and axial tension during neck flexion, has been proposed as a probable pathogenic mechanism for Hirayama disease. The lower cervical cord moves forward during neck flexion, comes into contact with the posterior surface of the vertebra, and becomes flattened at the contact segment [93]. Moreover, MRI demonstrates an anterior shift of the posterior dural sac and compression of the lower cervical cord consistent with "tight dural canal in flexion" [92, 94–97].

Nerve conduction studies often show low amplitude CMAPs at the median and ulnar nerves, but SNAPs are usually preserved. Typically, CMAPs of the ulnar nerve are more affected than those of the median nerve. Needle EMG shows evidence of fibrillation potentials, positive sharp waves, and signs of chronic reinnervation in the distribution of the C7, C8, and T1 myotomes. Electrophysiologic abnormalities may also be present in more proximal, non-atrophic muscles such as the deltoid and brachioradialis, and also in clinically unaffected contralateral hand muscles [91, 92, 98, 99]. Chronic denervation changes are most frequently found in the first dorsal interosseous (FDI) and flexor carpi ulnaris (FCU) muscles [100].

Infectious Etiologies

Occasionally, infectious diseases cause predominantly motor neuron degeneration with weakness. The sensory system is clinically spared. The term "acute flaccid myelitis" (AFM) is often used to refer to cases of acute flaccid weakness with spinal cord gray matter lesions on imaging or evidence of spinal cord motor neuron injury on electrodiagnostic testing (Table 16.3). AFM develops abruptly and progresses rapidly, usually after a prodromal febrile illness, with uniformly flaccid weakness involving one or more limbs and areflexia or hyporeflexia. Loss of bladder and bowel function may develop [101]. Poliomyelitis is the prototypical AFM; other subtypes include those associated with Hopkins syndrome, West Nile Virus, enteroviruses, and Japanese encephalitis.

In AFM, sensory responses are usually spared. CMAP amplitudes are consistently low after the first 3 weeks. After the first week, reduced recruitment and fibrillation potentials are seen, and this pattern persists for months [101].

Poliomyelitis

Until the mid-twentieth century, poliomyelitis was the most common human neurologic infection. With the introduction of polio vaccines, wild-type poliovirus infections were eliminated in most of the world with a major reduction in cases of more than 99% since 1988 [102], though occasional outbreaks still occur in a limited number of countries.

Paralytic poliomyelitis is seen in 1% or less of all poliovirus infection and shows the highest predilection for lumbar, cervical, and medullary anterior horn cells. Usually there is rapid evolution of flaccid paralysis, reaching a nadir in 1–2 days. After the plateau phase the patient is left with residual asymmetric flaccid paralysis, sometimes with leg length discrepancy. Usually patients who contract the disease in childhood have less severe weakness and paralysis compared to adults who contract the disease. Children with signs of prior poliomyelitis are occasionally seen in the EMG laboratory with evidence for chronic reinnervation [103].

An unusual late manifestation, post-polio syndrome, can occur 15–20 years or more after the acute illness, and is usually characterized by gradually progressive and persistent new muscle weakness, fatigue, pain and atrophy in the same muscle groups that were involved in the acute polio infection [104].

Asthma-Related Poliomyelitis Syndrome (Hopkins Syndrome)

In 1974, Hopkins reported a series of 10 children who developed flaccid paralysis 4–7 days after the onset of a moderate to severe asthma attack. Afterwards, several cases were reported around the world. The prognosis is usually poor, and most patients experience a permanent flaccid paralysis [105].

West Nile Virus

In a US-based study from 1999–2007, West Nile Virus neuro-invasive disease was reported in 443 children, comprising 30% of the total cohort of children with West Nile virus infection. Only 1% of them had isolated acute flaccid myelitis without encephalitis or meningitis. Similar to AFM from other viral etiologies, West Nile virus usually has rapid progression of flaccid paralysis with some residual paralysis, and the overall outcome is variable [106, 107].

Enterovirus

Enterovirus D68 and EV71 are suspected of causing AFM, though this association has not been definitively proven yet. Enterovirus D68 appeared to be associated with an extensive 2014 outbreak of AFM in the United States. Most of these AFM patients experience only partial recovery, with residual persistent weakness [108, 109]. Other enteroviruses, such as coxsackievirus and echovirus, have been less frequently reported in patients with flaccid paralysis and these associations are more tenuous.

Japanese Encephalitis Virus

AFM also has been described with Japanese encephalitis virus infection in endemic areas [110].

Conclusion

Despite the widespread availability of sophisticated genetic testing, EMG continues to be a valuable diagnostic tool in the assessment of motor neuron diseases. Infants with severe SMA may need respiratory support, and thus the first evaluation is often made in a critical care setting. EMG provides a rapid assessment and identifies neurogenic illness with a reasonably high degree of accuracy. Genetic testing, which even today, takes at least a week, often much longer, to yield results, can confirm a suspected diagnosis. Similarly, EMG is invaluable in atypical cases of 5q SMA as well as in non-5q SMAs. The wide variation of phenotypes in non-5q SMAs can be misleading, and EMG often helps the diagnostic process. Moreover, in non-genetic causes of motor neuron diseases, such as Hirayama and AFM, EMG is an essential part of the diagnostic investigation.

References

1. Arnold WD, Kassar D, Kissel JT. Spinal muscular atrophy: diagnosis and management in a new therapeutic era. Muscle Nerve. 2015;51(2):157–67.
2. Darras BT. Spinal muscular atrophies. Pediatr Clin N Am. 2015;62(3):743–66.
3. Ogino S, Wilson RB, Gold B. New insights on the evolution of the SMN1 and SMN2 region: simulation and meta-analysis for allele and haplotype frequency calculations. Eur J Hum Genet. 2004;12(12):1015–23.
4. Sugarman EA, Nagan N, Zhu H, Akmaev VR, Zhou Z, Rohlfs EM, et al. Pan-ethnic carrier screening and prenatal diagnosis for spinal muscular atrophy: clinical laboratory analysis of >72,400 specimens. Eur J Hum Genet. 2012;20(1):27–32.
5. Werdnig Z. Zwei fruihnfantile hereditare Falle von progressive Muskelatrophie unter dem Bilde der Dystrophie, aber auf neurotischer Grundlage. Arch Psychiat Neurol. 1891;22:437–81.
6. Hoffmann J. Ueber chronische spinale Muskelatrophie im Kindesalter, auf familiärer Basis. Deuts Zeitsch Nervenheilk. 1893;3:427–70.
7. Zerres K, Rudnik-Schoneborn S. 93rd ENMC international workshop: non-5q-spinal muscular atrophies (SMA)—clinical picture (6–8 April 2001, Naarden, The Netherlands). Neuromuscul Disord. 2003;13(2):179–83.
8. Dubowitz V. Chaos in the classification of SMA: a possible resolution. Neuromuscul Disord. 1995;5(1):3–5.
9. Iannaccone ST, Russman BS, Browne RH, Buncher CR, White M, Samaha FJ. Prospective analysis of strength in spinal muscular atrophy. DCN/spinal muscular atrophy group. J Child Neurol. 2000;15(2):97–101.
10. Wang CH, Finkel RS, Bertini ES, Schroth M, Simonds A, Wong B, et al. Consensus statement for standard of care in spinal muscular atrophy. J Child Neurol. 2007;22(8):1027–49.

11. Dubowitz V. Very severe spinal muscular atrophy (SMA type 0): an expanding clinical phenotype. Eur J Paediatr Neurol. 1999;3(2):49–51.
12. Bertini E, Burghes A, Bushby K, Estournet-Mathiaud B, Finkel RS, Hughes RA, et al. 134th ENMC international workshop: outcome measures and treatment of spinal muscular atrophy, 11-13 February 2005, Naarden, The Netherlands. Neuromuscul Disord. 2005;15(11):802–16.
13. Markowitz JA, Singh P, Darras BT. Spinal muscular atrophy: a clinical and research update. Pediatr Neurol. 2012;46(1):1–12.
14. Zerres K, Davies KE. 59th ENMC international workshop: spinal muscular atrophies: recent progress and revised diagnostic criteria 17–19 April 1998, Soestduinen, The Netherlands. Neuromuscul Disord. 1999;9(4):272–8.
15. Crawford TO. Spinal muscular atrophies. In: Jones HRJ, De Vivo DC, Darras BT, editors. Neuromuscular disorders of infancy, childhood, and adolescence: a clinician's approach. Philadelphia: Butterworth Heinemann; 2003. p. 145–66.
16. von Gontard A, Zerres K, Backes M, Laufersweiler-Plass C, Wendland C, Melchers P, et al. Intelligence and cognitive function in children and adolescents with spinal muscular atrophy. Neuromuscul Disord. 2002;12(2):130–6.
17. Kugelberg E, Welander L. Heredofamilial juvenile muscular atrophy simulating muscular dystrophy. AMA Arch Neurol Psychiatry. 1956;75(5):500–9.
18. Spiro AJ. Minipolymyoclonus: a neglected sign in childhood spinal muscular atrophy. Neurology. 1970;20(11):1124.
19. Zerres K, Rudnik-Schoneborn S, Forrest E, Lusakowska A, Borkowska J, Hausmanowa-Petrusewicz I. A collaborative study on the natural history of childhood and juvenile onset proximal spinal muscular atrophy (type II and III SMA): 569 patients. J Neurol Sci. 1997;146(1):67–72.
20. Kang PB, Krishnamoorthy KS, Jones RM, Shapiro FD, Darras BT. Atypical presentations of spinal muscular atrophy type III (Kugelberg-Welander disease). Neuromuscul Disord. 2006;16(8):492–4.
21. Bolton CF. Spinal muscular atrophies of childhood and adolescence. In: Jones HRJ, Bolton CF, Harper CM, editors. Pediatric clinical electromyography. Philadelphia/New York: Lippincott-Raven; 1996. p. 105–22.
22. Schwartz MS, Moosa A. Sensory nerve conduction in the spinal muscular atrophies. Dev Med Child Neurol. 1977;19(1):50–3.
23. Swoboda KJ, Prior TW, Scott CB, McNaught TP, Wride MC, Reyna SP, et al. Natural history of denervation in SMA: relation to age, SMN2 copy number, and function. Ann Neurol. 2005;57(5):704–12.
24. Kang PB, Gooch CL, McDermott MP, Darras BT, Finkel RS, Yang ML, et al. The motor neuron response to SMN1 deficiency in spinal muscular atrophy. Muscle Nerve. 2014;49(5):636–44.
25. Hausmanowa-Petrusewicz I. Spinal muscular atrophy. Infantile and juvenile type. Warsaw: National Center for Scientific, Technical and Economic Information; 1978.
26. Duman O, Uysal H, Skjei KL, Kizilay F, Karauzum S, Haspolat S. Sensorimotor polyneuropathy in patients with SMA type-1: electroneuromyographic findings. Muscle Nerve. 2013;48(1):117–21.
27. Rudnik-Schoneborn S, Goebel HH, Schlote W, Molaian S, Omran H, Ketelsen U, et al. Classical infantile spinal muscular atrophy with SMN deficiency causes sensory neuronopathy. Neurology. 2003;60(6):983–7.
28. Carpenter S, Karpati G, Rothman S, Watters G, Andermann F. Pathological involvement of primary sensory neurons in Werdnig-Hoffmann disease. Acta Neuropathol. 1978;42(2):91–7.
29. Ravid S, Topper L, Eviatar L. Acute onset of infantile spinal muscular atrophy. Pediatr Neurol. 2001;24(5):371–2.
30. Fernandez-Torre JL, Teja JL, Castellanos A, Figols J, Obeso T, Arteaga R. Spinal muscular atrophy type I mimicking critical illness neuropathy in a paediatric intensive care neonate: electrophysiological features. Brain Dev. 2008;30(9):599–602.

31. Galea V, Fehlings D, Kirsch S, McComas A. Depletion and sizes of motor units in spinal muscular atrophy. Muscle Nerve. 2001;24(9):1168–72.
32. Bromberg MB, Swoboda KJ. Motor unit number estimation in infants and children with spinal muscular atrophy. Muscle Nerve. 2002;25(3):445–7.
33. Gawel M, Kostera-Pruszczyk A, Lusakowska A, Jedrzejowska M, Ryniewicz B, Lipowska M, et al. Motor unit loss estimation by the multipoint incremental MUNE method in children with spinal muscular atrophy—a preliminary study. Neuromuscul Disord. 2015;25(3):216–21.
34. McComas AJ, Fawcett PR, Campbell MJ, Sica RE. Electrophysiological estimation of the number of motor units within a human muscle. J Neurol Neurosurg Psychiatry. 1971;34(2):121–31.
35. Gomez MR. Motor neuron diseases in children. In: Engel AG, Franzini-Armstrong C, editors. Myology: basic and clinical 2. 2nd ed. New York: McGraw-Hill; 1994. p. 1837–53.
36. Wadman RI, Vrancken AF, van den Berg LH, van der Pol WL. Dysfunction of the neuromuscular junction in spinal muscular atrophy types 2 and 3. Neurology. 2012;79(20):2050–5.
37. Shields RW Jr. Single fiber electromyography in the differential diagnosis of myopathic limb girdle syndromes and chronic spinal muscular atrophy. Muscle Nerve. 1984;7(4):265–72.
38. Buchthal F, Olsen PZ. Electromyography and muscle biopsy in infantile spinal muscular atrophy. Brain. 1970;93(1):15–30.
39. Hausmanowa-Petrusewicz I, Karwanska A. Electromyographic findings in different forms of infantile and juvenile proximal spinal muscular atrophy. Muscle Nerve. 1986;9(1):37–46.
40. Gath I, Sjaastad O, Loken AC. Myopathic electromyographic changes correlated with histopathology in Wohlfart-Kugelberg-Welander disease. Neurology. 1969;19(4):344–52.
41. Darras BT. Non-5q spinal muscular atrophies: the alphanumeric soup thickens. Neurology. 2011;77(4):312–4.
42. Pestronk A. Hereditary motor syndroms. St Louis MO: Washington University; 2013. http://neuromuscular.wustl.edu/synmot.html
43. Harms MB, Allred P, Gardner R Jr, Fernandes Filho JA, Florence J, Pestronk A, et al. Dominant spinal muscular atrophy with lower extremity predominance: linkage to 14q32. Neurology. 2010;75(6):539–46.
44. Guenther UP, Varon R, Schlicke M, Dutrannoy V, Volk A, Hubner C, et al. Clinical and mutational profile in spinal muscular atrophy with respiratory distress (SMARD): defining novel phenotypes through hierarchical cluster analysis. Hum Mutat. 2007;28(8):808–15.
45. Porro F, Rinchetti P, Magri F, Riboldi G, Nizzardo M, Simone C, et al. The wide spectrum of clinical phenotypes of spinal muscular atrophy with respiratory distress type 1: a systematic review. J Neurol Sci. 2014;346(1–2):35–42.
46. Eckart M, Guenther UP, Idkowiak J, Varon R, Grolle B, Boffi P, et al. The natural course of infantile spinal muscular atrophy with respiratory distress type 1 (SMARD1). Pediatrics. 2012;129(1):e148–56.
47. Stalpers XL, Verrips A, Poll-The BT, Cobben JM, Snoeck IN, de Coo IF, et al. Clinical and mutational characteristics of spinal muscular atrophy with respiratory distress type 1 in The Netherlands. Neuromuscul Disord. 2013;23(6):461–8.
48. Grohmann K, Varon R, Stolz P, Schuelke M, Janetzki C, Bertini E, et al. Infantile spinal muscular atrophy with respiratory distress type 1 (SMARD1). Ann Neurol. 2003;54(6):719–24.
49. Pitt M, Houlden H, Jacobs J, Mok Q, Harding B, Reilly M, et al. Severe infantile neuropathy with diaphragmatic weakness and its relationship to SMARD1. Brain. 2003;126(12):2682–92.
50. Sivakumar K, Kyriakides T, Puls I, Nicholson GA, Funalot B, Antonellis A, et al. Phenotypic spectrum of disorders associated with glycyl-tRNA synthetase mutations. Brain. 2005;128(10):2304–14.
51. Dubourg O, Azzedine H, Yaou RB, Pouget J, Barois A, Meininger V, et al. The G526R glycyl-tRNA synthetase gene mutation in distal hereditary motor neuropathy type V. Neurology. 2006;66(11):1721–6.

52. Goldfarb LG, Sivakumar K. GARS-associated axonal neuropathy. In: Pagon RA, Adam MP, Ardinger HH, Wallace SE, Amemiya A, LJH B, et al., editors. GeneReviews(R) [Internet]. Seattle, WA: University of Washington; 2006. p. 1993–2016. https://www.ncbi.nlm.nih.gov/books/NBK1242.
53. Auer-Grumbach M, Schlotter-Weigel B, Lochmuller H, Strobl-Wildemann G, Auer-Grumbach P, Fischer R, et al. Phenotypes of the N88S Berardinelli-Seip congenital lipodystrophy 2 mutation. Ann Neurol. 2005;57(3):415–24.
54. Rossor AM, Kalmar B, Greensmith L, Reilly MM. The distal hereditary motor neuropathies. J Neurol Neurosurg Psychiatry. 2012;83(1):6–14.
55. Harms MB, KM O-MK, Scoto M, Tuck EP, Bell S, Ma D, et al. Mutations in the tail domain of DYNC1H1 cause dominant spinal muscular atrophy. Neurology. 2012;78(22):1714–20.
56. Rossor AM, Oates EC, Salter HK, Liu Y, Murphy SM, Schule R, et al. Phenotypic and molecular insights into spinal muscular atrophy due to mutations in BICD2. Brain. 2015;138(2):293–310.
57. Fiorillo C, Moro F, Yi J, Weil S, Brisca G, Astrea G, et al. Novel dynein DYNC1H1 neck and motor domain mutations link distal spinal muscular atrophy and abnormal cortical development. Hum Mutat. 2014;35(3):298–302.
58. Fleury P, Hageman G. A dominantly inherited lower motor neuron disorder presenting at birth with associated arthrogryposis. J Neurol Neurosurg Psychiatry. 1985;48(10):1037–48.
59. DeLong R, Siddique T. A large New England kindred with autosomal dominant neurogenic scapuloperoneal amyotrophy with unique features. Arch Neurol. 1992;49(9):905–8.
60. Dyck PJ, Litchy WJ, Minnerath S, Bird TD, Chance PF, Schaid DJ, et al. Hereditary motor and sensory neuropathy with diaphragm and vocal cord paresis. Ann Neurol. 1994;35(5):608–15.
61. McEntagart M. TRPV4 axonal neuropathy spectrum disorder. J Clin Neurosci. 2012;19(7):927–33.
62. Echaniz-Laguna A, Dubourg O, Carlier P, Carlier RY, Sabouraud P, Pereon Y, et al. Phenotypic spectrum and incidence of TRPV4 mutations in patients with inherited axonal neuropathy. Neurology. 2014;82(21):1919–26.
63. Bosch AM, Stroek K, Abeling NG, Waterham HR, Ijlst L, Wanders RJ. The Brown-Vialetto-van Laere and Fazio Londe syndrome revisited: natural history, genetics, treatment and future perspectives. Orphanet J Rare Dis. 2012;7:83.
64. Ciccolella M, Catteruccia M, Benedetti S, Moroni I, Uziel G, Pantaleoni C, et al. Brown-Vialetto-van Laere and Fazio-Londe overlap syndromes: a clinical, biochemical and genetic study. Neuromuscul Disord. 2012;22(12):1075–82.
65. Voudris KA, Skardoutsou A, Vagiakou EA. Infantile progressive bulbar palsy with deafness. Brain Dev. 2002;24(7):732–5.
66. Dipti S, Childs AM, Livingston JH, Aggarwal AK, Miller M, Williams C, et al. Brown-Vialetto-van Laere syndrome; variability in age at onset and disease progression highlighting the phenotypic overlap with Fazio-Londe disease. Brain and Development. 2005;27(6):443–6.
67. Namavar Y, Barth PG, Poll-The BT, Baas F. Classification, diagnosis and potential mechanisms in pontocerebellar hypoplasia. Orphanet J Rare Dis. 2011;6:50.
68. Rudnik-Schoneborn S, Senderek J, Jen JC, Houge G, Seeman P, Puchmajerova A, et al. Pontocerebellar hypoplasia type 1: clinical spectrum and relevance of EXOSC3 mutations. Neurology. 2013;80(5):438–46.
69. Eggens VR, Barth PG, Niermeijer JM, Berg JN, Darin N, Dixit A, et al. EXOSC3 mutations in pontocerebellar hypoplasia type 1: novel mutations and genotype-phenotype correlations. Orphanet J Rare Dis. 2014;9:23.
70. La Spada AR, Wilson EM, Lubahn DB, Harding AE, Fischbeck KH. Androgen receptor gene mutations in X-linked spinal and bulbar muscular atrophy. Nature. 1991;352(6330):77–9.
71. Finsterer J. Perspectives of Kennedy's disease. J Neurol Sci. 2010;298(1–2):1–10.
72. Fratta P, Nirmalananthan N, Masset L, Skorupinska I, Collins T, Cortese A, et al. Correlation of clinical and molecular features in spinal bulbar muscular atrophy. Neurology. 2014;82(23):2077–84.

73. Rhodes LE, Freeman BK, Auh S, Kokkinis AD, La Pean A, Chen C, et al. Clinical features of spinal and bulbar muscular atrophy. Brain. 2009;132(12):3242–51.
74. Suzuki K, Katsuno M, Banno H, Takeuchi Y, Atsuta N, Ito M, et al. CAG repeat size correlates to electrophysiological motor and sensory phenotypes in SBMA. Brain. 2008;131(1):229–39.
75. Harding AE, Thomas PK, Baraitser M, Bradbury PG, Morgan-Hughes JA, Ponsford JR. X-linked recessive bulbospinal neuronopathy: a report of ten cases. J Neurol Neurosurg Psychiatry. 1982;45(11):1012–9.
76. Ramser J, Ahearn ME, Lenski C, Yariz KO, Hellebrand H, von Rhein M, et al. Rare missense and synonymous variants in UBE1 are associated with X-linked infantile spinal muscular atrophy. Am J Hum Genet. 2008;82(1):188–93.
77. Dlamini N, Josifova DJ, Paine SM, Wraige E, Pitt M, Murphy AJ, et al. Clinical and neuropathological features of X-linked spinal muscular atrophy (SMAX2) associated with a novel mutation in the UBA1 gene. Neuromuscul Disord. 2013;23(5):391–8.
78. Sreedharan J, Brown RH Jr. Amyotrophic lateral sclerosis: problems and prospects. Ann Neurol. 2013;74(3):309–16.
79. Hentati A, Bejaoui K, Pericak-Vance MA, Hentati F, Speer MC, Hung WY, et al. Linkage of recessive familial amyotrophic lateral sclerosis to chromosome 2q33-q35. Nat Genet. 1994;7(3):425–8.
80. Rabin BA, Griffin JW, Crain BJ, Scavina M, Chance PF, Cornblath DR. Autosomal dominant juvenile amyotrophic lateral sclerosis. Brain. 1999;122(8):1539–50.
81. Chance PF, Rabin BA, Ryan SG, Ding Y, Scavina M, Crain B, et al. Linkage of the gene for an autosomal dominant form of juvenile amyotrophic lateral sclerosis to chromosome 9q34. Am J Hum Genet. 1998;62(3):633–40.
82. Hentati A, Ouahchi K, Pericak-Vance MA, Nijhawan D, Ahmad A, Yang Y, et al. Linkage of a commoner form of recessive amyotrophic lateral sclerosis to chromosome 15q15-q22 markers. Neurogenetics. 1998;2(1):55–60.
83. Orlacchio A, Babalini C, Borreca A, Patrono C, Massa R, Basaran S, et al. SPATACSIN mutations cause autosomal recessive juvenile amyotrophic lateral sclerosis. Brain. 2010;133(2):591–8.
84. Vance C, Rogelj B, Hortobagyi T, De Vos KJ, Nishimura AL, Sreedharan J, et al. Mutations in FUS, an RNA processing protein, cause familial amyotrophic lateral sclerosis type 6. Science. 2009;323(5918):1208–11.
85. Kwiatkowski TJ Jr, Bosco DA, Leclerc AL, Tamrazian E, Vanderburg CR, Russ C, et al. Mutations in the FUS/TLS gene on chromosome 16 cause familial amyotrophic lateral sclerosis. Science. 2009;323(5918):1205–8.
86. Conte A, Lattante S, Zollino M, Marangi G, Luigetti M, Del Grande A, et al. P525L FUS mutation is consistently associated with a severe form of juvenile amyotrophic lateral sclerosis. Neuromuscul Disord. 2012;22(1):73–5.
87. Al-Saif A, Al-Mohanna F, Bohlega S. A mutation in sigma-1 receptor causes juvenile amyotrophic lateral sclerosis. Ann Neurol. 2011;70(6):913–9.
88. Luty AA, Kwok JB, Dobson-Stone C, Loy CT, Coupland KG, Karlstrom H, et al. Sigma nonopioid intracellular receptor 1 mutations cause frontotemporal lobar degeneration-motor neuron disease. Ann Neurol. 2010;68(5):639–49.
89. Butterfield RJ, Ramachandran D, Hasstedt SJ, Otterud BE, Leppert MF, Swoboda KJ, et al. A novel form of juvenile recessive ALS maps to loci on 6p25 and 21q22. Neuromuscul Disord. 2009;19(4):279–87.
90. Hirayama K, Toyokura Y, Tsubaki T. Juvenile muscular atrophy of unilateral upper extremity: a new clinical entity. Psychiatr Neurol Jpn. 1959;61:2190–7.
91. Hirayama K. Juvenile non-progressive muscular atrophy localized in the hand and forearm—observations in 38 cases. Rinsho Shinkeigaku. 1972;12(7):313–24.
92. Kikuchi S, Tashiro K. Juvenile muscular atrophy of distal upper extremity (Hirayama's disease). In: Jones Jr HR, De Vivo DC, Darras BT, editors. Neuromuscular disorders of infancy, childhood, and adolescence: a Clinician's approach. 1st ed. Philadelphia: Butterworth-Heinemann; 2003. p. 167–81.

93. Hirayama K, Tomonaga M, Kitano K, Yamada T, Kojima S, Arai K. Focal cervical poliopathy causing juvenile muscular atrophy of distal upper extremity: a pathological study. J Neurol Neurosurg Psychiatry. 1987;50(3):285–90.
94. Iwasaki Y, Tashiro K, Kikuchi S, Kitagawa M, Isu T, Abe H. Cervical flexion myelopathy: a "tight dural canal mechanism". Case report. J Neurosurg. 1987;66(6):935–7.
95. Huang YL, Chen CJ. Hirayama disease. Neuroimaging Clin N Am. 2011;21(4):939–50. ix-x
96. Kikuchi S, Shinpo K, Niino M, Higashi T, Tashiro K. Cervical myelopathy due to a "tight dural canal in flexion" with a posterior epidural cavity. Intern Med. 2002;41(9):746–8.
97. Kikuchi S, Tashiro K, Kitagawa M, Iwasaki Y, Abe H. A mechanism of juvenile muscular atrophy localized in the hand and forearm (Hirayama's disease)—flexion myelopathy with tight dural canal in flexion. Rinsho Shinkeigaku. 1987;27(4):412–9.
98. Ghosh PS, Moodley M, Friedman NR, Rothner AD, Ghosh D. Hirayama disease in children from North America. J Child Neurol. 2011;26(12):1542–7.
99. Lyu RK, Huang YC, YR W, Kuo HC, Ro LS, Chen CM, et al. Electrophysiological features of Hirayama disease. Muscle Nerve. 2011;44(2):185–90.
100. Liao MF, Chang HS, Chang KH, Ro LS, Chu CC, Kuo HC, et al. Correlations of clinical, neuroimaging, and electrophysiological features in Hirayama disease. Medicine (Baltimore). 2016;95(28):e4210.
101. Messacar K, Schreiner TL, Van Haren K, Yang M, Glaser CA, Tyler KL, et al. Acute flaccid myelitis: a clinical review of US cases 2012-2015. Ann Neurol. 2016;80(3):326–38.
102. Poliomyelitis: Fact Sheet. World Health Organization. 2016. http://www.who.int/mediacentre/factsheets/fs114/en/.
103. McMillan HJ, Darras BT, Kang PB, Saleh F, Jones HR. Pediatric monomelic amyotrophy: evidence for poliomyelitis in vulnerable populations. Muscle Nerve. 2009;40(5):860–3.
104. Gonzalez H, Olsson T, Borg K. Management of postpolio syndrome. Lancet Neurol. 2010;9(6):634–42.
105. Hopkins IJ, Shield LK. Letter: poliomyelitis-like illness associated with asthma in childhood. Lancet. 1974;1(7860):760.
106. Sejvar JJ, Bode AV, Marfin AA, Campbell GL, Pape J, Biggerstaff BJ, et al. West Nile virus-associated flaccid paralysis outcome. Emerg Infect Dis. 2006;12(3):514–6.
107. Lindsey NP, Hayes EB, Staples JE, Fischer M. West Nile virus disease in children, United States, 1999-2007. Pediatrics. 2009;123(6):e1084–9.
108. Greninger AL, Naccache SN, Messacar K, Clayton A, Yu G, Somasekar S, et al. A novel outbreak enterovirus D68 strain associated with acute flaccid myelitis cases in the USA (2012-14): a retrospective cohort study. Lancet Infect Dis. 2015;15(6):671–82.
109. Huang HI, Shih SR. Neurotropic Enterovirus infections in the central nervous system. Virus. 2015;7(11):6051–66.
110. Solomon T, Kneen R, Dung NM, Khanh VC, Thuy TT, Ha DQ, et al. Poliomyelitis-like illness due to Japanese encephalitis virus. Lancet. 1998;351(9109):1094–7.

Chapter 17
Radiculopathies and Plexopathies

Megan Crone and Hugh J. McMillan

Introduction

Nerve root compression or compromise is one of the most common reasons for electrodiagnostic testing in adults [1]. By comparison, radiculopathy is less common in childhood and adolescence but remains an important diagnostic consideration due to its debilitating symptoms and numerous etiological considerations in this age group [2]. This chapter will discuss pediatric radiculopathy, brachial and lumbar plexopathy with particular attention paid to neonatal brachial plexus palsies (previously known as obstetrical brachial plexus palsies).

Radiculopathies

Nerve Root and Spinal Anatomy

Anatomically, there are 31 pairs of spinal nerve roots that include: 8 cervical, 12 thoracic, 5 lumbar, 5 sacral and 1 coccygeal roots. The first seven cervical nerve roots exit above their numerically paired vertebral body. However, since there are 8 cervical nerve roots and only 7 cervical vertebrae, C8 exits below the C7 vertebrae, and then each of the thoracic, lumbar, sacral, and the coccygeal nerves exits below the corresponding numerical vertebral body. Spinal roots have a dorsal (somatic sensory)

M. Crone, MD, FRCPC (✉)
Alberta Children's Hospital, University of Calgary, Calgary, AB, Canada
e-mail: Megan.Crone@albertahealthservices.ca

H.J. McMillan, MD, MSc, FRCPC, FAAN (✉)
Division of Neurology, Children's Hospital of Eastern Ontario, University of Ottawa, Ottawa, ON, Canada
e-mail: hmcmillan@cheo.on.ca

© Springer International Publishing AG 2017

H.J. McMillan, P.B. Kang (eds.), *Pediatric Electromyography*,
DOI 10.1007/978-3-319-61361-1_17

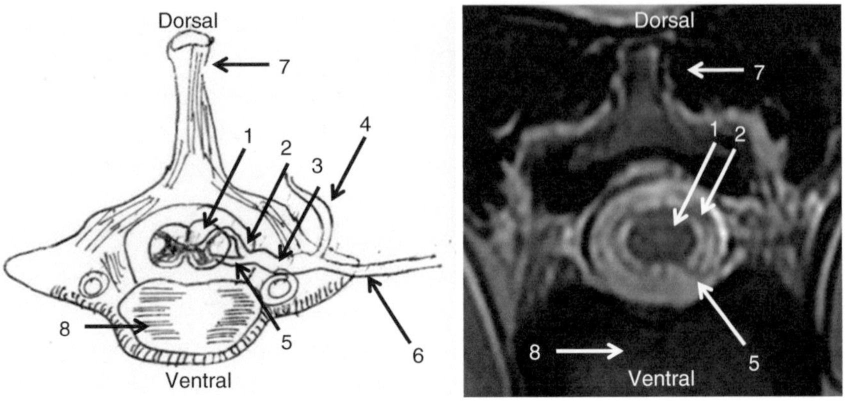

Fig. 17.1 Anatomy of the spinal cord, nerve root and vertebral body. Cross sectional (*axial*) view of the spine showing a sketch (*left*) and MRI T2-weighted image (*right*) revealing: (*1*) spinal cord (posterior columns); (*2*) dorsal root and dorsal root ganglion; (*3*) spinal nerve; (*4*) posterior primary ramus (continues to innervate paraspinal muscles); (*5*) ventral root; (*6*) anterior primary ramus (continues to form plexus); (*7*) vertebral spinous process; (*8*) vertebral body and intervertebral cartilaginous disc

and ventral (somatic motor) component. The motor nerve cell bodies, also known as motor neurons or anterior horn cells, are located within the ventral grey matter of the spinal cord. In contrast, the sensory nerve cell bodies, also known as dorsal root ganglia, are located outside of the spinal cord (Fig. 17.1). At each spinal level, the dorsal root and ventral root come together just proximal to the intervertebral foramen to form the spinal nerve. Sensory afferent and motor efferent fibers then travel together as the spinal nerve root. Just distal to the intervertebral foramen each spinal nerves divide into two, forming the posterior and anterior primary rami. The posterior ramus will innervate paraspinal muscles while the anterior ramus at the cervical and lumbosacral levels respectively, will give rise to the brachial and lumbosacral plexus.

The spinal vertebrae and its supporting ligamentous and muscular scaffolding affords protection to the spinal cord and exiting nerve roots while at the same time offering considerable mobility and flexibility. The vertebral body is located anterior to the spinal cord and in the thoracolumbar segments represents the familiar 'box-like' structure that is seen on radiographic images of the spine. Each vertebral body is separated by an intervertebral disc comprised of a viscous nucleus pulposus with an annulus fibrosus surrounding it in a circumferential manner. It is herniation of the nucleus pulposus that gives rise to most compressive radiculopathies in adults. The posterior spinous process and two posterolateral transverse processes represent three elongated bony projections to which stabilizing ligaments attach. The lateral pedicles connect each vertebral body to the posterior spinal and transverse processes. It is through the gap between each pedicle that spinal nerves exit in a space known as the intervertebral foramen.

Nerve roots are susceptible to the same injuries as peripheral nerves including compression, transection, infection, and infiltration. Congenital disorders of vertebral body development and alignment including hemivertebrae [3], spondylosis and scoliosis [4] can be associated with radiculopathy in the pediatric age group.

Clinical Symptoms

The key clinical features of a radiculopathy include: (1) severe back pain and paraspinal muscle spasm; (2) pain and paresthesia radiating in a dermatomal distribution; and (3) muscle weakness.

The dermatomal pattern of sensory symptoms must be differentiated from that of individual peripheral sensory nerves (Fig. 17.2). Dermatomes are areas of skin supplied by sensory neurons arising from a single spinal root. This pattern of sensory innervation is of early embryonic origin as paired blocks of mesodermal tissue (known as somites) give rise to sensory innervation to segments or regions of skin in a rostrocaudal or head-to-tail axis. Dermatomal areas have been mapped [5, 6] and differ from cutaneous nerve supply by individual peripheral sensory nerves.

Muscle weakness due to radiculopathy also occurs in a predictable pattern. Efferent motor fibers originating from a single spinal root level are collectively referred to as a myotome. Most muscles have contributions from two or more myotomes although typically, one level will predominate (Figs. 17.3 and 17.4). Muscle weakness that corresponds to a myotomal pattern, rather than that of a single peripheral nerve lesion, provides an opportunity to clinically and electrophysiological differentiate root lesions from peripheral nerve lesions. When clinically evaluating a patient with a suspected radiculopathy, physicians should become accustomed to evaluating a pattern of weakness, pattern of sensory deficit and integrity of deep tendon reflexes with a goal of differentiating a patient with a radiculopathy versus a peripheral nerve lesion. Muscle testing that is normal in one situation and abnormal in the other is ideal for helping to differentiate root versus nerve lesions (Fig. 17.5). Muscles that are normal or abnormal in both situations are not helpful for distinguishing between the two types of lesions.

Electrodiagnostic Testing

Lesions at the spinal nerve root can result in sensory and motor symptoms since both fibers travel together through the intervertebral foramen. However, in cases of radiculopathy due to disc herniation or spondylosis (causing ventral and/or dorsal nerve root compression), electrodiagnostic testing can help differentiate radiculopathies from more distal lesions. Lesions that are proximal to the dorsal root ganglion will result in clinical symptoms without any abnormality on sensory nerve conduction studies since the sensory nerve fibers remain in continuity with their dorsal root ganglia and thus do not degenerate. By comparison, given the intramedullary location of motor neurons in the ventral spinal cord, any compressive

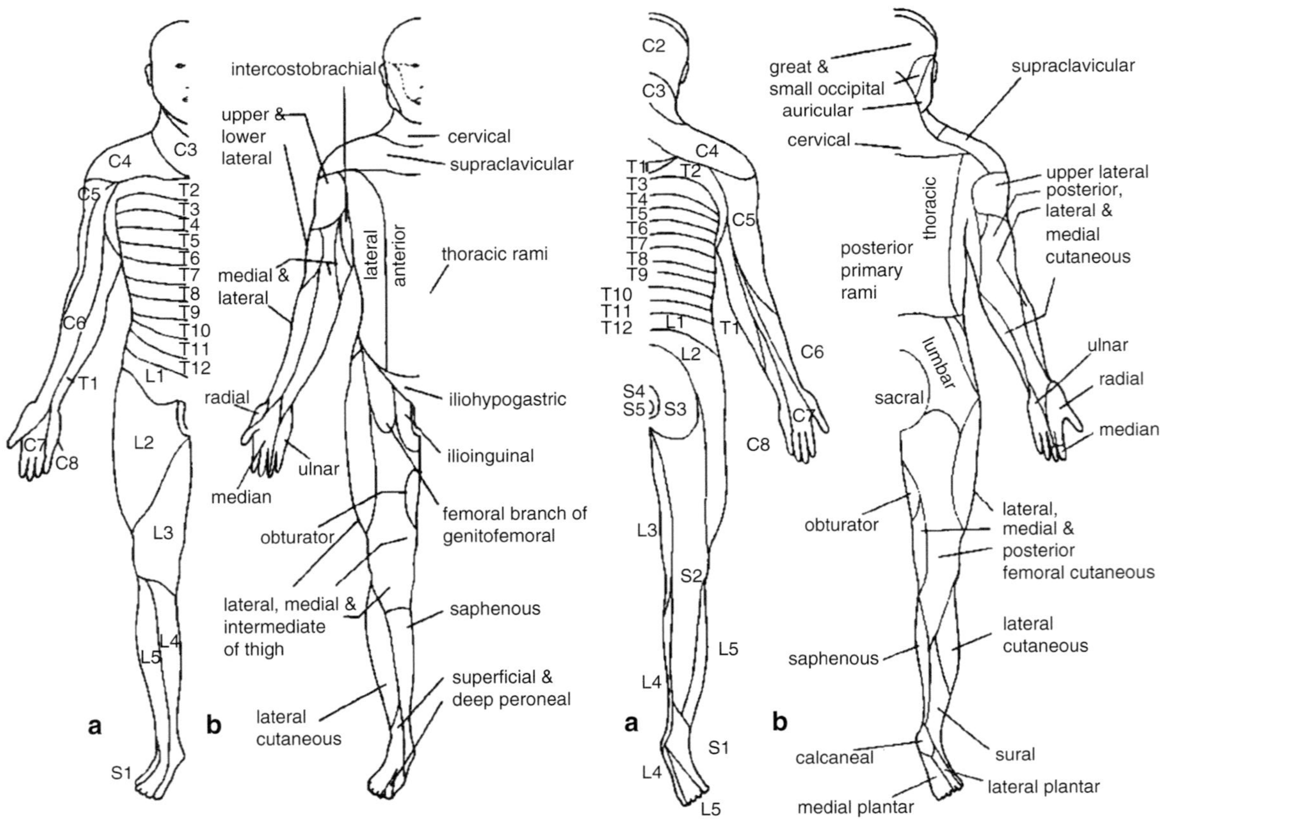

Fig. 17.2 Dermatomal (**a**) and peripheral sensory nerve (**b**) distributions of the ventral (*left*) and dorsal (*right*) body. Figure credit: J.A. Kiernan, University of Western Ontario [5]. Permission was obtained to use this figure

***Nerve* / Muscle**	**Myotome**	**Cord**	**Trunk**
Dorsal Scapular			
Rhomboids	C4**C5**C6		
Levator scapulae	C3C4C5		
Long Thoracic			
Serratus anterior	C5C6C7		
Long Pectoralis			
Pectoralis major (clavicular head)	**C5**C6	Lateral	Upper
Pectoralis major (sternal head)	C6**C7**C8T1	Medial	Lower
Pectoralis minor	C6C7C8	Medial	Middle
Suprascapular			
Supraspinatus	**C5**C6		Upper
Infraspinatus	**C5**C6		Upper
Subscapular			
Subscapularis	C5C6	Posterior	Upper
Teres Major	C5C6C7	Posterior	Upper
Thoracodorsal			
Latissimus Dorsi	C6**C7**C8	Posterior	All
Axillary			
Deltoid	**C5**C6	Posterior	Upper
Teres minor	C5C6	Posterior	Upper
Musculocutaneous			
Biceps brachii	C5**C6**	Lateral	Upper
Brachialis	C5C6	Lateral	Upper
Coracobrachialis	C6**C7**	Lateral	Upper
Radial			
Triceps	C6**C7**C8	Posterior	All
Brachioradialis	C5**C6**	Posterior	Upper
Extensor carpi radialis (longus/brevis)	C5**C6**	Posterior	Upper
Posterior interosseous			
Supinator	**C6**C7	Posterior	Upper + middle
Extensor carpi ulnaris	**C7**C8	Posterior	Middle + lower
Extensor digitorum communis	**C7**C8	Posterior	Middle + lower
Extensor digiti quinti	**C7**C8	Posterior	Middle + lower
Abductor pollicis longus	**C7**C8	Posterior	Middle + lower
Extensor pollicis (longus/brevis)	**C7**C8	Posterior	Middle + lower
Extensor indicis proprius	**C7**C8	Posterior	Middle + lower
Median			
Pronator teres	C6C7	Lateral	Middle + upper
Flexor carpi radialis	C6C7	Lateral	Middle + upper

Fig. 17.3 *Upper extremity*: differentiating *spinal root* versus *brachial plexus* versus *peripheral nerve* lesions. Bold = predominant innervation

Palmaris longus	C7**C8**T1	Medial	Middle + lower
Flexor digitorum superficialis	C7**C8**T1	Medial	Middle + lower
Flexor digitorum profundus (digit 2 & 3)	C7**C8**	Medial + lateral	Middle + lower
Abductor pollicis brevis	C8**T1**	Medial	Lower
Flexor pollicis brevis (longus/brevis)	C8**T1**	Medial	Lower
Opponens pollicis	C8**T1**	Medial	Lower
Lumbricals (I, II)	C8**T1**	Medial	Lower
Anterior Interosseus			
Flexor digitorum profundus (digits 2 & 3)	C7**C8**	Medial + lateral	Middle + lower
Flexor pollicis longus	C7**C8**	Medial + lateral	Middle + lower
Pronator quadratus	C7**C8T1**	Medial	Middle + lower
Ulnar			
Flexor carpi ulnaris	C7**C8**T1	Medial	Lower
Flexor digitorum profundus (digits 4 & 5)	C7**C8**T1	Medial + lateral	Middle + lower
Abductor digiti minimi	C8**T1**	Medial	Lower
Opponens digiti minimi	C8**T1**	Medial	Lower
Flexor digiti minimi	C8**T1**	Medial	Lower
Lumbricals (III, IV)	C8**T1**	Medial	Lower
Palmar interossei	C8**T1**	Medial	Lower
Flexor pollicis brevis (deep)	C8**T1**	Medial	Lower
Adductor pollicis	C8**T1**	Medial	Lower

Fig. 17.3 (continued)

lesion will disrupt communications between the motor neuron and the motor nerve. The key electrodiagnostic finding in classic radiculopathy that permits it to be differentiated from plexopathies and peripheral neuropathies is the finding of intact sensory nerve action potential (SNAP) amplitudes confirming the proximal site of injury. In radiculopathies, compound motor action potential (CMAP) amplitudes may be reduced, F waves at appropriate myotomes may be abnormal, and needle electromyography (EMG) findings will typically indicate a myotomal pattern of denervation. Caution must be taken in the case of diseases that infiltrate or extend into the intervertebral foramen (e.g., malignancy, infection) since dorsal root ganglia may be damaged in such cases, resulting in wallerian degeneration of sensory and motor fibers affecting both SNAP and CMAP amplitudes.

Case Example

A 15 year old young man suffered an injury after attempting to perform a backward somersault during which he landed awkwardly. Although he did not suffer any initial pain or symptoms, he developed severe, escalating back pain over the next 2 days that radiated bilaterally down the backs of both legs. He reported paraesthesias over the backs of his lower legs and the dorsal and plantar surfaces of both feet (L5 and S1 distributions). He had no bowel or bladder symptoms at any time and no saddle paresthesias. Due to increasing pain, he presented to the emergency room for evaluation. MRI of the spine (Fig. 17.6)

Nerves / Muscles	**Spinal Segments**
Obturator	
Obturator externus	**L2L**3L4
Adductor longus	**L2L3**L4
Adductor magnus	L2L3L4
Adductor brevis	L2L3L4
Gracilis	L2L3L4
Femoral	
Iliopsoas	**L1L2**L3
Rectus femoris	L2**L3L4**
Vastus lateralis/intermedius/medialis	L2**L3L4**
Pectineus	**L2L3**L4
Sartorius	**L2L3**L4
Sciatic	
Adductor magnus	L4L5S1
Semitendinosus	L5**S1**S2
Biceps femoris	L5**S1**S2
Semimenbranosus	L5**S1**S2
Tibial	
Gastrocnemius	**S1**S2
Plantaris	L4L5S1
Soleus	**S1**S2
Popliteus	L4L5S1
Tibialis posterior	L4**L5**
Flexor digitorum longus	L5**S1S2**
Flexor hallicis longus	L5**S1S2**
Small foot muscles	S1S2
Superificial peroneal	
Peroneus longus	**L5**S1
Peroneus brevis	**L5**S1
Deep Peroneal	
Tibialis anterior	**L4**L5
Extensor digitorum longus	**L5**S1
Extensor hallicis longus	**L5**S1
Peroneus tertius	L4**L5**S1
Extensor digitorum brevis	L5S1
Superior gluteal	
Gluteal medius/minimus	**L4L5**S1
Tensor fasciae latae	**L4L5**S1
Inferior gluteal	
Gluteus maximus	**L5S1**S2

Fig. 17.4 *Lower extremity*: differentiating *spinal root* versus *brachial plexus* versus *peripheral nerve* lesions. Bold = predominant innervation

confirmed a large central disc extrusion at L3/4 causing canal stenosis and impinging upon bilateral L5 and S1 nerve roots. He underwent L3 and L4 partial laminectomy with discectomy and excision of the apophyseal ring fragment. Post-operatively, his pain resolved but he was left with a persistent right foot drop. Neurology consultation 6 months after the injury confirmed the right foot

		Common peroneal neuropathy	
		Normal	**Abnormal**
L5 radiculopathy	**Normal**	Not helpful	None
	Abnormal	Gluteus medius Tensor facia latae Tibialis posterior L5 paraspinal muscle	Not helpful

Fig. 17.5 Clinical and electrophysiological testing used to differentiate an L5 root from a common peroneal nerve lesion. This example illustrates how muscles predicated to be normal in one situation and abnormal in the other are the most valuable for this assessment. Muscles that are normal or abnormal in both situations are not helpful

NERVE CONDUCTION STUDIES:

	Normal	Right	Left
SENSORY:			
Superficial peroneal nerve			
PL (msec)	< 3.8	2.6	2.6
SNAP (μV)	> 5.0	8.1	10.4
Sural nerve			
PL (msec)	< 4.2	3.3	3.3
SNAP (μV)	> 5	24.9	22.6
MOTOR:			
Peroneal nerve			
DML (ankle-EDB)	< 6.0	5.6	4.0
CMAP (mV)	> 2.4	0.1	0.7
CV (m/sec; fibula-ankle)	> 40	36	37
Tibial nerve			
DML (ankle-AH)	< 6.0	5.5	5.9
CMAP (mV)	> 3.9	2.1	0.8
CV (m/sec; knee-ankle)	> 4.0	34	43

ELECTROMYOGRAPHY:

Side	Muscle	Root	Fib	PSW	Amp	Dur	Poly	Recruit
Right	Peroneus longus	L5-S1	2+	2+	1+	1+	2+	3-
Right	Tibialis anterior	L4-5	2+	3+	2+	1+	3+	3-
Right	Biceps femoris (long)	L5-S2	2+	2+	Nml	Nml	Nml	1-
Right	Vastus lateralis	L2-4	Nml	Nml	Nml	Nml	Nml	Nml
Right	Gluteus medius	L4-S1	Nml	Nml	1+	1+	Nml	1-
Right	Gastrocnemius (med)	S1-2	2+	1+	1+	1+	2+	2-
Right	L5 Paraspinal	L4-S1	Nml	Nml	1+	1+	1+	1-

Right peroneal and tibial F-response absent. Bilateral tibial nerve H-reflexes were absent.

Abbreviations: PL = peak onset latency; SNAP = sensory nerve action potential; DML = distal motor latency; CMAP = compound motor action potential; EDB = extensor digitorum brevis; AH = abductor hallucis. Fib = fibrillation potential; PSW = positive sharp waves; Amp = amplitude; Dur = duration; Poly = polyphasic; Recruit = recruitment pattern.

Electrodiagnostic evidence for a severe bilateral (R>L) L5 and S1 radiculopathy.

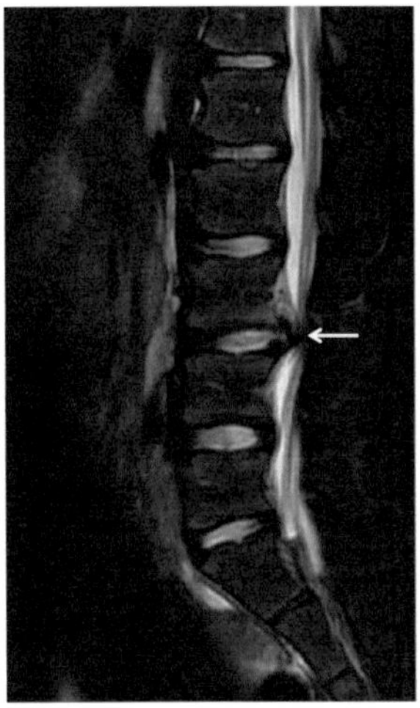

Fig. 17.6 MRI (T2-weighted imaging) and nerve conduction study findings in a 16-year-old male with central disc protrusion (*arrow*) causing bilateral L5 and S1 radiculopathies

drop. Muscle strength in his right leg (Medical Research Council scale): gluteus medius 5, gluteus maximus 5, iliopsoas 5, quadriceps 5, hamstrings 5-, tibialis anterior 2, peroneus longus 3, tibialis posterior 4-, gastrocnemius 4-, extensor hallicus longus 0. Strength testing of his left leg revealed: gluteus medius 5, gluteus maximus 5, iliopsoas 5, quadriceps 5, hamstrings 5-, tibialis anterior 4+, peroneus longus 4+, tibialis posterior 4+, gastrocnemius 4+, extensor hallicus longus 4. Reflexes were intact at the patellae but absent at both ankles. Sensory testing noted decreased pinprick sensation at the dorsal surfaces of both feet. Nerve conduction studies (Fig. 17.6) were consistent with severe bilateral (right > left) L5 and S1 radiculopathy. SNAP amplitudes were robust despite low CMAP amplitudes, indicating a proximal location of nerve root impingement. Late responses (bilateral tibial and peroneal F-responses and bilateral tibial H-reflexes) were absent. Needle EMG confirmed reinnervation in proximal L5/S1 muscles (e.g., gluteus medius) with ongoing denervation in distal muscles. Given that axonal continuity was demonstrated to all muscles studied, clinical improvement was predicted which was indeed observed in the following 12 months. This case illustrates some of the key electrophysiological findings that are seen in radiculopathies.

Etiology of Radiculopathies in Children

Pediatric radiculopathies are uncommon with no good epidemiological studies available to estimate the incidence of this problem. Adult population studies have estimated an annual incidence of cervical radiculopathy to be 107.3 per 100,000 for men and 63.5 per 100,000 for women [7]. The incidence of lumbar radiculopathies has been estimated to be 1–2% in the general population [8]. Pediatric case reports and case series have provided some insight into the varied etiology of this problem in childhood. These have included trauma with or without an underlying congenital spine abnormality (hemivertebrae, spondolithesis, congenital scoliosis or narrowing of the intervertebral foramen) [3, 4], infections or mechanical compression, tumor, or infiltrative lesion.

The likelihood of impingement of a specific spinal nerve root is largely dependent on the underlying etiology. Cervical radiculopathies are most commonly caused by disc calcification [9]. Over 300 pediatric cases of cervical disc calcification have been published, most commonly involving C5-C6 or C6-C7, with few cases involving the thoracic or lumbar nerve roots [10]. The etiology of disc calcification has yet to be determined, but trauma [11], infection, and inflammation [12] have been raised as possibilities. Although calcification may cause spinal stenosis and evidence of corticospinal tract involvement, less than 30% of children with cervical disc calcification will demonstrate clinical symptoms of radiculopathy [13]. Griesl syndrome is an uncommon non-traumatic complication of any inflammatory condition of the upper neck or otolaryngological procedure, which causes subluxation of the atlantoaxial joint. There may be an infectious, influenza-like prodrome, followed by significant neck and/or throat pain, torticollis and often atlantoaxial subluxation [14]. Approximately 15% of patients will experience neurological symptoms including a cervical radiculopathy [15]. Traumatic cervical radiculopathies are most commonly caused by high-speed motor vehicle accidents with seat belt injuries, in which high velocity traction injuries are also likely to damage the brachial plexus causing avulsions of the cervical roots which will be discussed below.

Pediatric thoracic root disease is the least common site of a radiculopathy and when present, is most commonly caused by spinal arachnoid cysts. One large case series of patients with spinal arachnoid cysts including 31 pediatric patients noted 36% (11/31) to involve thoracic nerve root(s), 19% (6/31) thoracolumbar, 13% (4/31) lumbrosacral, 13% (4/31) thoracocervical, 10% (3/31) sacral, 7% (2/31) lumbar, and 3% (1/31) cervical [16]. Another one case series found 5 of 15 patients with spinal arachnoid cysts to be children [17]. All five children had thoracic spinal arachnoid cysts; 2/3 of the 15 patients had associated radiculopathies with their arachnoid cyst; however, this was not reported for specific age groups. In pediatric patients, unlike the general population, spinal arachnoid cysts are more often intradural.

The most common cause of pediatric lumbosacral radiculopathies is disc disease, usually due to an intra-canal or intra-foraminal herniated nucleus pulposus [18]. Under the age of 15 years, the frequency of radiculopathy ranges from 0.05% in a population-based study based upon 6500 patients seen at the Mayo Clinic [19], to as high as 42% when comparing children referred to for disc disease at a tertiary-care pediatric hospital [20]. The reported incidence in Japanese children who underwent operation for back pain was 15.4% in patients under 20 years of age and 4.6% under 15 years [21]. Newer studies have reported an incidence ranging from 1 to 5% in patients under the age of 20 years [22–24]. In one series, 91.4% of adolescent patients with lumbar disc disease complained of back and leg pain [25], congruent with another study in which 85.1% of adolescent patients had both complaints [26]. There is no clear gender predominance of disc herniation. Risk factors for developing lumbar disc disease include: family history, lumbar load (similar to our case presented above), strenuous exercise, and obesity [27]. Since disc herniation is relatively rare in children, other etiologies should be considered. These include: non-spondylotic etiologies such as juxta-facet cysts, and spondylolytic causes, commonly seen in athletes, with symptomatology from spondylolisthesis, ragged-edge osteophytes, periosteal edema, and hematomas [18]. The rare possibility of an intraspinal or vertebral tumor must also be considered. These most commonly occur in the lumbrosacral regions and can include Ewing's sarcoma [28], osteoblastoma [29], childhood chordoma [30], neurofibromatosis [31], schwannoma [32], and Langerhans histiocytosis-X [33].

Discal cysts can be located anywhere along the lengths of the spinal cord and produce radiculopathies. Characteristics of discal cysts may include: symptoms of unilateral single nerve root compression; lesions occurring at a slightly younger age and at a higher intervertebral disc level than the typical disc herniation; minimal degeneration of the involved disc on imaging studies; communication between the cyst and the corresponding intervertebral disc; intralesional, bloody-to-clear serous fluid content of the cyst; and, an absence of either disc material inside the cyst [34]. About 75% of patients (all-ages) with discal cysts will have symptoms of sciatica [35].

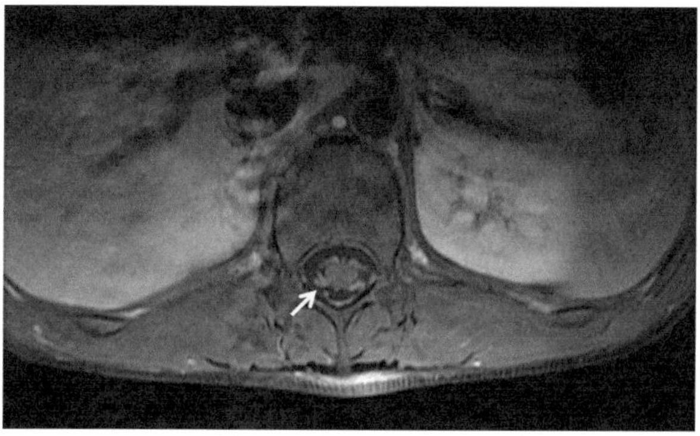

Fig. 17.7 MRI coronal STIR T2-weighted image of the brachial plexus in a 16-year-old patient with chronic inflammatory demyelinating polyradiculoneuropathy (CIDP) showing nerve root thickening (*arrow*)

Radiculopathy symptoms including back pain and paresthesias with nerve root thickening can be seen in systemic inflammatory disorders. Chronic inflammatory demyelinating polyradiculoneuropathy (CIDP) is associated with MRI evidence of root thickening and gadolinium enhancement (Fig. 17.7) in approximately 40% of affected children [36] and 60% of adults [37] although the majority of such patients will not complain of any clinical symptoms of nerve root involvement. Adults with CIDP have occasionally been reported to demonstrate symptoms of a painful polyradiculopathy that has been attributed to spinal nerve root impingement secondary to root inflammation and thickening that on rare occasions may be so severe as to cause lumbar stenosis [38] and even produce symptoms of spinal cord compression [39]. Nerve root thickening is by no means unique to CIDP. Homogeneous nerve root enlargement is also reported in patients with Charcot-Marie-Tooth disease [40, 41], Guillain-Barré syndrome [42], and infectious causes including HIV and CMV [43]. Polyradiculopathy without nerve root thickening is also reported with: neurobrucellosis [44], herpes simplex virus [45], cytomegalovirus [46], herpes zoster virus [47] and Lyme disease [48]. Nodular nerve root thickening can be seen in neurofibromatosis-related nerve sheath tumors [49], neoplasias (e.g., neurolymphomatosis) [50] and granulomatous disease [51]. Infiltrative etiologies can also occur at any spinal level. These can include hematological malignancies as acute lymphoblastic leukemia or lymphoma but can also be seen with solid tumors such as osteosarcoma [52, 53].

Plexopathies

The brachial and lumbosacral plexi arise from mixed spinal nerves after they emerge from the intervertebral foramina and give rise to three main nerve trunks. The word plexus arises from the Latin word *plectere* meaning braid or twine. Neurologists and neurophysiologists must have a thorough working knowledge of plexus anatomy in order to correctly localize lesions within these structures. Schematic diagrams of the brachial plexus (Fig. 17.8) and lumbosacral plexus (Fig. 17.9) are particularly useful as physicians can draw or visualize these structures when attempting to differentiate root from plexus from nerve lesions [54, 55].

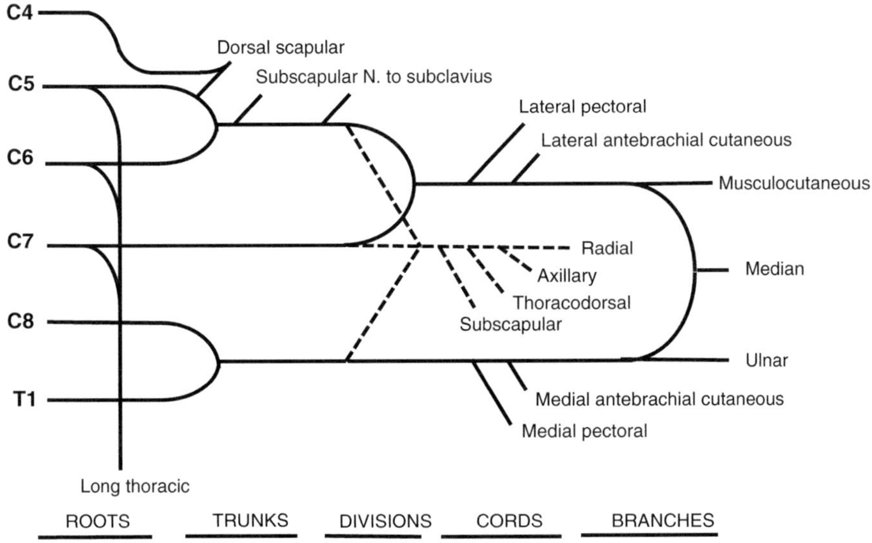

Fig. 17.8 Schematic figure of the brachial plexus (adapted from Blumenfeld [54])

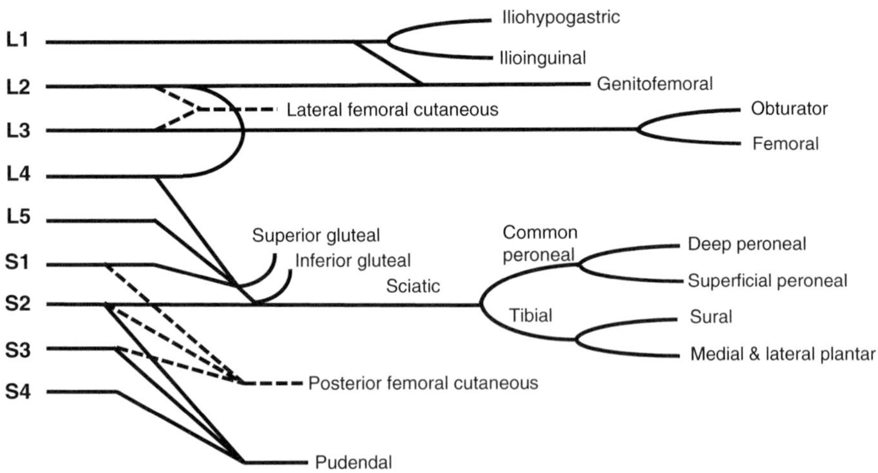

Fig. 17.9 Schematic figure of the lumbosacral plexus (adapted from Blumenfeld [54])

Brachial Plexus Anatomy

The brachial plexus is located between the base of the neck and the axilla. It is divided into roots, trunks, divisions, cords, and nerves, although roots and nerves are not considered part of the actual plexus. The brachial plexus arises mainly from 4 cervical and 1 thoracic anterior primary rami or roots (C5 to T1). The C4 spinal root does provide nerve fibers to the dorsal scapular nerve which (like the long thoracic nerve) arises directly from roots, although the C4 root is not traditionally considered to be a contributor to the brachial plexus (Fig. 17.8). Two upper cervical roots (C5, C6) fuse to form the upper trunk; the middle root (C7) forms the middle trunk; and two lower cervical roots (C8, T1) form the lower trunk. Two nerves, the suprascapular and subclavian, arise from the upper trunk. Each trunk then divides into divisions: anterior and lateral. Divisions then unite to form three cords: medial, posterior and lateral before finally dividing into multiple terminal nerves. Careful clinical and electrodiagnostic testing can help to localize a lesion within the brachial plexus.

Clinical Symptoms

Brachial plexopathies can have varied presentations depending on the site of the lesion and underlying etiology. Since the brachial plexus eventually gives rise to all sensory and motor nerves of the arm and hand, lesions within the plexus cause areas of numbness and paresthesia, along with specific patterns of muscle weakness. Pain can be a predominant clinical feature for some etiologies, including trauma and compressive or infiltrative lesions. Other diseases such as genetic disorders, including hereditary neuropathy with liability to pressure palsy (HNPP), may give rise to painless weakness and sensory loss. Etiologies will be discussed in greater detail below. Like all peripheral neural elements, an intact plexus is essential for normal limb growth. The long-term sequela of plexus injuries early in life can include limb length discrepancy and orthopedic complications such as joint contractures and restricted range of motion, as well as malpositioned joints that heighten the risk of uneven wear and arthritis. Upper trunk lesions at birth (Erb palsy) in particular can give rise to malposition of the glenohumeral joint that requires long-term orthopedic monitoring and can respond to successful relocation of the humeral head [56]. Lower trunk lesions (Klumpke paralysis) due to traumatic root avulsion or tumor infiltration can give rise to an ipsilateral Horner syndrome, which manifests clinically as a triad of ptosis, miosis, and anhidrosis. This is generally attributed to injury of sympathetic preganglionic neurons at T1 that innervate the superior cervical ganglion; there are reports of children with C7, C8 and/or T1 root avulsions presenting with this syndrome [57]. Early injury to sympathetic fibers (typically as neonatal brachial plexus injury) can manifest as iris heterochromia as the sympathetic fibers play an important role in normal changes in eye color change in the first few months of life.

Electrodiagnostic Testing

When evaluating a patient with a potential plexopathy, neurophysiologists must perform sensory and motor nerve conduction studies as well as needle electromyography. Absent or reduced sensory nerve responses can provide important clues to the location of plexus lesions (Fig. 17.10) as well as to differentiate plexus lesions (where SNAP amplitudes are reduced or absent) from radiculopathies (where SNAP amplitudes

Nerve conduction studies: assisting with localization within the brachial plexus

Sensory:

Brachial plexus		Peripheral nerve
Trunk	Cord	
Upper	Lateral	Lateral antebrachial cutaneous
Upper	Lateral	Median to (first/second digit)
Upper	Posterior	Radial (to base of first digit)
Middle	Posterior	Posterior antebrachial cutaneous
Middle	Lateral	Median (to second digit)
Middle	Lateral	Median (to third digit)
Lower	Medial	Ulnar (to fifth digit)
Lower	Medial	Dorsal ulnar cutaneous
Lower	Medial	Medial antebrachial cutaneous

Motor:

Brachial plexus		Peripheral nerve
Trunk	Cord	
Upper	Lateral	Musculocutaneous (to biceps)
Upper	Posterior	Axillary (to deltoid)
Middle	Posterior	Radial (to EDC or EIP)
Lower	Medial	Median (to APB)
Lower	Medial	Ulnar (to ADM or FDI)

From Dumitru and Zwarts Chapter 19 Brachial plexopathies and Proximal mononeuropathies.

Fig. 17.10 Sensory and motor nerve conduction studies to assist localizing a lesion within the brachial plexus

remain intact). Nerve conduction studies and even more importantly needle EMG can accurately localize lesions within the plexus and aid in differentiating patterns of denervation from that seen in lesions affecting roots or peripheral nerves (Fig. 17.3).

Etiology of Brachial Plexopathy in Children

The potential causes of brachial plexopathies even after their localization are numerous. Trauma particularly that associated with birth injuries (described below) is a common cause. Physicians must remain alert to non-accidental injuries, particularly in infants and toddlers, who may not be developmentally capable of recounting the circumstances of their injury [58]. Immune causes of brachial plexus neuropathy, also known as Parsonage-Turner syndrome can give rise to severe, abrupt-onset shoulder girdle pain followed by muscle weakness and amyotrophy. Although this is more common in adults, it has been described in children as young as 3 months old [59]. Other inflammatory causes of brachial plexus lesions can include Lewis-Sumner syndrome or multifocal acquired demyelinating sensory and motor neuropathy (MADSAM), an asymmetrical form of chronic inflammatory demyelinating polyneuropathy (CIDP) that is occasionally reported in childhood. This disorder may respond to intravenous immunoglobulin (IVIg) therapy [60, 61].

Hereditary brachial plexus neuralgia or hereditary neuralgic amyotrophy (HNA) is an autosomal dominant disorder resulting from *SEPT9* gene mutations. HNA can mimic Parsonage-Turner syndrome. Although the initial presentation of hereditary neuralgic amyotrophy can occur as early as the toddler years [62], it is more common in late adolescence [63]. Hereditary neuropathy with liability to pressure palsies (HNPP) is an autosomal dominant disorder resulting from a deletion or, less commonly, a point mutation of *PMP22*. About 20% of patients with HNPP may present with a brachial plexopathy. Onset is typically seen around adolescence and is typically characterised by episodes of painless muscle weakness and paresthesias that result from focal demyelination. Pain and muscle atrophy—dominant features of hereditary neuralgic amyotrophy and immune brachial plexitis are not seen or are less severe in children with HNPP [64]. Electrodiagnostic testing is key since nerve conduction studies can demonstrate focal conduction block even in asymptomatic nerves [65]. Pediatric brachial plexopathy can also occur from extrinsic compression or infiltration from various primary or metastatic tumors including neurofibroma, sarcoma, neuroblastoma, lymphoma or infantile myofibromatosis [66, 67]. Although symptom onset can be insidious, it can also be present at birth mimicking neonatal brachial plexus palsy.

Neonatal Brachial Plexus Palsy

Neonatal brachial plexus palsy (NBPP), previously referred to as obstetrical brachial plexus palsy, results from injury to the brachial plexus at or around the time of birth. Given the location and structure of the brachial plexus it is susceptible to traction or compression injury. Although NBPP is often attributed to traumatic and/or difficult delivery (e.g., shoulder dystocia, breech delivery, difficult vaginal extraction of a large infant) [68] the most significant risk factor for NBPP appears to be large infant size, specifically birth weight ≥4 kg [69, 70]. However, non-traumatic causes may in some cases be associated, including: uterine anomalies and fetal malposition (i.e., compression against maternal sacral promontory) [71, 72]. NBPP has been well described in deliveries with no evidence of trauma or fetal distress, including routine and/or early Caesarean section [73].

The incidence of NBPP is about 1.5–4 per 1000 live births [74, 75]. The majority of infants (66–85%) with NBPP exhibit mild, transient symptoms resulting from neurapraxia or 'bruising' of the nerve fibers within the plexus; such infants will demonstrate a complete clinical recovery by around 1 month and require no intervention beyond routine physical therapy [76–79]. However, a smaller subset of infants with NBPP (15–33%) will suffer a more severe injury attributable to axonotmesis (partial tearing of the nerve), neurotmesis (complete tearing of the nerve) or the most severe, nerve root avulsion where the nerve root is torn out of the spinal cord (Fig. 17.11). Patients with NBPP can therefore be thought to exist along a continuum with more severe nerve damage not surprisingly associated with a lower likelihood of spontaneous recovery and a higher risk of long-term deficits.

Brachial plexopathies have been classified into four categories by Narakas and Birch [80, 81], depending upon the levels involved: Group I, C5-C6 paralysis of the shoulder and biceps; Group II, C5-C7 paralysis of the shoulder, biceps, and forearm

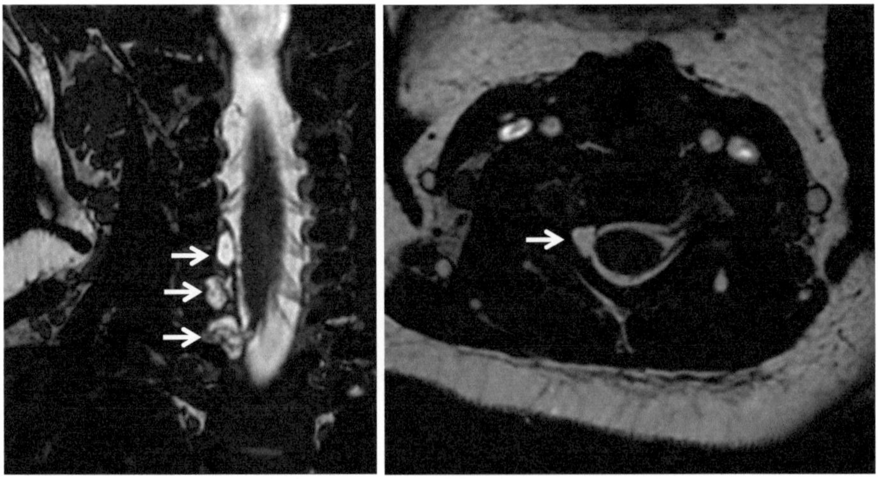

Fig. 17.11 MRI of the spinal roots, coronal T2-weighted image sequence shows pseudomeningocoeles involving the right C6, C7 and C8 nerve root levels (*white arrows*). Axial T2-weighted image at the *right* C6 level confirms root avulsion as no nerve roots can be seen compared to the unaffected *left side*. With severe traction injuries the nerve root is pulled into the intervertebral foramina with associated meningeal tearing leading to nerve root edema and pseudomeningoceles

extensors; Group III, C5-T1 complete paralysis of the limb and; Group IV, complete paralysis of the limb with Horner's syndrome.

Although clinical examination may provide insight into the levels involved, it is not possible to initially differentiate neuropraxia, axonotmesis or neurotmesis. The true severity of NBPP becomes more apparent in 3–6 months after birth. Infants with moderate-to-severe OBPP due to axonotmesis or neurotmesis present a challenge to clinicians and surgeons. Care must be taken not to operate in cases where nerve regeneration is underway, however, yet similarly, surgery should be offered as soon as it becomes clear that spontaneous recovery is unlikely. There is substantial evidence that early repair of nerve lesions improves results [82]. Infants with profound proximal arm weakness at 3 months and are unlikely to show any meaningful spontaneous recovery may be offered early surgical intervention (i.e., microsurgical reconstruction and nerve transfer) [83] since infants with severe biceps weakness (i.e., inability to flex elbow against gravity) at 3 months show a high probability of severe residual neurological deficits [79, 84].

Nerve conduction studies and electromyography may be used to assist decision-making with regard to surgery, however, several limitations are noted. EMG of infant muscle can provide an overly optimistic view of axonal connectivity. There are several reasons for the discrepancy between EMG findings and clinical outcome in some infants. First, the muscle fiber diameter of a 3-month old infant is only 17 μm^3 which is more than threefold smaller than the adult muscle fiber diameter. Due to this smaller cross-sectional area, the muscle of an infant contains 11 times more motor units compared to an adult. An EMG needle will therefore "listen" to the activity of many more motor units when determining the recruitment pattern of a muscle (an indicator of the connection between nerve and muscle). Thus, EMG in an infant may over-estimate how well the actual connection and eventual recruitment pattern will be when the muscles enlarge and mature [85]. Furthermore, the disruption of nerve fibers (particularly sensory fibers) at a critical stage of development may increase the likelihood of developmental apraxia caused by impaired motor programming in early infancy [86].

Nerve conduction studies (NCS) can also provide important information. However, this testing is also more challenging in infants due to several technical factors. Infants typically have more subcutaneous fat, which insulates nerves. This can make the test less sensitive and more difficult to perform due to the need for higher stimulation intensity to elicit certain responses. The shorter limbs of infants also increase the potential for artifact, since co-stimulation of adjacent nerves can occur when stimulus intensity is increased. Overall, NCS/EMG can be more difficult to interpret in NBPP. Despite these limitations, there remains a role for NCS. A recent study found that when bilateral NCS were completed in infants with unilateral NBPP between day 10 and 60 of life, the side-to-side difference in motor amplitude correlated with clinical outcome [87]. It is important for EMG studies in these infants to be performed in an EMG laboratory where the personnel are experienced with examining children.

Case Example

A 3–1/2 month old girl was evaluated for right arm weakness after a difficult delivery. Her primiparous mother had gestational diabetes in the final month of pregnancy. Delivery was via an induced vaginal birth at 39 weeks. Vacuum assistance was required for delivery. Shoulder dystocia occurred and the infant was vigorous at birth with no resuscitation required. Birth weight was 9 lb., 1 oz. There was no clavicular or humeral fracture at birth. However, decreased movement of her right arm was noted after birth. Parents recall that initially she had essentially no movement of her right arm and hand, including very little grasp with her right hand in the first few days of life. Her right hand strength improved in the first several weeks but no change was noted in proximal arm movement. She was bringing her left arm to her mouth but was not doing the same on the right. When maintained in a relaxed supine position, she tended to keep her right elbow extended and her right wrist and fingers flexed in the characteristic waiter's tip position. Physical exam was notable for weakness of her right proximal upper extremity. She showed no clinically evident active movement of her right deltoid, biceps or triceps. She showed partial antigravity activity of wrist extension and finger extension; however, she could not fully extend her right arm or fingers. Right finger flexion was preserved. No contractures were noted. EMG confirmed little to no axonal connection to upper-trunk innervated muscles. Her right deltoid and triceps revealed no discernable motor units; however, abundant fibrillation potentials and positive sharp waves were seen. The right biceps and infraspinatus each displayed one or two motor units. MRI spine and brachial plexus confirmed root avulsions at C6, C7, and C8 (Fig. 17.11). Subsequent surgical exploration and brachial plexus reconstruction surgery confirmed this finding and also noted that the C5 nerve root entered a neuroma in continuity.

Lumbosacral Plexus Anatomy

The lumbosacral plexus is formed by the ventral rami of the lumbar and sacral spine (L1 to S4) and gives rise to several large nerves in the pelvis and lower extremities (Fig. 17.9). The lumbosacral plexus serves as a pathway for all sensory and motor connections extending into the lower extremities.

Clinical and Electrodiagnostic Considerations

Lumbosacral plexopathy can be a source of severe disability for affected children. Symptoms may include weakness, sensory loss, and/or debilitating pain. Functional impairment can be severe as independent ambulation may be lost. Neurological abnormality associated with lesions in the lumbosacral plexus almost always extend well beyond the distribution of a single nerve root or peripheral nerve and symptoms can be quite debilitating. Careful examination of proximal hip muscles (e.g., gluteus medius, gluteus maximus) is essential at differentiating lower plexus lesions from isolated sciatic neuropathy. Similarly, evaluating hip adductor muscles can be important for differentiating a lumbar plexus lesion from an isolated femoral neuropathy. Electrodiagnostic testing principles are similar to what has been described for the brachial plexus. Namely, loss of sensory and motor amplitudes are expected in plexus lesions which may be an important differentiating feature from a proximal, preganglionic nerve root injury such as compressive radiculopathies where sensory responses remain intact. Compared to the upper extremity, there are fewer sensory and motor nerves easily accessible for study in the leg. As such, careful electromyography is critical for localizing lesions and directing imaging studies in the lower extremities.

Etiology of Lumbosacral Plexopathy in Children

Lumbosacral plexopathies are exceedingly rare in childhood. Similar to the brachial plexus, lumbosacral plexopathies can result from a range of genetic and acquired conditions. Most cases will result from traumatic injury [88], including rare reports of birth related injury attributed to precipitous breech delivery [89]. The lumbosacral plexus lies in close proximity to pelvic muscles and viscera making it susceptible to compression from pelvic malignancy [90]. Children with neurocutaneous syndromes are at risk of intrinsic, expansive nerve tumors such as neurofibromas and malignant nerve sheath tumors [91]. Inflammatory disorders, infection, and post-infectious plexitis [92, 93] have also been reported.

MR imaging and ultrasonography have proven to be very helpful at imaging the brachial and lumbosacral plexus in infants and children [94, 95]. Despite these advances there is still an important role for electrodiagnostic testing in infants and children. Electromyography is essential for localizing and narrowing the field of likely injury, thereby enabling the surgeon to focus on a smaller area for exploration and thus reducing the duration of anesthetic required. Moreover, electromyography can provide important information as to whether anatomical abnormalities seen on imaging (e.g., foramen narrowing, mild disc bulge) are or are not causing functional impingement of nerve roots. Finally, it plays an essential role in decision making and prognostication by providing information regarding axonal continuity and nerve regeneration that cannot be obtained by imaging studies alone.

References

1. Dumitru D, Zwarts M. Radiculopathies. In: Dumitru D, Amato AA, Zwarts MJ, editors. Electrodiagnostic medicine. Philadelphia, PA: Hanley & Belfus Inc.; 2002. p. 713–76.
2. Jones HR. Plexus and nerve root lesions. In: Jones HR, Bolton CF, Harper CM, editors. Pediatric clinical electromyography. Philadelphia, PA: Lippincott-Raven Publishers; 1996. p. 123–69.

3. Vialle R, Charosky S, Padovani JP, Rigault P, Glorion C. Surgical treatment of high-grade lumbosacral spondylolisthesis in childhood, adolescent and young adult by the 'double-plate' technique: a past experience. Eur Spine J. 2006;15(8):1210.
4. Guo J, Chen D, Cho D. Child hemivertebra combined with butterfly vertebra of the cervicothoracic junction mimicking traumatic burst fracture. Spine J. 2016;16(2):45–6.
5. Kiernan J. 2016. Distribution of spinal nerve roots and cutaneous nerves. http://publish.uwo.ca/~jkiernan/dermator.gif. Accessed 24 Oct 2016.
6. Foerster O. The dermatomes in man. Brain. 1933;56:1–39.
7. Radhakrishnan K, Litchy W, O'Fallon W. Epidemiology of cervical radiculopathy. A population-based study from Rochester, Minnesota, 1976 through 1990. Brain. 1994;117(2):325–35.
8. Schoenfeld A, Laughlin M, Bader J, Bono C. Characterization of the Incidence and Risk Factors for the Development of Lumbar Radiculopathy. J Spinal Disord Tech. 2012;25:163–7.
9. Imagama S, Wakao N, Ando K, Tauchi R, Tsuboi A, Ishiguro N. Conservative treatment for cervical radiculopathy due to extensive foraminal disc calcification in children. J Bone Joint Surg Am. 2011;93(16):e93 1–5. doi:10.2106/JBJS.K.00053.
10. Tsutsumi S, Yasumoto Y, Ito M. Idiopathic intervertebral disk calcification in childhood: a case report and review of literature. Childs Nerv Syst. 2011;27:1045–51.
11. Wong CC, Pereira B, Pho RW. Cervical disc calcification in children. A longterm review. Spine. 1992;17:139–44.
12. Coventry MB. Calcification in a cervical disc with anterior protrusion and dysphagia. A case report. J Bone Joint Surg Am. 1970;52:1463–6.
13. Dai L, Ye H, Qian Q. The natural history of cervical disc calcification in children. J Bone Joint Surg. 2004;86:467–72.
14. Mathern G, Batzdorf U. Grisel's syndrome. Cervical spine clinical, pathologic, and neurologic manifestations. Clin Orthop Relat Res. 1989;244:131–46.
15. Nozaki F, Kusunoki T, Tomoda Y. Grisel syndrome as a complication of Kawasaki disease: a case report and review of the literature. Eur J Pediatr. 2013;172:119–21.
16. Bond A, Zada G, Bowen I, McComb J, Krieger M. Spinal arachnoid cysts in the pediatric population: report of 31 cases and a review of the literature: clinical article. J Neurosurg Pediatr. 2012;9:432–41.
17. Qi W, Zhao L, Fang J, Chang X, Xu Y. Clinical characteristics and treatment strategies for idiopathic spinal extradural arachnoid cysts: a single-center experience. Acta Neurochir. 2015;157:539–45.
18. Sairyo K, Sakai T, Amari R, Yasui N. Causes of radiculopathy in young athletes with spondylolysis. Am J Sports Med. 2010;38:357.
19. Webb J, Svien H, Kennedy R. Protruded lumbar intervertebral discs in children. JAMA. 1954;154:1153–4.
20. Gennuso R, Humphreys R, Hoffman H, Hendrick E, Drake J. Lumbar intervertebral disk disease in the pediatric population. Pediatr Neurosurg. 1992;18:282–6.
21. Kurihara A, Kataoka O. Lumbar disc herniation in children and adolescents. A review of 70 operated cases and their minimum 5-year follow-up studies. Spine (Phila Pa 1976). 1980;5:443–51.
22. Bradbury N, Wilson L, Mulholland R. Adolescent disc protrusions. A longterm follow-up of surgery compared to chymopapain. Spine (Phila Pa 1976). 1996;21:372–7.
23. Lee J, Ernestus R, Schröder R, Klug N. Histological study of lumbar intervertebral disc herniation in adolescents. Acta Neurochir. 2000;142(10):1107.
24. Kumar R, Kumar V, Das NK, Behari S, Mahapatra AK. Adolescent lumbar disc disease: findings and outcome. Childs Nerv Syst. 2007;23:1295–9.
25. Kuh S, Kim Y, Cho Y, Yoon Y, Jin B, Kim K. Surgical treatments for lumbar disc disease in adolescent patients; chemonucleolysis/microsurgical discectomy/PLIF with cages. Yonsei Med J. 2005;46:125–32.
26. Wang H, Cheng J, Xiao H, Li C, Zhou Y. Adolescent lumbar disc herniation: Experience from a large minimally invasive treatment centre for lumbar degenerative disease in Chongqing, China. Clin Neurol Neurosurg. 2013;115:1415–9.

27. Mattila V, Saarni L, Parkkari J, Koivusilta L, Rimpelä A. Early risk factors for lumbar discectomy: an 11-year follow-up of 57,408 adolescents. Eur Spine J. 2008;17:1317–23.
28. Song X, Choi J, Rao C, Nallu S, Nicastri AD. Primary Ewing sarcoma of lumbar spine with massive intraspinal extension. Pediatr Neurol. 2008;38:58–60.
29. Zileli M, Cagli S, Basdemir G, Erashin Y. Osteoid osteomas and osteoblastomas of the spine. Neurosurg Focus. 2003;15(5):E5.
30. Coffin C, Swanson P, Wick M, Dehner L. Chordoma in childhood and adolescence. A clinicopathologic analysis of 12 cases. Arch Pathol Lab Med. 1993;117:927–33.
31. Pollack I, Colak A, Fitz C. Surgical management of spinal cord compression from plexiform neurofibromas in patients with neurofibromatosis 1. Neurosurgery. 1998;43:248–55.
32. Salvant J, Young H. Giant intrasacral schwannoma: an unusual cause of lumbosacral radiculopathy. Surg Neurol. 1994;41:411–3.
33. Padovani R, Cavallo M, Tonelli M. Histiocytosis-X: a rare cause of radiculopathy. Neurosurgery. 1998;22:1077–9.
34. Chiba K, Toyama Y, Matsumoto M, Maruiwa H, Watanabe M, Nishizawa T. Intraspinal cyst communicating with the intervertebral disc in the lumbar spine: discal cyst. Spine. 2001;26(19):2112–8.
35. Aydin S, Abuzayed B, Yildirim H, Bozkus H, Vural M. Discal cysts of the lumbar spine: report of five cases and review of the literature. Eur Spine J. 2010;19:1621–6. doi:10.1007/s00586-010-1395-9.
36. McMillan HJ, Kang PB, Jones HR, Darras BT. Childhood chronic inflammatory demyelinating polyradiculoneuropathy: combined analysis of a large cohort and eleven published series. Neuromuscul Disord. 2013;23:103–11.
37. Duggins A, McLeod J, Pollard J, Davies L, Yang F, Thompson E. Spinal root and plexus hypertrophy in chronic inflammatory demyelinating polyneuropathy. Brain. 1999;122:1383–90.
38. Ginsberg L, Platts A, Thomas P. Chronic inflammatory demyelinating polyneuropathy mimicking a lumbar spinal stenosis syndrome. J Neurol Neurosurg Psychiatry. 1995;59:189–91.
39. Schady W, Goulding P, Lecky B, King R, Smith C. Massive nerve root enlargement in chronic inflammatory demyelinating polyneuropathy. J Neurol Neurosurg Psychiatry. 1996;61:636–40.
40. Haubrich C, Krings T, Senderek J, Zuchner S, Schroder JM, Noth J. Hypertrophic nerve roots in a case of Roussy-Levy syndrome. Neuroradiology. 2002;44:933–7.
41. Choi SK, Bowers RP, Buckthal PE. MR imaging in hypertrophic neuropathy: a case of hereditary motor and sensory neuropathy, type I (Charcot-Marie-Tooth). Clin Imaging. 1990;14:204–7.
42. Yikilmaz A, Doganay S, Gumus H, Per H, Kumandas S, Coskun A. Magnetic resonance imaging of childhood Guillain-Barré syndrome. Childs Nerv Syst. 2010;26(8):1103–8.
43. Borgstein BJ, Koster PA, Portegies P, Peeters FL. Myelography in patients with acquired immuno deficiency syndrome. Indications and results. Neuroradiology. 1989;326(30):31.
44. Baumann M, Birnbacher R, Koch J, Strobl R, Rostásy K. Uncommon manifestations of neuroborreliosis in children. Eur J Paediatr Neurol. 2010;14:274–7.
45. De Fine OB, Buhl M. Herpes simplex virus and Guillain-Barré. Br Med J. 1975;1:192–3.
46. Sohal A, Riordan A, Malleaw M, Solomon T, Kneen R. Successful treatment of cytomegalovirus polyradiculopathy in a 9-year-old child with congenital human immunodeficiency virus infection. J Child Neurol. 2009;24:215–8.
47. Braverman D, Ku A, Nagler W. Herpes zoster polyradiculopathy. Arch Phys Med Rehabil. 1997;78:880–2.
48. Scelsa S, Herskovitz S, Berger A. A predominantly motor polyradiculopathy of Lyme disease. Muscle Nerve. 1996;19:780–3.
49. Lin J, Martel W. Cross-sectional imaging of peripheral nerve sheath tumors: characteristic signs on CT, MR imaging, and sonography. AJR Am J Roentgenol. 2001;76:75–82.
50. Grisariu S, Avni B, Batchelor TT, van den Bent MJ, Bokstein F, Schiff D. Neurolymphomatosis: an International Primary CNS Lymphoma Collaborative Group report. Blood. 2010;115:5005–11.

51. Smith JK, Matheus MG, Castillo M. Imaging manifestations of neurosarcoidosis. AJR Am J Roentgenol. 2004;182:289–95.
52. Vazquez E, Lucaya J, Castellote A, Piqueras J, Sains P, Olive T, Sanchez-Toledo J, Ortega JJ. Neuroimaging in pediatric leukemia and lymphoma: differential diagnosis. Radiographics. 2002;22:1411–28.
53. Yamamoto T, Fujita I, Kurosaka M, Mizuno K. Sacral radiculopathy secondary to multicentric osteosarcoma. Spine. 2001;26:1729–32.
54. Blumenfeld H. Major plexuses and peripheral nerves. In: Blumenfeld H, editor. Neuroanatomy through clinical cases. Sunderland, MA: Sinauer Associated Inc Publishers; 2002. p. 338–65.
55. Ferrante MA, Wilbourn AJ. Plexopathies. In: Levin K, Luders HO, editors. Philadelphia, PA: WB Saunders Co; 2000. p. 201–14.
56. Pöyhiä T, Lamminen A, Peltonen J, Willamo P, Nietosvaara Y. Treatment of shoulder sequelae in brachial plexus birth injury. Acta Orthop. 2011;82:482–8.
57. Huang YG, Chen L, Gu YD, Yu GR. Histopathological basis of Horner's syndrome in obstetric brachial plexus palsy differs from that in adult's brachial plexus injury. Muscle Nerve. 2008;37:632–7.
58. McMillan HJ, Yang M, Jones HR. Brachial plexopathy and nonaccidental injury: role of the neurologist. J Child Neurol. 2010;25:1–3.
59. Tsairis P, Dyck PJ, Mulder DW. Natural history of brachial plexus neuropathy: report of 99 patients. Arch Neurol. 1972;27:109–17.
60. McDonald DG, Farrell MA, McMenamin JB. Focal upper limb neuropathy in a child. Eur J Paediatr Neurol. 2000;4:283–7.
61. Dionne A, Brunet D. A case of Lewis-Sumner Syndrome with conduction abnormalities only in the brachial plexus and roots. Muscle Nerve. 2006;34:489–93.
62. Dunn HG, Daube JR, Gomez MR. Heredofamilial brachial plexus neuropathy (hereditary neuralgic amyotrophy with brachial predilection) in childhood. Dev Med Child Neurol. 1978;20:109–17.
63. Klein CJ, Dyck PJ, Friedenberg SM, et al. Inflammation and neuropathic attacks in hereditary brachial plexus neuropathy. J Neurol Neurosurg Psychiatry. 2002;73:45–50.
64. Verhagen WI, Gabreels-Festen AA, van Wensen PJ, Joosten EM, Vingerhoets HM, Gabreels FJ, de Graaf R. Hereditary neuropathy with liability to pressure palsies: a clinical electroneurophysiological and morphological study. J Neurol Sci. 1993;116:176–84.
65. Mouton P, Tardieu S, Gouider R, Birouk N, Maisonobe T, Dubourg O, Brice A, LeGuern E, Bouche P. Spectrum of clinical and electrophysiologic features in HNPP patients with the 17p11.2 deletion. Neurology. 1999;52:1440–6.
66. Tierney TS, Tierney BJ, Rosenberg AE, Krishnamoorthy KS, Butler WE. Infantile myofibromatosis: a nontraumatic cause of neonatal brachial plexus palsy. Pediatr Neurol. 2008;39:276–8.
67. Alfonso I, Papazian O, Prieto G, Alfonso DT, Melnick SJ. Neoplasm as a cause of brachial plexus palsy in neonates. Pediatr Neurol. 2000;22:309–11.
68. Mehta SH, Gonik B. Neonatal brachial plexus injury: obstetrical factors and neonatal management. J Pediatr Rehabil Med. 2011;4:113–8.
69. Gilbert WM, Nesbitt TS, Danielsen B. Associated factors in 1611 cases of brachial plexus injury. Obstet Gynecol. 1999;93:536–40.
70. McFarland LV, Raskin M, Daling JR, Benedetti TJ. Erb/Duchenne's palsy: a consequence of fetal macrosomia and method of delivery. Obstet Gynecol. 1986;68:784–8.
71. Dunn DW, Engle WA. Brachial plexus palsy: intrauterine onset. Pediatr Neurol. 1985;1:367–9.
72. Gherman RB, Ouzounian JG, Goodwin TM. Brachial plexus palsy: an in utero injury? Am J Obstet Gynecol. 1999;180:1303–7.
73. Gherman RB, Goodwin TM, Ouzounian JG, Miller DA, Paul RH. Brachial plexus palsy associated with cesarean section: an in utero injury? Am J Obstet Gynecol. 1997;177:1162–4.
74. Foad SL, Mehlman CT, Ying J. The epidemiology of neonatal brachial plexus palsy in the United States. J Bone Joint Surg Am. 2008;90:1258–64.

75. Hoeksma AF, ter Steeg AM, Nelissen RG, van Ouwerkerk WJ, Lankhorst GJ, de Jong BA. Neurological recovery in obstetric brachial plexus injuries: an historical cohort study. Dev Med Child Neurol. 2004;46:76–83.
76. Gordon M, Rich H, Deutschberger J, Green M. The immediate and long-term outcome of obstetric birth trauma. Brachial plexus paralysis. Am J Obstet Gynecol. 1973;117:51–6.
77. Sjoberg I, Erichs K, Bjerre I. Cause and effect of obstetric (neonatal) brachial plexus palsy. Acta Paediatr Scand. 1988;77:357–64.
78. Greenwald AG, Schute PC, Shiveley JL. Brachial plexus birth palsy: a 10-year report on the incidence and prognosis. J Pediatr Orthop. 1984;4:689–92.
79. Waters PM. Comparison of the natural history, the outcome of microsurgical repair, and the outcome of operative reconstruction in brachial plexus birth palsy. J Bone Joint Surg Am. 1999;81:649–59.
80. Narakas AO. Injuries to the brachial plexus. In: Bora FW, editor. The pediatric upper extremity: diagnosis and management. Philadelphia: WB Saunders; 1986. p. 247–58.
81. Birch R, Bonney G, Wynn Parry CB. Birth lesions of the brachial plexus. In: Surgical disorders of the peripheral nerves. Philadelphia, PA: WB Saunders Co; 1998. p. 209–33.
82. Malessy MJ, Pondaag W. Nerve surgery for neonatal brachial plexus palsy. J Pediatr Rehabil Med. 2011;4:141–8.
83. Narakas AO. Thoughts on neurotization or nerve transfers in irreparable nerve lesions. Clin Plast Surg. 1984;11:153–9.
84. Fisher DM, Borschel GH, Curtis CG, Clarke HM. Evaluation of elbow flexion as a predictor of outcome in obstetrical brachial plexus palsy. Plast Reconstr Surg. 2007;120:1585–90.
85. Van Dijk JG, Malessy MJ, Stegeman DF. Why is the electromyogram in obstetric brachial plexus lesions overly optimistic? Muscle Nerve. 1998;21:260–1.
86. Brown T, Cupido C, Scarfone H, Pape K, Galea V, McComas A. Developmental apraxia arising from neonatal brachial plexus palsy. Neurology. 2000;55:24–30.
87. Heise CO, Siqueira MG, Martins RS, Gherpelli JL. Motor nerve-conduction studies in obstetric brachial plexopathy for a selection of patients with a poor outcome. J Bone Joint Surg Am. 2009;91:1729–37.
88. Egel RT, Cueva JP, Adair RL. Posttraumatic childhood lumbosacral plexus neuropathy. Pediatr Neurol. 1995;12:62–4.
89. Hope EE, Bodensteiner JB, Thong N. Neonatal lumbar plexus injury. Arch Neurol. 1985;42:94–5.
90. Planner A, Donaghy M, Moore N. Causes of lumbrosacral plexopathy. Clin Radiol. 2006;61(12):987–95.
91. Pratap A, Nepal P, Agrawal A, Singh M, Pandey S. Giant malignant nerve sheath tumor of lumbosacral plexus with intraspinal extension in a child with neurofibromatosis type 1. Pediatr Neurosurg. 2007;43(5):410–3.
92. Sander JE, Sharp FR. Lumbosacral plexus neuritis. Neurology. 1981;31:470–3.
93. Awerbuch G, Nigro M, Dabrowski E, Levin J. Childhood lumbrosacral plexus neuropathy. Pediatr Neurol. 1989;5(5):314–6.
94. Birchansky S, Altman N. Imaging the brachial plexus and peripheral nerves in infants and children. Semin Pediatr Neurol. 2000;7(1):15–25.
95. Kirchmair L, Enna B, Mitterschiffthaler G, Morigal B, Greher M, Marhofer P, Kapral S, Gassner I. Lumbar plexus in children, a sonographic study and its relevance to pediatric regional anesthesia. Anesthesiology. 2004;101(2):445–50.

Chapter 18
Acquired and Hereditary Neuropathies

Monique M. Ryan and Hugh J. McMillan

Introduction

Peripheral neuropathies result from dysfunction of one or more components of the peripheral nervous system including direct damage to axons or myelin, or damage to Schwann cells which are responsible for myelinating segments of peripheral nerves. Compared to adults, peripheral neuropathies are less common in childhood and typically present with weakness, gross motor delay, gait abnormalities and/or sensory abnormalities.

Genetic neuropathies account for 30–70% of all pediatric peripheral nerve disease, thus it is not entirely clear whether inherited or acquired neuropathies are more common in childhood. The prevalence of hereditary peripheral neuropathy (Charcot-Marie-Tooth (CMT) disease) is approximately 1 in 2,500 [1–3] and is typically characterized by symmetrical neurologic deficits which slowly progress over time. Acquired neuropathies in childhood may be caused by a variety of insults, including trauma, but are most often inflammatory in origin, and can be either acute or chronic in their temporal course. In contrast to adults, children rarely have chronic neuropathies related to systemic diseases such as diabetes or side-effects of medication. This chapter will provide a practical approach to the clinical and electrodiagnostic evaluation of the child with suspected neuropathy.

M.M. Ryan, M Med, BS, FRACP (✉)
Murdoch Childrens Research Institute, The Royal Children's Hospital,
University of Melbourne, Melbourne, VIC, Australia
e-mail: monique.ryan@rch.org.au

H.J. McMillan, MD, MSc, FRCPC, FAAN (✉)
Division of Neurology, Children's Hospital of Eastern Ontario, University of Ottawa,
Ottawa, ON, Canada
e-mail: hmcmillan@cheo.on.ca

© Springer International Publishing AG 2017

H.J. McMillan, P.B. Kang (eds.), *Pediatric Electromyography*,
DOI 10.1007/978-3-319-61361-1_18

Approach to the Childhood Neuropathies

The evaluation of a child with suspected neuropathy requires an organized, stepwise approach which takes into consideration the broad spectrum of metabolic, genetic and acquired disorders that can give rise to peripheral neuropathies. The clinical history is helpful, giving an idea of the age and distribution of onset of symptoms. Parents and children rarely describe weakness, as such, at presentation; rather, they describe functional difficulties such as tripping, difficulty with running or climbing stairs, and changes in appearance of their child's feet or ankles. Thus, the physical examination is key to neuroanatomical localization in such children. In the genetic neuropathies, sensory changes usually consist of 'negative' phenomena; numbness, loss of joint position sense and predisposition to trophic injuries. In acquired neuropathies 'positive' sensory phenomena—paraesthesia, pain, and/or burning sensations—often predominate. With a detailed history, physical examination, electrophysiological testing and as appropriate, biochemical testing, genetic testing, cerebrospinal fluid analysis, and/or neuroimaging studies, clinicians will increase the diagnostic yield in this broad and complex array of diseases (Table 18.1).

Anatomical Site(s) Involved

Children with suspected neuropathy will often show clinical findings in other areas of the central or peripheral nervous system. By identifying abnormalities elsewhere along the neuraxis, one can obtain important clues to narrow the differential diagnosis and direct investigations.

Proper localization mandates a detailed neurologic examination with characterisation of the pattern of weakness, the extent and location of sensory loss, changes in the deep tendon reflexes, and presence of cerebellar signs such as ataxia and dysdiadochokinesia.

Concomitant central nervous system involvement, including cognitive deficits or regression, seizures and/or psychiatric symptoms may point to systemic, genetic or metabolic causes of neuropathy [4, 5]. Several rare hereditary disorders of metabolism present during infancy or early childhood with peripheral nerve involvement and varying degrees of involvement of the central nervous system. These conditions include Krabbe disease, metachromatic leukodystrophy, peroxisomal disorders, Cockayne syndrome, giant axonal neuropathy, infantile neuroaxonal dystrophy and hereditary tyrosinemia. Central nervous system symptoms often overshadow the concomitant peripheral neuropathy in these conditions, but identification and characterization of the neuropathy can be helpful in narrowing the differential diagnosis. MRI of the brain is indicated in such cases, with additional metabolic testing to investigate for leukodystrophies, mitochondrial disorders (e.g., *POLG* mutations), peroxisomal disorders, Brown-Vialetto-Van Laere (BVVL) syndrome and/or toxin exposure.

Table 18.1 Approach to the child with suspected peripheral neuropathy

1.	*Anatomical site(s) that are clinically involved*:
–	Brain
–	Cranial nerve(s)
–	Spine
–	Nerve plexus
–	Sensory ganglia
–	Nerve root(s)
–	Motor neuron
–	Peripheral nerve(s)
2.	*Non-neurological findings*
–	Non-neurological organ involvement
–	Concomitant diseases (auto-immune disease, cardiac disease)
–	Toxin/medication exposures
–	Family history, consanguinity
3.	*Age at symptom onset*
4.	*Time course of neuropathy: acute, sub-acute or chronic*
5.	*Pattern of peripheral nerve involvement*
–	Polyneuropathy
–	Mononeuropathy
–	Mononeuritis multiplex
6.	*Peripheral nerve type(s) and fiber size(s) involved*:
–	Motor
–	Sensory, large fiber (vibration, proprioception, two-point discrimination)
–	Sensory, small fiber (pain, temperature, light touch)
–	Autonomic
7.	*Neurophysiologic features*
–	Axonal versus demyelinating
–	Uniform versus non-uniform

Pertinent family history can provide further insight, including information pertaining to inheritance patterns. In some cases a focused examination of family members can be helpful in children with suspected neuropathies.

When cranial neuropathies are the first or dominant manifestation of a peripheral neuropathy, the differential diagnosis may often be narrowed accordingly. Diphtheria remains an important world-wide cause of acquired neuropathy with outbreaks reported [6]. Patients initially present with pharyngitis that is often associated with a grayish-white pseudomembrane in the throat. About 15% of patients develop neurological complications with the first neurological symptoms being bulbar dysfunction caused by diphtheria toxin-mediated cranial nerve paralysis. Almost all patients who develop a demyelinating polyneuropathy will have preceding cranial nerve involvement, making this an important diagnostic clue [6]. Other infectious causes including Lyme disease, which often presents with a unilateral facial nerve palsy and less commonly with other cranial nerve involvement [7, 8]. Children with the Miller-Fisher variant of Guillain-Barré syndrome will present with a triad of ophthalmoplegia, ataxia and areflexia [9]. It is important to note that cranial neuropathies may be present in traditional cases of Guillain-Barré syndrome; it is only when the cranial nerves constitute the predominant region of peripheral nerve involvement that Miller-Fisher syndrome should be considered.

Spinal cord involvement is differentiated from peripheral neuropathies by the well demarcated sensory level and presence of sphincter (bowel, bladder) dysfunction. Peripheral neuropathies by contrast show a degree of nerve injury that is proportion to axon length, where longer axons show more severe changes relatively earlier in the disease course. As a result, weakness and sensory loss resulting from peripheral neuropathy are initially seen in the distal lower extremities, though patchy radicular involvement may occur in the setting of inflammatory neuropathies, giving rise to a mixed distal/myotomal pattern in some patients. Deep tendon reflexes are typically depressed or absent in peripheral neuropathies, while the plantar responses remain flexor. Extensor plantar responses in the setting of depressed or absent deep tendon reflexes reflect spinal or cerebral involvement, as seen in Friedreich ataxia and metachromatic leukodystrophy.

Non-neurological Findings

Non-neurological symptoms and signs can provide the clinician with important clues to the diagnosis of many peripheral neuropathies. Involvement of organs such as the liver, spleen, heart, skin and lymphatic tissues increases the likelihood of specific underlying diseases in children with polyneuropathy. The general physical examination should include the skin, abdomen and cardiorespiratory systems, looking for clues suggestive of storage disorders or other inborn errors of metabolism. Non-neurological symptoms and signs suggestive of the aetiology of pediatric neuropathies are summarised in Table 18.2.

Autonomic symptoms—cardiac arrhythmias, hypotension or hypertension, abnormal sweating and trophic skin changes, bowel and bladder dysfunction—may be seen in specific acquired and genetic neuropathies. One classic example, described in Chap. 17, is the Horner syndrome seen in cases of traumatic nerve root avulsion at the neck/shoulder.

Age at Symptom Onset

Age of first symptom onset is a helpful clue to determining the underlying cause of childhood neuropathies (Table 18.3). Many hereditary or metabolic causes of polyneuropathy are symptomatic from birth, causing hypotonia, hypo- or areflexia,

Table 18.2 Non-neurological findings suggestive of causation of pediatric neuropathies

Sign/symptom		
Ocular	Optic atrophy	Mitochondrial disease (Friedreich ataxia, OPA1), CMT2A, CMT4A
	Retinis pigmentosa	Peroxisomal diseases, mitochondrial disorders, ataxia with vitamin E deficiency
	Ophthalmoplegia	Mitochondrial disorders, Miller Fisher syndrome
Ear	Hearing loss	Brown-Vialetto-van Laere syndrome, CMT1B, CMTX, Cockayne syndrome
Throat	Pharyngitis	Diphtheria
	Discoloured, enlarged tonsils	Tangier disease
Skin	Hypopigmentation	Leprosy
	Hyperpigmentation	Adrenoleukodystrophy (buccal), diabetes (acanthosis nigricans)
	Angiokeratomas	Fabry disease
	Purpura	Henoch-Schonein purpura
	Discoid rashes	Systemic lupus erythematosus
	Photosensitivity	Systemic lupus erythematosus, Cockayne syndrome, xeroderma pigmentosum
	Desquamation	Arsenic poisoning
	Nail changes (Mees' lines)	Arsenic and thallium poisoning
Hair	Alopecia	Thallium poisoning
	Curly, kinking hair	Giant axonal neuropathy
Cardiac	Cardiomyopathy	Mitochondrial disorders, Friedreich ataxia, ataxia with vitamin E deficiency
	Conduction defects	Mitochondrial disorders, glue/solvent abuse
Respiratory	Diaphragmatic weakness	Spinal muscular atrophy with respiratory distress, Brown-Vialetto-van Laere syndrome
Gastro-intestinal	Abdominal pain	Mitochondrial disorders, Fabry disease, arsenic and lead poisoning
	Pseudo-obstruction	Mitochondrial disorders
Systemic	Lymphadenopathy	Lymphoma
	Hepatomegaly	Tyrosinemia, hemophagocytic syndromes
Extremities	Arthritis	Lyme disease, Farber disease
	Xanthomas	Cerebrotendinous xanthomatosis
Cerebral	Cognitive regression	Leukodystrophies, mitochondrial syndromes, peroxisomal disorders, lead toxicity
	Seizures	Merosin-deficient congenital muscular dystrophy

contractures of major joints (arthrogryposis multiplex congenita), feeding difficulties, and/or motor or global developmental delay. Early-onset peripheral neuropathies may be isolated (e.g., congenital hypomyelinating neuropathy, which is a severe form of Charcot-Marie-Tooth disease) or can be associated with combined peripheral and central nervous system findings (e.g., Krabbe disease,

Table 18.3 Age and temporal pattern of symptom onset in pediatric neuropathies

	Congenital and infancy	Childhood to adolescent onset
Acute onset	Guillain-Barré syndrome	Guillain-Barré syndrome
	Mitochondrial disorders	Hereditary neuropathy with tendency to pressure palsies (HNPP)
	Brown-Vialetto-van Laere syndrome	Mitochondrial neuropathies
		Toxic neuropathies
		Porphyria
		Diphtheria neuropathy
		Tyrosinemia
		Tangier disease
		Infectious neuropathies
Sub-acute or chronic	Early-onset forms of CMT (Congenital hypomyelinating neuropathy, Déjerine-Sottas disease)	Charcot-Marie-Tooth disease
	Brown-Vialetto-van Laere syndrome	Chronic inflammatory demyelinating neuropathy
	Mitochondrial neuropathies	Brown-Vialetto-van Laere syndrome
	Neuropathies associated with lysosomal storage disorder (Krabbe, MLD)	Mitochondrial neuropathies
	Neuropathies associated with other inborn errors of metabolism/genetic disorders—giant axonal neuropathy, Cockayne disease, merosin-deficient congenital muscular dystrophy, etc.	Friedreich ataxia
	Hereditary sensory and autonomic neuropathies	Neuropathies associated with lysosomal storage disorder (Krabbe, MLD, Fabry disease)
		Neuropathies associated with other inborn errors of metabolism/genetic disorders—giant axonal neuropathy, Cockayne disease, merosin-deficient congenital muscular dystrophy, etc.
		Hereditary sensory and autonomic neuropathies

metachromatic leukodystrophy, giant axonal neuropathy, and mitochondrial diseases). The severity of the disease phenotype can also vary significantly, particularly with inborn errors of metabolism.

Historically, infants with congenital hypo- or demyelinating neuropathies were diagnosed as having Déjerine-Sottas disease or CMT type 3 (CMT3). With advances in molecular genetics it has become apparent that mutations in genes causative of CMT1 (autosomal dominant demyelinating CMT), CMT2 (autosomal dominant axonal CMT), and CMT4 (autosomal recessive CMT) (Table 18.4) are allelic with these severe congenital neuropathies, suggesting that these neuropathies lie in a spectrum of severity rather than in distinct phenotypic categories.

Table 18.4 Classification of Charcot-Marie-Tooth disease

CMT type 1: Autosomal dominant, demyelinating, 60% of all CMT			
CMT1A	*PMP22* duplication	70–80% of all CMT1	Pes cavus
CMT1B	*MPZ* mutation	5–10% of all CMT1	More severe weakness than CMT1A
CMT1C	*LITAF* mutation	1–2% of all CMT1	Early onset
CMT1D	*EGR2* mutation	1–2% of all CMT1	
CMT1E	*PMP22* point mutation	<5% of all CMT1	
CMT1F	*NEFL* mutation	<5% of all CMT1	
HNPP	*PMP22* deletion	<10% of all CMT1	Tendency to pressure palsies
CMT type 2: Autosomal dominant, axonal, 20% of all CMT cases			
CMT2A1	*KIF1B* mutation	Rare	
CMT2A2	*MFN2* mutation	20–30% of CMT2	
CMT2B	*RAB7* mutation	Rare	
CMT2B1	*LMNA* mutation	Rare	
CMT2C	*TRPV4* mutation	Rare	
CMT2D	*GARS* mutation	Rare	
CMT2E	*NEFL* mutation	Rare	
CMT2F	*HSPB1* mutation	Rare	
CMT2G	Unknown	Rare	
CMT2H/K	*GDAP1* mutation	Rare	
CMT2I/J	*MPZ* mutation	Rare	
CMT2L CMT2M DNM2 Rare CMT2N AARS Rare CMT2O DYNC1H1 Rare CMT2P LRSAM1 Rare CMT2Q DHTKD1 Rare CMT2R TRIM2 Rare CMT2S IGHMBP2 Rare CMT2T DNAJB2 Rare CMT2U MARS Rare CMT2V NAGLU Rare CMT2W HARS Rare	*HSPB8* mutation	Rare	
CMT type X: X-linked, intermediate demyelinating/axonal			
CMTX1	*GJB1* (*Cx32*) mutation	90% of CMTX	
CMTX2		<10% of CMTX	
CMTX3		<10% of CMTX	
CMTX5	*PRPS1* mutation	<5% of CMTX	
CMT type 4: Autosomal recessive, total 5–10% of all CMT cases			
CMT4A	*GDAP1* mutation	25% of all CMT4	
CMT4B1	*MTMR2* mutation	Rare	
CMT4B2	*SBF2* mutation	Rare	
CMT4C	*SH3TC2* mutation	Rare	
CMT4D	*NDRG1* mutation	Rare	

Table 18.4 (continued)

CMT4E	*EGR2* mutation	Rare	
CMT4F	*PRX* mutation	Rare	
CMT4H	*FGD4* mutation	Rare	
CMT4J	*FIG4* mutation	Rare	

Time Course of the Neuropathy (Acute, Sub-acute or Chronic)

Polyneuropathies can be subdivided according to how rapidly a patient's symptoms progress (Table 18.3). Acute-onset neuropathies such as Guillain-Barré syndrome, vasculitic neuropathies, trauma, and some metabolic neuropathies (e.g., hereditary tyrosinemia and porphyria) can become symptomatic within days to weeks.

Guillain-Barré syndrome (GBS) is the most common form of acute flaccid paralysis in childhood [10]. GBS is an acute-onset, autoimmune disorder in which T lymphocytes invade peripheral nerves and Schwann cells, activating antibody and complement deposition within these structures [11]. GBS is subclassified, on the basis of its clinical and neurophysiological findings, as acute inflammatory demyelinating polyradiculoneuropathy (AIDP), Miller-Fisher syndrome (MFS), or acute motor axonal neuropathy (AMAN). AIDP is the most common subset of pediatric GBS in the Western world, while well-documented outbreaks of AMAN occur in some Asian countries. MFS occurs in children but is rare in that age group. Children with GBS present with rapidly evolving, symmetrical muscle weakness, often associated with pain or paraesthesias, and with diminished or absent muscle tendon reflexes. Symptoms typically develop over several days. Children may complain of limb pain or paraesthesias, and these may be the primary complaints in some cases. The degree of weakness varies. Respiratory failure and autonomic instability are common complications of pediatric GBS [10].

Metabolic causes of acute weakness include hereditary tyrosinemia and porphyria. Hereditary tyrosinemia is a rare autosomal recessive disease, usually presenting with liver disease and Fanconi syndrome, in which some children have acute neurological crises that may include an acute painful axonal polyneuropathy [12]. Acute intermittent porphyria (AIP) is the most common form of porphyria in childhood, presenting with acute episodes of neuropathy and/or paralysis and respiratory failure, sometimes after exposure to particular medications [13]. AIP may also have a GBS-like presentation in some patients [14].

Infections are an uncommon cause of neuropathy in childhood. A generalized motor-sensory demyelinating polyneuropathy mimicking AIDP is rarely seen after severe throat or skin infections with *Corynebacterium diphtheria*. Diphtheria is very uncommon in countries with universal vaccination programs [6]. Lyme disease follows infection with *Borrelia burgdorferi*, a spirochete spread by the bite of infected *Ixodes* ticks. Aside from the classic facial palsy, peripheral neuropathy is much less common in children than in adults with Lyme disease, and when it occurs it is usually transient [7]. Leprosy, the most common cause of neuropathy worldwide, remains endemic in Southeast Asia and Mexico. Lepromatous neuropathy can be associated with both segmental demyelination and axonal degeneration, and classically presents with a mononeuritis multiplex pattern. Other infections occasionally associated with neuropathy include rabies and trypanosomiasis [15, 16].

Brown-Vialetto-van Laere (BVVL) syndrome and Fazio-Londe disease are clinically overlapping motor neuron diseases involving primarily the lower cranial nerves and presenting with ponto-bulbar palsy, sensorineural deafness and respiratory failure, often in association with upper motor neuron signs. Most cases present in childhood or adolescence. BVVL and Fazio-Londe disease are caused by mutations in riboflavin transporter genes, and are, in some cases, reversible with high-dose riboflavin therapy [17].

Slower onset, more chronic pediatric polyneuropathies include the various forms of Charcot-Marie-Tooth (CMT) disease and chronic inflammatory demyelinating polyneuropathy (CIDP). The presenting symptoms include a combination of gait abnormalities, difficulty running, foot drop and sensory changes. Progression can be insidious, and it may be difficult to pinpoint the precise onset of disease. Many children are first referred because of orthopaedic problems such as toe walking from shortened Achilles tendons, cavus or planus foot deformities, and hammer toes.

Chronic inflammatory demyelinating polyradiculoneuropathy (CIDP) is distinguished from GBS by its more chronic nature; children with CIDP demonstrate progressive or relapsing-remitting weakness, usually with minimal sensory deficits, which evolves over no less than 4 weeks [18]. Occasional children have more rapidly progressive weakness mimicking GBS [19].

CMT, also known as hereditary motor and sensory neuropathy (HMSN), is the most common cause of hereditary polyneuropathy, with disease prevalence (for all CMT types) of approximately 1 in 2500 people [20]. More than 80 genes have been linked to CMT, which is classified on the basis of inheritance pattern and neurophysiologic subtype (Table 18.4).

CMT1 shows predominantly "demyelinating" features (i.e., severe slowing of nerve conduction), while CMT2 shows predominantly "axonal" features (i.e., low-amplitude sensory and motor responses, with normal conduction velocities, accompanied by signs of denervation and/or reinnervation on needle examination). CMT1 accounts for about 60% of all patients with CMT [21]. Six subtypes have been described, involving five genes (Table 18.4). CMT1A, which results from a 1.5-Mb duplication at 17q11.2 involving the peripheral myelin protein 22 (*PMP22*) gene, accounts for 70–80% of all CMT1 cases. CMT1B (5–10% of all CMT1 cases) results from point mutations in the myelin protein zero (*MPZ)* gene. Other CMT1 subtypes are uncommon.

CMT type 2, the predominantly axonal form of CMT disease, also exhibits autosomal dominant inheritance. The overall prevalence of CMT2 is about half that of CMT1. The age of onset varies from childhood to late adulthood [22]. A large number of clinical subtypes, involving a similarly large number of genes, have been described (Table 18.4) [23]. The most common form of CMT, CMT type 2A2, is caused by a mutation in the mitofusin 2 (*MFN2*) gene, an important mediator of mitochondrial fusion. The remaining CMT2 genes are individually rare.

CMTX accounts for 15% of CMT cases [21]. The most common form of CMTX, CMTX1, is caused by mutations in the gap junction beta-1 (*GJB1*) gene. Affected males show a phenotype similar to, or more severe than, CMT1A, although weakness is often of slightly later onset than in CMT1A. Female heterozygotes may be unaffected or may have very mild-moderate clinical symptoms.

Genetic testing for CMT can be complex. Algorithms for sequential gene testing are available but have, to some extent, been overtaken by the increasing availability of gene panels and other forms of next generation sequencing [24]. Nevertheless it is important to remember that mutations in the four genes named above, *PMP22*, *MPZ*, *MFN2*, and *GJB1*, account for the vast majority of cases. Nerve biopsies are rarely required in patients suspected to have CMT, except for rare cases with unusual clinical features raising concern about vasculitic neuropathy, or inflammatory neuropathy superimposed on underlying genetic conditions.

Although all forms of CMT typically demonstrate a chronic disease course, disease onset can be more rapid in some cases, particularly in CMT patients exposed to neurotoxic agents such as chemotherapeutic drugs (e.g., vincristine), or prolonged therapy with certain antibiotics (e.g., metronidazole, nitrofurantoin) [25]. Thus, it is important to consider the potential neurotoxicity of medications that are prescribed for these patients.

Pattern of Peripheral Nerve Involvement

There are three common patterns of peripheral nerve injury; mononeuropathies, mononeuritis multiplex and polyneuropathies.

Mononeuropathies are characterized by sensory and/or motor symptoms and signs limited to the distribution of a single peripheral nerve. Most mononeuropathies in children result from traumatic nerve injury or—less commonly—extrinsic compression, and will be covered in Chap. 20.

Mononeuritis multiplex is defined by sensory and/or motor symptoms involving two or more peripheral nerves, and separated in space and/or time. Hereditary neuropathy with liability to pressure palsies (HNPP) is the most common cause of mononeuritis multiplex in childhood. Other causes of mononeuritis multiplex—such as vasculitic neuropathies—are extremely rare in childhood, though leprosy is a common cause of this pattern of neuropathy in some regions of the world [26].

Polyneuropathy is the third general pattern of peripheral nerve disease. Most polyneuropathies are sensorimotor, symmetrical and length-dependent, affecting the longest nerves first in a "glove and stocking" distribution. The feet are affected first, the upper extremities being unaffected until weakness and sensory loss have extended rostrally from the feet towards the knees. Affected children typically present with gait abnormalities and clumsiness, usually with minimal sensory deficits, with their physical examination showing length-dependent weakness and loss of the deep tendon reflexes. Children with longstanding weakness often develop characteristic foot deformities—pes cavus or (less commonly) pes planus. As symptoms progress, the hands become involved, resulting in loss of grip strength and atrophy of the intrinsic hand muscles.

Autonomic nerve dysfunction can also be seen in some chronic polyneuropathies affecting small-fiber sensory nerves (e.g., diabetic neuropathies), with patients complaining of cold hands and feet, hypo- or hyperhidrosis, and sometimes symptoms related to hypo-or hypertension.

Peripheral Nerve Type(s) and Fiber Size(s) Involved

Although most peripheral nerves are mixed, containing all fiber types, hereditary diseases can show a predilection for specific fiber types. Clinicians must ascertain if the patient's symptoms point to predominant dysfunction of sensory fibers, motor fibers, both sensory and motor fibers (sensorimotor), and/or autonomic fibers.

Sensory-predominant neuropathies can result from large- or small-fiber nerve dysfunction. Standard neurophysiologic testing selectively evaluates the large fiber sensory afferents, which are myelinated and conduct much more quickly than small fiber sensory afferents. Large fiber sensory afferents carry information about vibration, proprioception, and two-point discrimination along large, myelinated Aα fibers. Patients with large fiber sensory dysfunction typically complain of gait unsteadiness and clumsiness, and have difficulty with tasks requiring intact proprioception. A useful physical finding in these patients is the presence of a positive Romberg sign. Pediatric diseases associated with predominantly large-fiber sensory loss include diseases such as the autosomal recessive sensory ataxia of Charlevoix-Saguenay (ARSACS) [27], abetalipoproteinemia [28], and Friedreich ataxia [29].

Small fiber sensory afferents include unmyelinated C-type and poorly myelinated Aδ-type fibers, which carry information about pain, temperature, and light touch. Small fiber sensory disease must be identified on the basis of the clinical history and physical examination, since nerve conduction studies and electromyography cannot evaluate the function of small fibers. Patients with small fiber sensory dysfunction may complain of dysesthesia (spontaneous pain), hyperesthesia (a heightened perception of a stimulus), allodynia (a sensation of pain elicited by a stimulus that is not normally painful), paresthesia (pins and needles), or hypesthesia (decreased perception).

Hereditary sensory and autonomic neuropathies (HSAN) are genetic disorders affecting nerve small fibers, resulting in varying degrees of autonomic fiber dysfunction. Affected patients present with complications of sensory loss, such as painless self-mutilation—for example, that caused by biting their own lips or fingers while teething. Painless finger and foot ulceration may result from pressure injuries or unnoticed trauma. Affected children may have decreased or absent pain from long bone fractures or skin lacerations. Due to their selective involvement of small fibers in sensory nerves, most HSANs are associated with normal neurophysiologic testing, depending on the subtype. Clinicians therefore need to have a high index of suspicion for these conditions. Nerve biopsy may reveal selective loss of specific subpopulations of small unmyelinated nerve fibers. Genetic testing is now commercially available for most of the HSANs.

Autonomic fibers innervate many visceral organs. Autonomic neuropathy can present with a range of clinical symptoms including orthostatic hypotension, syncope, sudomotor symptoms (impaired or excessive sweating), gastrointestinal symptoms (dysphagia, early satiety, nausea, vomiting, decreased appetite and/or weight loss due to impaired gastric emptying, constipation), and urinary symptoms (frequent micturition, impaired bladder emptying). Erectile dysfunction may be seen in adolescent and adult males. Nerve conduction studies cannot be used to evaluate the integrity of autonomic nerves so, similarly to small-fiber sensory neuropathy, autonomic neuropathy is largely diagnosed by a careful history. Assessments of autonomic function, such as tilt table testing and assessment of the quantitative sudomotor axon reflex, can be performed at some highly specialized pediatric centers.

Some disorders give rise to a pure autonomic neuropathy, but in most there is overlap with sensory and/or motor neuropathies. HSAN type 3 (Riley-Day syndrome) is associated with significant autonomic dysfunction in addition to its sensory findings. Dysautonomia is also seen in 20–40% of patients with childhood Guillain-Barré syndrome [10], as well as some toxic neuropathies (e.g., those associated with vincristine and amiodarone).

Motor-predominant neuropathies are uncommon in childhood, in contrast to motor neuron diseases. Most children with painless progressive muscle weakness will eventually be found to have a disease of motor neurons or anterior horn cells, such as spinal muscular atrophy (SMA). Inflammatory nerve disorders, such as the Guillain-Barré syndrome variant acute motor axonal neuropathy (AMAN), show selective involvement of motor nerves. AMAN is more common in some Asian countries and is often associated with antecedent Campylobacter jejuni gastroenteritis [10]. Distal hereditary motor neuropathies (dHMNs) are an emerging group of hereditary disorders affecting motor nerves and showing clinical and genetic overlap with Charcot-Marie-Tooth disease (CMT) type 2, distal spinal muscular atrophies (dSMAs) and hereditary spastic paraplegia (HSP) syndromes [30]. Motor-predominant neuropathy may develop after exposure to such medications as amiodarone, dapsone and tacrolimus [31]. Lead poisoning causes a motor neuropathy in adults, but in children is more likely to cause an encephalopathy with irritability and cognitive decline.

Sensorimotor polyneuropathy is the most common form of neuropathy in children, in whom it has an extensive differential diagnosis.

Neurophysiological Features

Nerve conduction studies (NCS) have several important functions. First, they confirm or exclude the presence of large-fiber peripheral nerve disease. Importantly, NCS selectively study large myelinated nerve fibers and therefore cannot exclude a small-fiber neuropathy, which requires other testing modalities for diagnosis (see Chap. 19). Second, NCS confirm the fiber types involved: sensory, motor or both. Third, it provides an assessment of the severity of an underlying neuropathy, including whether or not axonal continuity is present. This is particularly important for children who have suffered a traumatic nerve injury in whom it is necessary to make decisions regarding the timing and need for operative repair. Finally, NCS allows neurophysiologists to characterize if the neuropathy is demyelinating or axonal in nature, or has features of both. As focal neuropathies are the subjects of Chaps. 17 and 20, localization will not be discussed here.

Features suggestive of peripheral nerve demyelination include prolongation of distal latencies and slowing of nerve conduction to <75% of the normal values for age: in adults, this equates to conduction velocities of <38 m/s in the upper limbs,

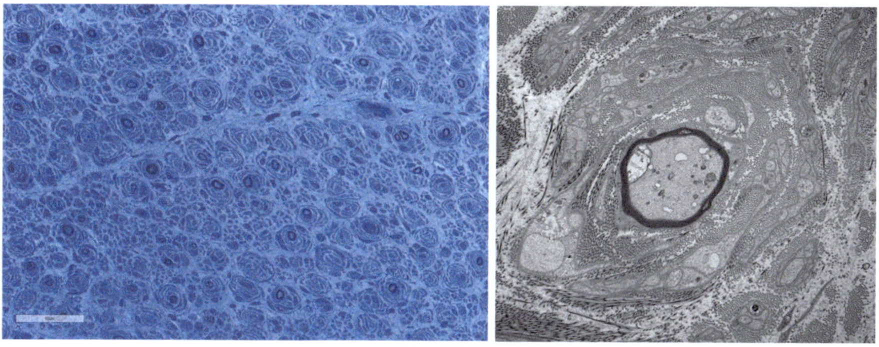

Fig. 18.1 Sural nerve biopsy of an adolescent with CMT1A. *Left: toluidine blue* staining shows hypertrophic neuropathy that shows uniform, homogenous involvement of all axons. Stains for inflammatory cells (not shown) revealed no significant infiltration. *Right:* concentric Schwann cell processes surrounding a remyelinated axon. The thickness of the myelin coat is much less than that of a normal healthy nerve. Photo credit: Dr. Jean Michaud, Department of Pathology, Children's Hospital of Eastern Ontario

and <30 m/s in the lower limbs. Normal values for nerve conduction parameters in childhood have been established (see Chap. 24). Slowing of peripheral nerve conduction may be uniform or non-uniform. Uniform slowing is characterized by a similar degree of demyelination in all nerves as well as at all points along each nerve that is studied. Uniform slowing is characteristic of most patients with hereditary neuropathies. Although biopsy is rarely performed for patients suspected of having CMT, it typically demonstrates homogeneous or uniform involvement of all axons (Fig. 18.1). Since the demyelination is similar from fiber-to-fiber, the signal is conducted in an equally slow manner along all nerve fibers. In contrast, non-uniform slowing reflects variable changes in nerve fibers at different points along their lengths. Some fibers may also be more affected than other fibers. This gives rise to neurophysiological phenomena known as temporal dispersion where different fibers conduct at different rates depending upon the degree to which they have been affected (Fig. 18.2). Non-uniform slowing is more commonly seen with acquired, inflammatory demyelinating disorders (such as GBS or CIDP). Although rarely performed, and not required for the diagnosis of pediatric CIDP [18], the uneven or patchy demyelination is apparent on nerve biopsy of CIDP patients (Fig.18.3). Non-uniform slowing is not specific to inflammatory neuropathies and has been reported with some hereditary nerve disorders, such as CMTX [32] and metachromatic leukodystrophy. In such conditions, peripheral nerve demyelination may be more marked or more apparent at their most proximal sites as evidenced by the loss of F-waves. Distal demyelination is reflected in the prolongation of distal motor latencies.

Conduction block is an extreme example of non-uniform slowing, in which the nerve action potential is partially or wholly blocked from transmitting (Fig. 18.4). This is associated with a drop in amplitude of the compound muscle action potential recorded from that nerve across the site of the conduction block (i.e., the amplitude drops with proximal stimulation compared to distal stimulation). Conduction block is also often a sign of acquired (typically inflammatory) neuropathies, but can also

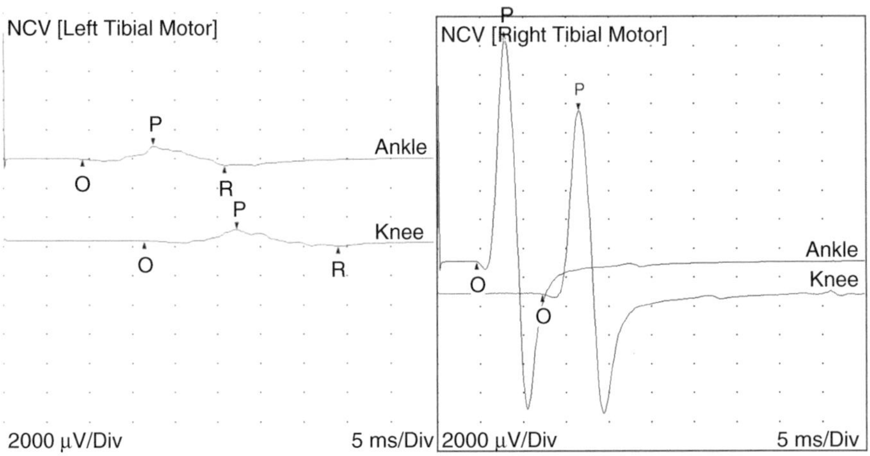

Fig. 18.2 Temporal dispersion noted in a patient with an acute demyelinating polyradiculoneuropathy (AIDP) or Guillain-Barre syndrome (GBS). Tibial nerve motor responses are shown in a child (8 years) with AIDP (*left*) and are compared to a healthy child (*right*). Nerve conduction studies of the median nerve (recorded at the abductor hallicus) in the child with AIDP shows a prolonged distal latency (9.3 ms). The compound motor action potential (CMAP) amplitude when stimulated at the ankle was 1.0 mV and when stimulated at the popliteal fossa was 0.9 mV. The duration of the CMAP amplitude was 138% longer when stimulated at the more proximal site consistent with temporal dispersion. Conduction velocity was 24 ms. In the healthy child, distal latency of 4.6 ms and distal compound motor action potential (CMAP) amplitude 15.4 mV and conduction velocity 48 ms. The sensitivity and sweep speeds are identical between the two tracings

be seen with hereditary neuropathy with liability to pressure palsies (HNPP) and after toxin exposures (such as gasoline sniffing [33]) and diphtheria [34].

Features suggestive of axonal loss include low or absent sensory and motor nerve action potential amplitudes. Patients may show mild slowing of conduction velocity although this is typically still >75% of the lower limit of normal.

Pediatric NCS are typically performed using a hand-held stimulator and surface electrodes to record peripheral nerve responses in the same way that this testing is undertaken in adults. Electrodiagnostic testing in children requires specific considerations (see Chap. 3). Recording electrodes should be selected to conform to small hand and foot size (see Chaps. 4 and 5). Caution must be taken to ensure that limb temperature is monitored since anxiety and/or small limb size can increase the risk of limb cooling and temperature-related artifacts that may arise during testing. Skin temperature should be at least 32°C in the upper limb and 30°C in the lower limb at the time of recording [35] (see Chap. 11).

Nerve conduction testing typically begins with sensory nerve studies, as these require lower stimulation intensities and are better tolerated by children. Normal values are grouped by age, with conduction velocities and amplitudes increasing with advancing age, particularly over the first 2 years of life (Chap. 24). The selection of peripheral nerves amenable to NCS in infants is more limited, due to short limb and digit length, and a relative increase in subcutaneous fat compared to older children.

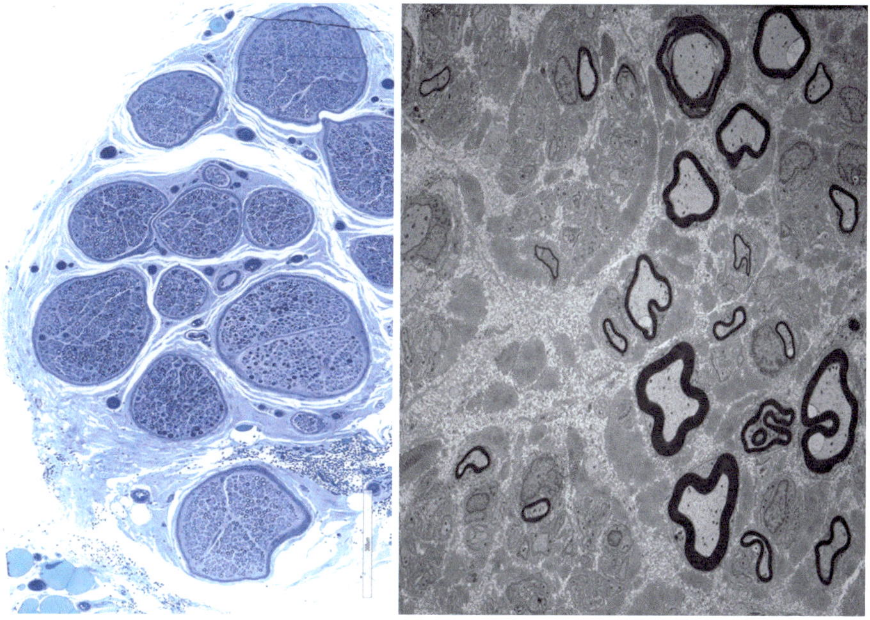

Fig. 18.3 Patient with confirmed chronic inflammatory demyelinating polyradiculoneuropathy (CIDP). *Left: toluidine blue* stained semi-thin section shows patchy population of myelinated fibers from one fascicle to another and within some fascicles. *Right*: ultrastructural study shows the unequal loss of myelinated fibers. Photo credit: Dr. Jean Michaud, Department of Pathology, Children's Hospital of Eastern Ontario

The sensory nerves typically studied in infants include the median, ulnar, and medial plantar nerves. Sural responses are difficult to record in small babies and infants. Motor nerves generally studied in infants include median (recording at abductor pollicus brevis), ulnar (recording at abductor digiti minimi), peroneal (recording at extensor digitorum brevis), and tibial (recording at abductor hallucis). The common peroneal nerve response can be difficult to elicit in newborns due to the small size of the extensor digitorum brevis. This becomes technically easier after the first 12 months of age.

In children with acquired neuropathies such as GBS, the diagnostic gain of neurophysiologic studies may be increased by recording late responses, such as F waves, which can reveal proximal demyelination that might not be identified on recording nerve conduction studies exclusively from distal peripheral nerve segments [10].

Electromyography is a vital part of the assessment of traumatic injury in children. Specific injuries are commonly linked to certain mononeuropathies (e.g., axillary neuropathy after anterior shoulder dislocation and radial neuropathy after supracondylar fracture), reflecting the mechanism of injury and proximity of nerve to the site of trauma in each case. In this context, nerve conduction studies and EMG provide important information regarding whether or not axonal continuity exists, as well as the presence and degree of spontaneous reinnervation, which can help predict the likelihood and time course of spontaneous recovery.

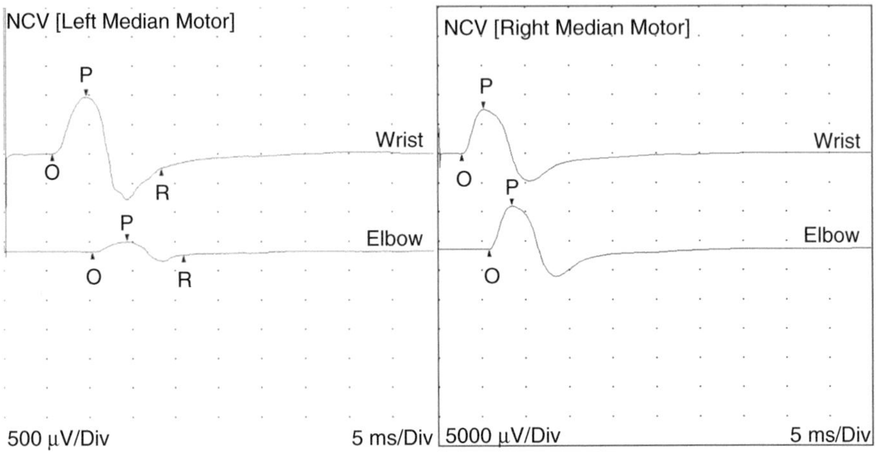

Fig. 18.4 Conduction block noted in a patient with an acute demyelinating polyradiculoneuropathy (AIDP) or Guillain-Barre syndrome (GBS). Median nerve motor responses are shown in an adolescent with AIDP (*left*) and a healthy child (*right*). Nerve conduction studies of the median nerve (recorded at the abductor pollicis brevis) in the child with AIDP shows a prolonged distal latency (5.7 ms). The compound motor action potential (CMAP) amplitude when stimulated at the wrist was 1.0 mV and when stimulated at the antecubital fossa was 0.2 mV, consistent with conduction block (i.e., >50% amplitude drop between distal and proximal stimulation sites). In the healthy child, there is a distal latency of 2.7 ms, distal compound motor action potential (CMAP) amplitude 7.5 mV and conduction velocity 63 ms. Note that the sensitivity is 10× greater on the *left* indicating the lower CMAP amplitudes. The sweep speed is identical between the two tracings

Needle EMG must be interpreted with some caution when evaluating neonates and infants with traumatic neuropathies. In children with neonatal brachial plexus palsies (NBPP), EMG may provide an overly optimistic view of potential for recovery. There are several reasons for the discrepancy between EMG findings and clinical outcome in infants. One is that the average muscle fiber diameter of a 3-month-old infant is only 17 μm, which is more than three-fold smaller than the adult muscle fiber diameter. Due to this smaller cross-sectional area, the muscle of an infant contains 11 times more motor units compared to an adult. An EMG needle will therefore "listen" to many more motor units when recording the recruitment pattern of an infant's muscle, which may lead the electromyographer to overestimate the normality of that pattern in small children [36].

Additional Considerations

Traumatic Nerve Injuries

Seddon proposed a classification system to categorize the severity of focal nerve injuries into one of three groups: neurapraxia, axonotmesis, and neurotmesis [37].

Neurapraxia, the least severe form of peripheral nerve injury, involves an area of segmental demyelination due to local traumatic and/or compression injury. The myelin is disrupted, and affected fibers do not convey afferent sensory or efferent motor signals, but axons remain intact. Clinically, neurapraxic injury cannot be distinguished—in the acute phase—from more serious nerve injuries. Long-term outcome is typically favourable, however, as the viable Schwann cells can repair the damaged segment (assuming the offending cause has been removed). Clinical and electrodiagnostic evidence of segmental demyelination may also be seen in patients with acquired (e.g., GBS) and hereditary neuropathies (e.g., HNPP). Some forms of drug abuse (gasoline or glue sniffing, or "huffing") have also been reported to cause conduction block upon a superimposed sensorimotor polyneuropathy with demyelinating features [33].

In axonotmesis, an intermediate form of nerve injury, some or all axons within a nerve fiber are transected. When an axon is cut, the segment of the axon that has been separated from its cell body (located in the dorsal root ganglion for sensory fibers, or in the anterior horn for motor fibers), degenerates through a process known as Wallerian degeneration. While axonotmesis is most commonly seen with trauma, it can also be associated with a traumatic nerve injuries, such as inflammatory neuropathies, vasculitides, and toxin exposures. Although the patient's clinical symptoms are immediately apparent, it takes time for the changes of denervation to become detectable on EMG: anywhere from days to 3–4 weeks, depending upon the length of the nerve and the site of injury [38]. During the Wallerian degeneration phase, the nerve fibers distal to the site of transection die back. During the recovery phase, the axon of the proximal segment regenerates, forming nerve twigs which grow distally, into and through the surviving neurilemmal tubes of Schwann cell basement membranes. The regenerating axons are then myelinated by the Schwann cells. With axonotmesis, some components of the nerve, including Schwann cells and potentially a percentage of the total nerve fibers, remain intact, subsequently acting as a conduit or path along which the regenerating nerve may grow. The fact that this path remains in place increases the likelihood that regenerating nerve fibers will locate and accurately reinnervate their target muscles distal to the site of nerve injury. Nerve regeneration proceeds at a slow pace, approximately 1 mm per day, or 1 inch per month [39].

Needle EMG suggest axonotmesis in situations where active denervation is noted (fibrillation potentials or positive sharp waves) accompanied by some evidence of ongoing axonal continuity (motor unit action potentials under volitional control). When no axonal continuity is noted, the electromyographer cannot distinguish axonotmesis from the most severe form of nerve injury, neurotmesis.

Neurotmesis, the most severe form of nerve injury, is characterized by complete transection of all nerve elements. In this situation the likelihood of spontaneous and meaningful reinnervation is low, as there is no path to guide the regenerating nerves.

Mononeuropathies

Mononeuropathies are rare in children, accounting for fewer than 10% of pediatric referrals for electromyographic (EMG) testing [40]. In children, focal neuropathies affect the median, ulnar, radial, peroneal, and sciatic nerves with more evenly distributed proportions than in adults, in whom 65% of focal neuropathies affect the median nerve, mainly due to carpal tunnel syndrome (CTS). Trauma is the most common cause of pediatric mononeuropathies, most often due fractures and lacerations, many of which are related to sports injuries. Compressive lesions are the second most common mechanism for pediatric mononeuropathies, while nerve entrapment is relatively uncommon, in contrast to adults.

The history is generally indicative of the etiology of pediatric mononeuropathies, while a targeted physical examination confirms the clinical suspicion of a peripheral nerve lesion and localizes focal deficits. The neurophysiologic examination enables exclusion of generalized neuropathies, plexopathy and radiculopathy. A detailed electromyographic examination is particularly useful in localizing focal lesions in idiopathic mononeuropathies. Nerve imaging, by ultrasound or magnetic resonance (MR) neurography, is an invaluable adjunct to the clinical and electrodiagnostic examinations [41]. In children with idiopathic mononeuropathies, nerve imaging rules out extrinsic compression by adjacent tumors or soft tissue lesions, as well as intrinsic nerve lesions such as perineuriomas, schwannomas, and neurofibromata. Imaging can also be a useful accompaniment to electrodiagnostic testing in guiding the specific site of nerve biopsy, when it is not immediately evident that a standard site of biopsy such as the sural nerve at the ankle will be adequate. Ultrasound may be even more sensitive than MRI in identifying focal nerve lesions when performed by a skilled technician in sonographically accessible regions [42]. Soft tissue changes—such as high-signal changes in atrophic muscles on STIR- and T2-weighted MR images- infer axonal injury rather than neurapraxia or conduction block, the presence of which may affect management [41]. Both ultrasound and MRI can be useful to guide fascicular biopsy in mononeuropathies in which the diagnosis remains unclear; fascicular biopsy reduces the risk that sampling a mixed nerve will result in iatrogenic paralysis of the innervated muscles.

Neuroimaging in Childhood Polyneuropathies

Magnetic resonance imaging (MRI) and ultrasound can be useful complementary tests to NCS/EMG in children with peripheral neuropathy. Both modalities give excellent soft tissue resolution, are non-invasive, and do not involve ionizing radiation. Both can be very useful in characterising pediatric mononeurpathies, as described above.

MRI is being increasingly used as a tool to aid in the diagnosis of suspected acute or chronic inflammatory polyradiculoneuropathies, including Guillain-Barré syndrome and chronic inflammatory demyelinating polyradiculoneuropathy (CIDP). MRI shows thickening of the cauda equina and/or thickening and gadolinium enhancement of the spinal nerve roots in 90–95% of children and adults with GBS [43, 44]. Nerve root thickening or enhancement is seen in approximately 40% of children with CIDP [19, 45]. While the finding of nerve root enlargement and thickening can support a diagnosis of inflammatory neuropathy in the right clinical context, it is by no means specific to this disease, since nerve root thickening can also be seen in CMT [46] and neurofibromatosis [47], among other diseases. Characteristic cervical spine and posterior fossa abnormalities are noted in older children and adolescents with inherited ataxias associated with neuropathies, including ARSACS (autosomal recessive ataxia of Charlevoix-Saguenay). MR imaging of affected patients may show thinning of the upper cervical spinal cord and progressive cerebellar atrophy particularly affecting the superior cerebellar folia. In contrast, patients with Friedreich ataxia have either normal cerebellar structures or show mild, non-specific abnormalities.

References

1. Hagberg B, Westerberg B. The nosology of genetic peripheral neuropathies in Swedish children. Dev Med Child Neurol. 1983;25:3–18.
2. Evans OB. Polyneuropathy in childhood. Pediatrics. 1979;64:96–105.
3. Ouvrier RA, McLeod JG. Chronic peripheral neuropathy in childhood: an overview. Aust Paediatr J. 1988;24(Suppl 1):80–2.
4. Sedel F, Barnerias C, Dubourg O, Desguerres I, Lyon-Caen O, Saudubray JM. Peripheral neuropathy and inborn errors of metabolism in adults. J Inherit Metab Dis. 2007;30:642–53.
5. Sedel F, Baumann N, Turpin JC, Lyon-Caen O, Saudubray JM, Cohen D. Psychiatric manifestations revealing inborn errors of metabolism in adolescents and adults. J Inherit Metab Dis. 2007;30:631–41.
6. Logina I, Donaghy M. Diphtheritic polyneuropathy: a clinical study and comparison with Guillain-Barre syndrome. J Neurol Neurosurg Psychiatry. 1999;67:433–8.
7. Belman AL, Iyer M, Coyle PK, Dattwyler R. Neurologic manifestations in children with North American Lyme disease. Neurology. 1993;43:2609–14.
8. Steere AC. Lyme disease. N Engl J Med. 2001;345:115–25.
9. Lin JJ, Hsia SH, Wang HS, Lyu RK, Chou ML, Hung PC, et al. Clinical variants of Guillain-Barre syndrome in children. Pediatr Neurol. 2012;47:91–6.
10. Ryan MM. Guillain-Barre syndrome in childhood. J Paediatr Child Health. 2005;41:237–41.
11. Dalakas MC. Basic aspects of neuroimmunology as they relate to immunotherapeutic targets: present and future prospects. Ann Neurol. 1995;37(Suppl 1):S2–13.
12. Mitchell G, Larochelle J, Lambert M, Michaud J, Grenier A, Ogier H, et al. Neurologic crises in hereditary tyrosinemia. N Engl J Med. 1990;322:432–7.
13. Albers JW, Fink JK. Porphyric neuropathy. Muscle Nerve. 2004;30:410–22.
14. McEneaney D, Hawkins S, Trimble E, Smye M. Porphyric neuropathy--a rare and often neglected differential diagnosis of Guillain-Barre syndrome. J Neurol Sci. 1993;114:231–2.
15. Sheikh KA, Ramos-Alvarez M, Jackson AC, Li CY, Asbury AK, Griffin JW. Overlap of pathology in paralytic rabies and axonal Guillain-Barre syndrome. Ann Neurol. 2005;57:768–72.
16. Genovese O, Ballario C, Storino R, Segura E, Sica RE. Clinical manifestations of peripheral nervous system involvement in human chronic Chagas disease. Arq Neuropsiquiatr. 1996;54:190–6.
17. Bosch AM, Stroek K, Abeling NG, Waterham HR, Ijlst L, Wanders RJ. The Brown-Vialetto-Van Laere and Fazio Londe syndrome revisited: natural history, genetics, treatment and future perspectives. Orphanet J Rare Dis. 2012;7:83.
18. Nevo Y, Topaloglu H. 88th ENMC international workshop: childhood chronic inflammatory demyelinating polyneuropathy (including revised diagnostic criteria), Naarden, The Netherlands, December 8-10, 2000. Neuromuscul Disord. 2002;12:195–200.
19. McMillan HJ, Kang PB, Jones HR, Darras BT. Childhood chronic inflammatory demyelinating polyradiculoneuropathy: combined analysis of a large cohort and eleven published series. Neuromuscul Disord. 2013;23:103–11.
20. Skre H. Genetic and clinical aspects of Charcot-Marie-Tooth's disease. Clin Genet. 1974;6:98–118.
21. Ionasescu VV, Ionasescu R, Searby C. Screening of dominantly inherited Charcot-Marie-Tooth neuropathies. Muscle Nerve. 1993;16:1232–8.

22. Bienfait HM, Baas F, Koelman JH, de Haan RJ, van Engelen BG, Gabreels-Festen AA, et al. Phenotype of Charcot-Marie-Tooth disease Type 2. Neurology. 2007;68:1658–67.
23. Zuchner S, Vance JM. Molecular genetics of autosomal-dominant axonal Charcot-Marie-Tooth disease. NeuroMolecular Med. 2006;8:63–74.
24. Saporta AS, Sottile SL, Miller LJ, Feely SM, Siskind CE, Shy ME. Charcot-Marie-Tooth disease subtypes and genetic testing strategies. Ann Neurol. 2011;69:22–33.
25. Weimer LH, Podwall D. Medication-induced exacerbation of neuropathy in Charcot Marie Tooth disease. J Neurol Sci. 2006;242:47–54.
26. Ryan MM, Tilton A, De GU, Darras BT, Jones HR Jr. Paediatric mononeuritis multiplex: a report of three cases and review of the literature. Neuromuscul Disord. 2003;13:751–6.
27. Peyronnard JM, Charron L, Barbeau A. The neuropathy of Charlevoix-Saguenay ataxia: an electrophysiological and pathological study. Can J Neurol Sci. 1979;6:199–203.
28. Lowry NJ, Taylor MJ, Belknapp W, Logan WJ. Electrophysiological studies in five cases of abetalipoproteinemia. Can J Neurol Sci. 1984;11:60–3.
29. Fogel BL, Perlman S. Clinical features and molecular genetics of autosomal recessive cerebellar ataxias. Lancet Neurol. 2007;6:245–57.
30. Rossor AM, Kalmar B, Greensmith L, Reilly MM. The distal hereditary motor neuropathies. J Neurol Neurosurg Psychiatry. 2012;83:6–14.
31. Venance SL, Strong MJ. Toxic motor neuronopathies and neuropathies. In: Eisen A, editor. Handbook of clinical neurophysiology. Amsterdam: Elsevier; 2004. p. 437–50.
32. Ryan MM, Jones HR Jr. CMTX mimicking childhood chronic inflammatory demyelinating neuropathy with tremor. Muscle Nerve. 2005;31:528–30.
33. Burns TM, Shneker BF, Juel VC. Gasoline sniffing multifocal neuropathy. Pediatr Neurol. 2001;25:419–21.
34. Creange A, Meyrignac C, Roualdes B, Degos JD, Gherardi RK. Diphtheritic neuropathy. Muscle Nerve. 1995;18:1460–3.
35. Kang PB. Pediatric nerve conduction studies and EMG. In: Blum AS, Rutkove SB, editors. Clinical neurophysiology primer. Totowa: Humana Press Inc; 2007. p. 369–89.
36. VAN Dijk JG, Malessy MJ, Stegeman DF. Why is the electromyogram in obstetric brachial plexus lesions overly optimistic? Muscle Nerve. 1998;21:260–1.
37. Seddon HJ. A Classification of Nerve Injuries. Br Med J. 1942;2:237–9.
38. Gooch CL, Weimer LH. The electrodiagnosis of neuropathy: basic principles and common pitfalls. Neurol Clin. 2007;25:1–28.
39. Seddon HJ, Medawar PB, Smith H. Rate of regeneration of peripheral nerves in man. J Physiol. 1943;102:191–215.
40. Ryan MM, Jones HR. Mononeuropathies. In: Darras BT, Jones HR, Ryan MM, De Vivo DC, editors. Neuromuscular disorders of infancy, childhood and adolescence: a clinician's approach. 2nd ed. San Diego: Elsevier; 2014. p. 243–73.
41. Cortes C, Ramos Y, Restrepo R, Restrepo JA, Grossman JA, Lee EY. Practical magnetic resonance imaging evaluation of peripheral nerves in children: magnetic resonance neurography. *Radiol Clin N Am*. 2013;51:673–88.
42. Zaidman CM, Seelig MJ, Baker JC, Mackinnon SE, Pestronk A. Detection of peripheral nerve pathology: comparison of ultrasound and MRI. Neurology. 2013;80:1634–40.
43. Yikilmaz A, Doganay S, Gumus H, Per H, Kumandas S, Coskun A. Magnetic resonance imaging of childhood Guillain-Barre syndrome. Childs Nerv Syst. 2010;26:1103–8.
44. Smith N, Pereira J, Grattan-Smith P. Investigation of suspected Guillain-Barre syndrome in childhood: what is the role for gadolinium enhanced magnetic resonance imaging of the spine? J Paediatr Child Health. 2014;50:E72–6.
45. McMillan HJ, Miller E. Cranial nerve hypertrophy in pediatric chronic inflammatory demyelinating polyradiculoneuropathy. *Pediatr Radiol*. 2010;40(Suppl 1):S176.
46. Haubrich C, Krings T, Senderek J, Zuchner S, Schroder JM, Noth J, et al. Hypertrophic nerve roots in a case of Roussy-Levy syndrome. Neuroradiology. 2002;44:933–7.
47. Lin J, Martel W. Cross-sectional imaging of peripheral nerve sheath tumors: characteristic signs on CT, MR imaging, and sonography. AJR Am J Roentgenol. 2001;176:75–82.

Chapter 19
Diagnosis and Evaluation of Small Fiber Peripheral Neuropathy in Children

Nancy L. Kuntz

Introduction

Clinical neurophysiologists who evaluate infants and children need to have a special skill set and knowledge base. This is due to the fact that the differential diagnosis of neurologic disorders, including small fiber neuropathies, is much broader in young patients and includes rare, inherited, congenital onset disorders which present primarily at birth or during the early years of life. In addition, the ability of infants and children to communicate their experience or explain themselves is limited by their life experiences, their cognition/perception and their vocabulary/language skills.

Signs and symptoms of small fiber peripheral neuropathy depend on the exact type of nerve fiber targeted, the severity of the loss of nerve fiber function and the age of the child. "Small fiber" peripheral neuropathy refers to those processes which damage or limit the function of small unmyelinated A delta and unmyelinated C fibers. These fibers mediate nociception (pain), temperature and autonomic functions. The types of autonomic dysfunction which can occur due to lack of functioning small nerve fibers include: dry eyes, dry mouth, orthostatic lightheadedness through a spectrum to syncope, palpitations, abnormal sweating, overheating, erectile dysfunction, nausea, vomiting, constipation, early satiety, urinary frequency, nocturia and others [1].

In some of the inherited sensory and autonomic peripheral neuropathies, the residual function of sensory nerves mediating pain or temperature is so poor that tissue mutilation occurs without perceived pain: corneal scarring from rubbing the eyes; amputation of parts of the tongue post emergence of teeth; Charcot joints and fractures of the long bones since these children lack the normal perception of pain that is required to negatively reinforce activities which injure tissues during play.

N.L. Kuntz, M.D.
Northwestern Feinberg School of Medicine, Ann & Robert H Lurie Children's Hospital of Chicago, Chicago, IL, USA
e-mail: NKuntz@luriechildrens.org

© Springer International Publishing AG 2017

H.J. McMillan, P.B. Kang (eds.), *Pediatric Electromyography*,
DOI 10.1007/978-3-319-61361-1_19

With less severe loss of small nerve fibers, symptoms tend to appear at an older age. For example, one young school-aged boy was diagnosed with HSAN IV after being seen in a local ER for a lesion in one calf which was draining purulent material. An X-ray of the leg demonstrated the presence of two full length sewing needles buried in his calf muscles. The patient denied pain and stated he had no clue about how the needles got into his leg. It was strongly suspected that, because it didn't hurt, the patient placed the needles in his leg muscle out of curiosity. He had already developed classical Charcot joints in both knees at the time of presentation.

Various pathologic insults preferentially impact different types of nerve fibers. The reasons for this are not always known. If both large and small fibers are affected simultaneously, it is easiest to confirm the peripheral nerve involvement by standard motor and sensory nerve conduction studies which document the large fiber involvement and then to use the clinical symptoms to infer additional impact on the small fibers. However, if the symptoms are limited to small fiber involvement, then more specialized testing, as outlined in the rest of this chapter, is necessary to confirm the diagnosis.

Signs and Symptoms of Small Fiber Peripheral Neuropathy

Clinical symptoms relating to dysfunction of small nerve fibers can be non-descript. The younger the patient, the less specific the complaints may be. Children with acquired small fiber nerve injury causing allodynia or hyperpathia tend to manifest behavior somewhere between irritable to hysterical, refusing to move or be touched; but they do not always complain of pain. Children with pain due to acquired small nerve fiber dysfunction can have neurologic examinations that are considered completely normal with preserved strength, muscle stretch reflexes, coordination and sense of touch. Standard "neurologic" tests including motor and sensory nerve conduction studies, MRI of brain and spine and cerebrospinal fluid examination can be normal, leading a clinical team to suspect an underlying conversion disorder or other mental health problem. A number of children with acquired inflammatory small fiber disorders have been placed in psychiatric facilities for evaluation prior to consideration of small fiber dysfunction and neuropathic pain as the cause of their monumental distress [2]. One patient, a 6-year-old boy, was completely unable or unwilling to describe his pain until the neuropathic pain was under control. Then he told the treating team: "There's two things. A medium pain that's always there. And bad pain like rockets blasting through my hands".

When a peripheral neuropathy is limited to small nerve fibers, muscle tone, strength and muscle stretch reflexes are normal on examination. Touch, position sense, vibration and coordination are normal by observation and on direct examination. Temperature and pain perception should be found to be abnormal if they can be examined or if the level of function can be inferred by observation. With chronic small fiber dysfunction, skin can become dry, cracked or shiny [3]. Autonomic dysfunction can cause the skin to lose its ability to wrinkle in response to immersion in water (pruniness) [4] (Fig. 19.1).

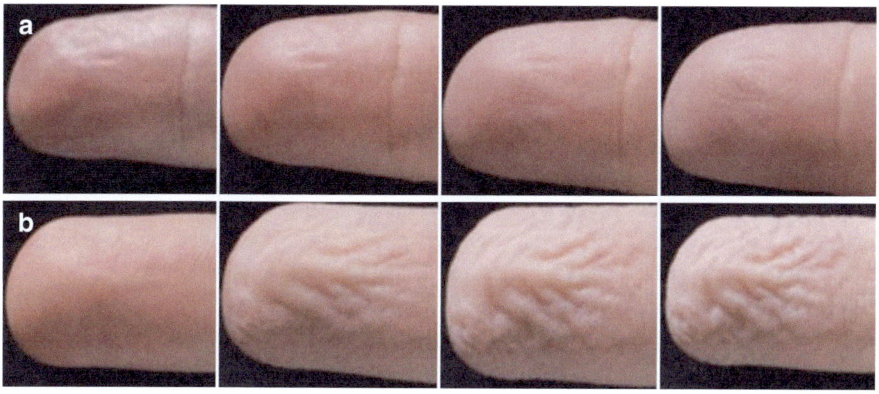

Fig. 19.1 Finger immersion test of vasomotor sympathetic function. Hand is immersed for 30 min in a heated water bath. Digital pictures are taken (*from left to right*) at baseline and after 5, 15 and 30 min of immersion. Pictures in (**a**) reflect changes in subject with small fiber peripheral neuropathy. Pictures in (**b**) are from normal control

Methods of Testing

Clinical

Quantitative sensory testing: The younger a child is, the more difficult it can be to accomplish a reliable or quantitative sensory examination. When cooperation and focused attention allow quantitative testing of clinical sensory thresholds (thermal thresholds for small fiber function), normal results are helpful. However, it has been demonstrated that abnormal thermal thresholds can be feigned; therefore, abnormal quantitative thermal thresholds are less reliable [5]. The frequency of false negative results for subjective pinprick thresholds in patients with objective evidence of SFN has been reported at 19%, higher than one might anticipate in adults [6]. Common sense suggests that reliability would be even less in children. Computer-assisted sensory examinations are used in adult patients but the same caveats apply with respect to false positive results, particularly with younger patients who tend to be more distractable.

Neurophysiologic

Nerve Conduction Studies: Sensory nerve conduction studies assess the function of large myelinated sensory nerve fibers. Some disorders may affect all types of nerve fibers; however, if the abnormality is limited to small nerve fibers, standard sensory nerve conduction studies will be normal.

Contact Heat Evoked Potential (CHEP): This technique applies cycles of heating and cooling using a heat foil thermode placed over glabrus skin on an extremity while recording the evoked potential over a CZ scalp electrode. This evoked potential is mediated by A delta fibers and demonstrates increased latency and decreased amplitude in subjects with documented small fiber neuropathy as compared to normal adult controls [7]. This causes no tissue injury and is considered non-invasive but does involve a minor degree of discomfort. There are no published reports using this technique in children.

Microneurography: A technique has been developed to record impulse traffic within peripheral nerves using specialized coated tungsten electrodes. The burst frequencies from single unmyelinated afferent and efferent fibers tend to be relatively uniform within an individual over time. However, there are wide variations between individuals which make it difficult to establish reference ranges. The technique is time-consuming and requires a skilled evaluator. Movement interferes with the recording which is likely why this has not been applied to children. At present, this technique functions more as a research tool than a clinical diagnostic test [8].

Autonomic Testing

While autonomic testing is relatively new, experience is being gained with the use of these techniques in children and adolescents. Normative data is being systematically gathered and it will be very helpful when this process is complete with results published.

Adrenergic: Short duration Head Up Tilt tests (HUT) are performed to assess the adrenergic support of heart rate and blood pressure in response to orthostatic stress. Protocols for autonomic tilt testing are simpler and shorter, and do not use infusions of vasoactive drugs, in contrast to cardiac tilt testing. A preceding interval of 10–30 minutes of supine rest is required followed by passive elevation to a 70° HUT on a motorized tilt table. Heart rate, blood pressure and clinical well-being are monitored for 10 minutes. Other parameters such as end-tidal CO2, oxygen saturation, respiratory rate and regional cerebral perfusion are also monitored in our laboratory. With the data obtained, other causes of dizziness, such as occult hyperventilation or isolated cerebral hypoperfusion, can be identified. Adolescents frequently present with dizziness and data have been gathered on healthy controls to demonstrate that the range of normal heart rate responses to HUT is broader in adolescents than adults [9]. Normative data from larger groups of adolescents are being collected at present and will be useful for clinical correlation. Adrenergic function can also be assessed from evaluation of blood pressure responses during a Valsalva maneuver. The rebound increase of blood pressure during phase II of the Valsalva maneuver and the phase IV overshoot of blood pressure both rely on adrenergic support (Fig. 19.2).

Cardiovagal: The heart rate response to deep breathing (HR_{DB}) is a quantification of the variation in heart rate that occurs during normal breathing— "sinus arrhythmia". It is easy to perform, requiring children to use visual or auditory cues to pace deep breathing at 6 cycles per minute while their heart rate is recorded. The

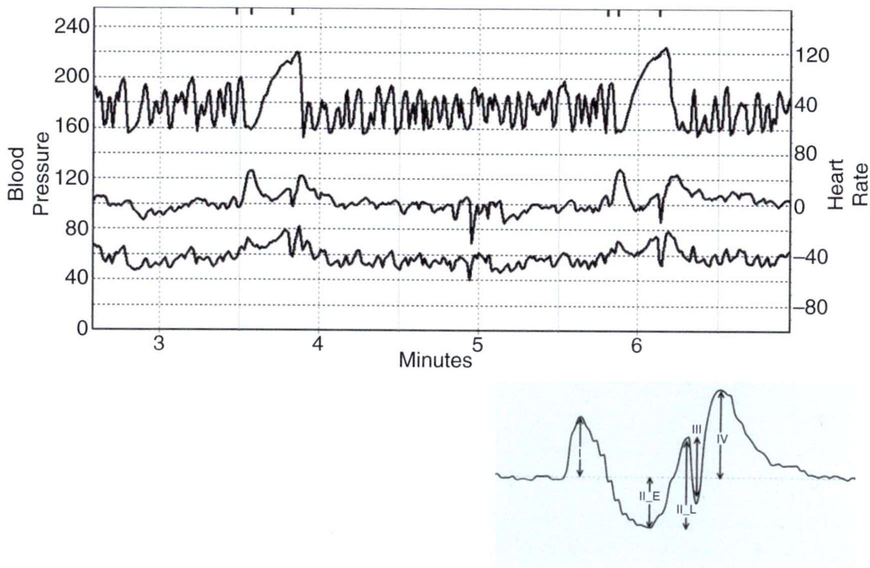

Fig. 19.2 Heart rate (*upper tracing*) and blood pressure responses (*lower two traces*) for a 7 year old girl performing Valsalva maneuver. Timing of Valsalva pressure indicated by *solid bar above top graph*. Cartoon below physiologic tracing identifies components of the blood pressure response to Valsalva maneuver

mean is calculated from the maximal excursions of heart rate during the largest five consecutive responses. Normal values have been collected from 9 years of age and older with an inverse relationship between age and HR_{DB} [10, 11]. Valsalva Ratio (VR) is vagally mediated and is the ratio of the highest heart rate occurring during a 15 second Valsalva maneuver (performed on a mouthpiece with an air leak) to the lowest heart rate occurring within 30 seconds of completion. Normal values in adults are between 1.5 and 2.9 and several studies [10, 11] have documented very similar findings 6–17 year olds. It is difficult to get younger children to sustain pressure on the mouthpiece long enough to accomplish this measurement. Cardiovagal responses can be obtained by other maneuvers including squat to stand, assuming a squat or forcefully coughing; however, reference ranges have not been adequately established for these responses in either adults or children.

Electrochemical Skin Impedance: A device that uses reverse iontophoresis and chronoamperometry to assess sweating on the palms and soles has been demonstrated to correlate with epidermal nerve fiber density. The Sudoscan device uses stainless steel plates against which palms and soles are placed for a 3 minute scan with the subject in a standing position [12]. This is a recently developed device so, despite the relative simplicity of use, there are no reports describing the use of this technique in children.

Heart rate variability: Measures of heart rate variability (HRV) are obtained by monitoring the electrocardiogram (ECG) for intervals of time between 5 minutes and 24 hours, analyzing sequential R-R intervals. Heart rate variability

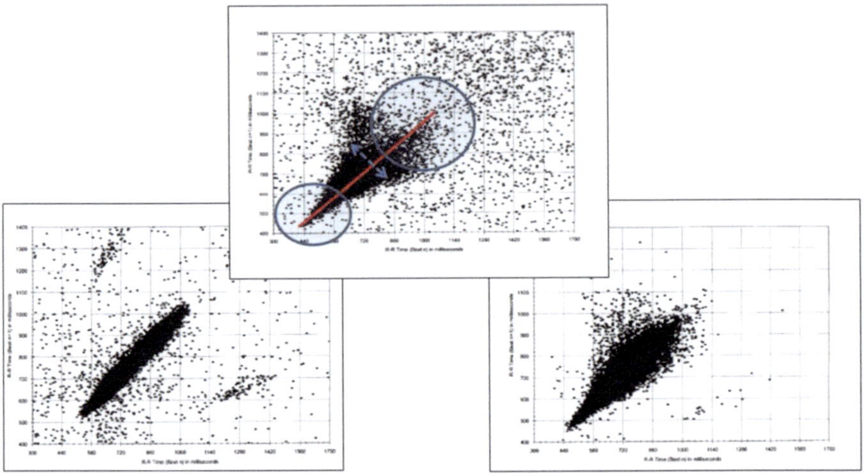

Fig. 19.3 Poincaré plots of heart rate variability. Normal (*middle graph*): "ice cream cone" shaped plot with labels indicating higher heart rates in *circle to left*, lower heart rates in *circle to right*, "line of identity" in *red*. ROHHAD (Rapid onset Obesity, Hypoventilation, Hypothalamic Dysfunction and Autonomic Dysregulation) (*right graph*): narrow plot, note decreased heart rate variability at lower heart rates. CCHS (Congenital Central Hypoventilation Syndrome) (*left graph*): narrow "cigar" shaped plot indicating decreased heart rate variability

is created by the naturally opposing influences of sympathetic and parasympathetic tone on the sinoatrial node (cardiac pacemaker). Physiologic state and age affect the degree of variability [13, 14]. While cardiologists report variables relating to time domain and frequency parameters, a scatter plot of successive R-R intervals (Poincaré plot) creates an immediate visual image of HRV (Fig. 19.3). Decreased variability appears as a cigar-shaped pattern with robust heart rate variability appearing in the shape of an ice-cream cone.

Pupillometry: Basal size of the pupils and velocity of change in size reflect a balance between sympathetic and parasympathetic tone. Normal values have been collected [15]. The ambient light, medications and presence of any ocular disease must be taken into consideration when testing pupillary function. In addition, any stimuli that might trigger sudden anxiety or fear should be avoided as alterations in the sympathetic/parasympathetic balance will affect pupil function.

Sudomotor: Production of sweat in response to heat stress or emotional stress is a sympathetically-mediated autonomic function that is mediated by acetylcholine as the neurotransmitter. Function at the level of the peripheral axon reflex can be measured with quantitative sudomotor axon reflex testing (QSART/QSWEAT). A plastic capsule is used to focally place acetylcholine onto a patch of skin. A small electric current is used to iontophorese the acetylcholine through the skin where it stimulates the sweat glands. A retrograde impulse through the small nerves innervating the sweat gland reflexively stimulates an adjacent sweat gland and the amount of reflex sweating generated onto an adjacent patch of skin is measured. Four capsules are placed along the limbs in a length-dependent fashion (foot, distal

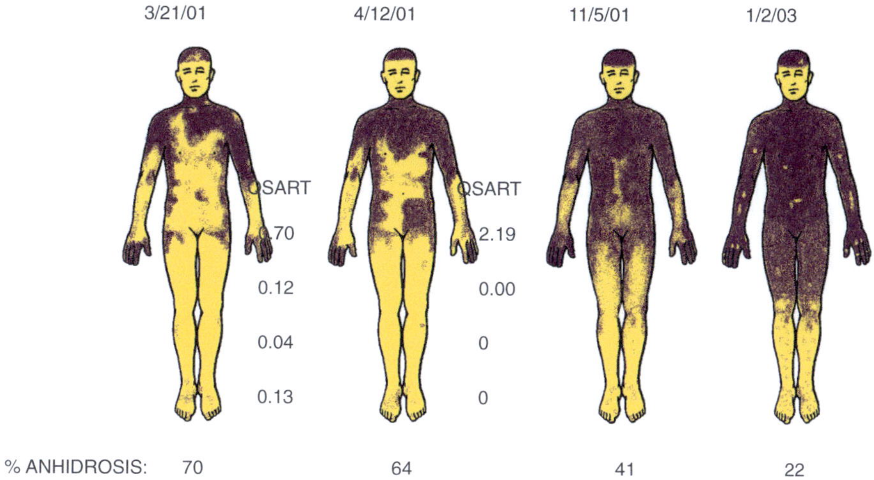

Fig. 19.4 TST (Thermoregulatory Sweat Test) performed serially in a 6 year old boy with small fiber peripheral neuropathy to demonstrate ongoing clinical improvement

leg, proximal thigh and distal forearm) and stimulated simultaneously [10]. This technique has been used in toddlers and young children successfully; however, normative data are sparse under 10 years of age [11]. A different technique can be used to evaluate the entire central to peripheral sudomotor apparatus: thermoregulatory sweat testing (TST). An individual who is well-hydrated and who is not taking any antihistamine or other medication that suppresses sweating is placed in a controlled hot and humid environment. It takes 45–60 minutes in such a setting to increase core temperature by 1°C or to 38.0°C (whichever is higher). All individuals without disease will sweat under these conditions. A moisture sensitive powder is placed over the ventral surface of cheeks, trunk and extremities. A color-coded response is evident, indicating where the individual subject was able to sweat [10]. Lesions from the hypothalamus through the spinal cord and out to focal/generalized nerve distributions can interfere with sweating. The disadvantage of the TST is that it requires that a special chamber or environment be fabricated to warm the patient. The advantage is that this procedure is non-invasive and can be repeated over time to follow the course of a disease (Fig. 19.4). Also, the entire ventral surface of the body is being studied and focal and/or strictly length dependent abnormalities can be outlined (Fig. 19.5). In 2011, a decade's worth of experience obtaining TSTs in children at Mayo Clinic Rochester was reviewed. Children between 2 and 18 years of age were examined with valid, clinically useful results obtained in 94% of studies [16].

Sympathetic Skin Response (SSR): Surface electrodes placed over the palm and sole of the feet are used to record sympathetic skin responses (SSR) [17]. A number of types of sensory stimuli can be used to provoke this response in sympathetic nerves: auditory, tactile, electrical. A novel use of SSR was described by Pereon and colleagues when they used auditory signals of varying intensity to determine the

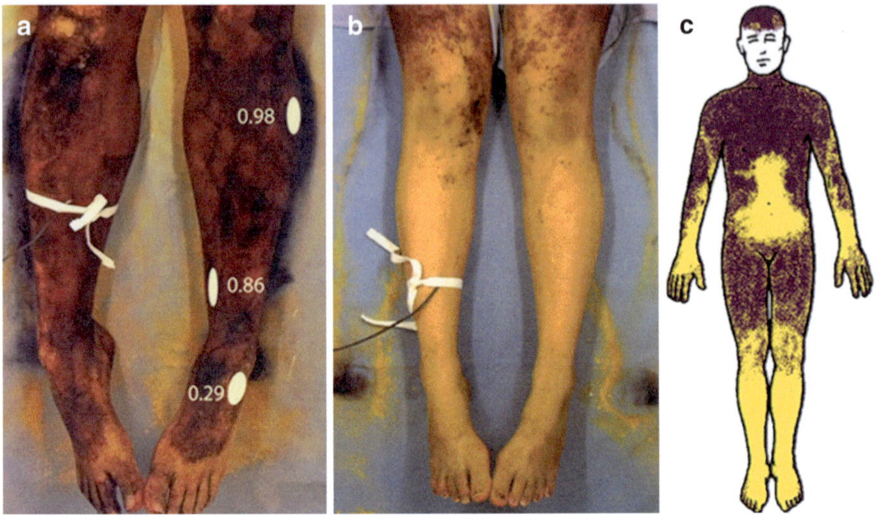

Fig. 19.5 TST (thermoregulatory sweat test). (**a**) Demonstrates involvement of only the distal foot/toes that was not detected by standard QSART testing which assesses proximal foot as most distal site. (**b**) Demonstrates length dependent anhidrosis involving both lower extremities. (**c**) A cartoon of the sweat pattern on the entire body, for the subject in (**b**), demonstrating trunk and upper extremity involvement as well

hearing threshold for a child post cochlear implant [18]. SSR is non-invasive but habituates quickly to repeated sensory stimuli. It is usually judged on its presence or absence.

Vasomotor: Vasoreactivity has not been studied extensively with techniques that are clinically applicable. One simple test that has been developed is to look for wrinkling or "pruning" of the skin in response to timed water immersion or application of a topical anesthetic under an occlusive dressing. Development of pruny skin is a sympathetically mediated vasoconstrictive phenomenon [4] (Fig. 19.1). Skin changes have been subjectively graded.

Pathologic

Standard Nerve Histology: Peripheral nerve biopsies are a "gold standard" for evaluating the constituent elements of nerves. However, biopsies are invasive, require general anesthesia in children and leave a small functional sensory or motor deficit. Sural sensory nerves are traditionally biopsied just proximal to the lateral malleolus in diffuse or generalized processes and the ensuing clinical sensory deficit is minimal and generally well-tolerated. Nevertheless, the invasive nature of this procedure, and the difficulties inherent in repeating such a biopsy to assess response to treatment, have led to development of less invasive testing methods.

Intraepidermal Nerve Fiber Density (IEFND): Small nerve fibers can be seen (and quantified) in the epidermis and in sweat glands. In adults, 3 mm full thickness skin biopsies are obtained under local anesthesia with a skin punch biopsy tool. Samples are usually taken at five sites along the limbs. Normal values for epidermal nerve fiber density, nerve fiber length and nerve branching density have been obtained from 18 to 90 years of age [19]. McArthur and colleagues obtained 3 mm skin punch biopsies under local anesthesia for 98 patients, eight of whom were between 13 and 19 years of age (mean 18 years). The IENFD at the level of the thigh and distal leg were both higher than in other controls aged 20–79 years of age. However, the thigh/distal leg ratio was the same as in all other controls up to 60 years of age [20]. While this type of biopsy is less invasive than a standard nerve biopsy, it is still invasive and more difficult to justify performing without clear normal values for young children and adolescents, especially at multiple sites.

Sweat Gland Nerve Fiber Density: Sweat glands are incidentally obtained in most of the skin punch biopsies done to determine IEFND [21]. Normative values are available for adults but not yet for children and adolescents.

Corneal Confocal Microscopy (CCM): A non-invasive method for evaluating nerve integrity, corneal confocal microscopy, has been used to quantify corneal nerve fiber density, corneal nerve fiber length and corneal nerve branch density in various medical conditions prone to small fiber neuropathy such as diabetes mellitus. Chen and colleagues evaluated a cohort of 63 patients with type I diabetes mellitus between 14 and 85 years of age and an equivalent number of age-matched controls. Motor and sensory nerve conduction studies, IENFD and CCM were performed on all subjects. While IEFND has been shown to detect early small nerve fiber injury when nerve conduction studies and quantitative sensory testing are still normal, CCM was shown in this study to have a slightly better sensitivity and specificity. CCM is non-invasive and can be scored in an automated manner that provides rapid results. Obtaining corneal tomographic images does not require undue cooperation from children and adolescents so it is a promising biomarker of early diabetic neuropathy [22, 23].

Imaging

MR Neurography (MRN) with Dorsal Root Ganglion Imaging: An MRN protocol has been developed that allows imaging of bilateral dorsal root ganglia. This has been used to evaluate patients with Sjögren syndrome when other quantitative sensory physiologic tests were unrevealing [24]. The imaging demonstrated enlargement of the dorsal root ganglia in affected individuals that was reversed after immunotherapy. The limitation for this procedure in children is the time required for them to be motionless during imaging, as in other magnetic resonance imaging studies; therefore, it would likely require anesthesia in younger children.

Ultrasound: 25 adults with small fiber peripheral neuropathy confirmed by IEFND and age/BMI-matched controls were studied by ultrasound. Cross-sectional areas of superficial peroneal sensory and sural sensory nerves was increased in the subjects with SFPN as compared to controls. This technique does not provide much information regarding the specific etiology but may serve as a non-invasive, low cost initial screening approach [25].

Genetic

If the phenotypic presentation and/or family history strongly suggest a Mendelian disorder and a gene test (or affordable gene test panel) is available to confirm that diagnosis, proceeding directly to genetic testing may be a minimally-invasive and cost efficient approach. There are circumstances when physiologic testing, in conjunction with the clinical findings, will significantly narrow the differential diagnosis. For example, findings on nerve conduction studies and/or pupillometry can focus the diagnostic possibilities to the spectrum of inherited peripheral neuropathies [26].

Causes of Small Fiber Peripheral Neuropathy in Children

Inherited

Hereditary Sensory and Autonomic Neuropathies (HSAN): There are six different types of HSAN which have been described and for each of which one or more gene mutations have been identified. HSAN I is an autosomal dominant neuropathy that presents during adolescence or early adulthood with painless injuries. Affected individuals develop length-dependent motor and sensory loss over time. Neuropathic pain in the lower extremities, sensorineural hearing loss, and abnormalities on motor and sensory NCS usually develop over time. HSAN I has been linked to mutations in the *SPTLC1* gene [27]. All other HSAN subtypes demonstrate autosomal recessive inheritance. HSAN II presents at birth or early childhood with a significant loss of pain, temperature and touch sensation with variable autonomic involvement (excess sweating, tonic pupils or urinary incontinence). Nerve biopsies demonstrate no small myelinated fibers and decreased numbers of unmyelinated fibers. Mutations in several genes have been identified as causative: *WNK1*, *FAM134G*, *KIF1A*, and *SCN9A*, with the *FAM134G*-associated cases demonstrating the most prominent autonomic symptoms [28]. HSAN III is referred to as familial dysautonomia or Riley-Day Syndrome and occurs in individuals of Ashkenazi Jewish descent. Symptoms are present from birth, including gastrointestinal dysmotility, decreased pain and temperature sensation, and cardiovascular instability. The size and number of neurons in the dorsal root, sympathetic and parasympathetic ganglia are decreased at birth and progressively decline over time.

Nearly half of individuals with HSAN III experience clinical crises relating to recurrent vomiting, blood pressure instability or cardiac dysrhythmia. Absence of fungiform papillae on the tongue, absence of emotionally triggered overflow tears after 6 months of age, absence of the axon flare response after intradermal histamine injection and pupillary hypersensitivity to parasympathomimetic agents are findings suggestive of this diagnosis [29]. HSAN IV is also known as Congenital Insensitivity to Pain with Anhidrosis (CIPA) and is related to mutations in *NTRK1*. Sural nerve biopsy demonstrates a complete absence of unmyelinated axons and a decrease in small myelinated neurons with normal density of myelinated fibers. The symptoms, predictably, include anhydrosis and no response to painful stimuli with preserved muscle stretch reflexes and muscle strength. Mutilation of the tongue, lips, biting of the fingertips, recurrent bony fractures leading to joint and limb deformity and corneal injury are common and begin early in life [30]. HSAN V is clinically similar to HSAN IV with decreases in small myelinated and unmyelinated nerve fibers due to mutations in *NGF*. HSAN VI has been documented in one family with a mutation in *DST* causing severe dysautonomia with absent muscle stretch reflexes, weakness with contractures and severe psychomotor retardation [28].

Paroxysmal Extreme Pain Syndromes: A number of mutations in *SCN9A* cause loss of function for individuals who then lack pain or temperature perception [31]. Historically, some of these individuals have performed in the circus demonstrating their ability to tolerate pinsticks and other insults without pain. Other mutations in this gene cause gain-of-function mutations in the sodium channels which lead to prolonged action potentials on small sensory fibers and the subjective experience of prolonged sharp pain with sensory activation. Paroxysms of pelvic and rectal pain are amongst the most frequently described symptoms. [32].

Erythromelalgia: This clinical syndrome likely includes several different discrete disorders that are unified by episodes of bright red, hot and intensely painful distal extremities, sometimes accompanied by edema (Fig. 19.6). Sensory nerve

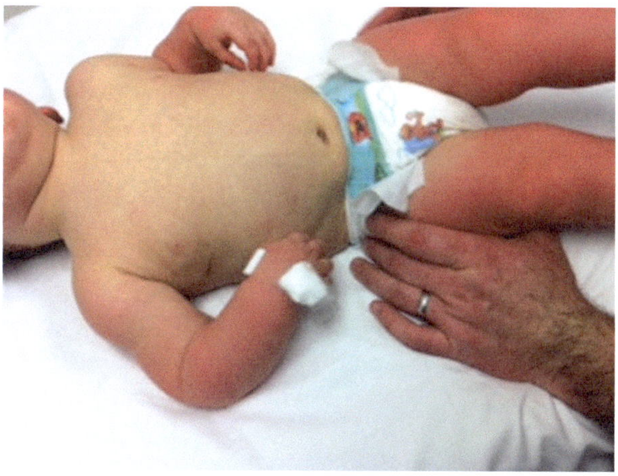

Fig. 19.6 Severe erythromelalgia in a 2 year old male. Erythema and hyperpathia were present in all four extremities in a length dependent fashion. Photograph courtesy of Dr. Anthony J Mancini

conduction studies are normal but the majority of affected children demonstrate abnormal IEFND, QSWEAT and TST results. Some, but not all, of the children with this presentation have been found to have mutations in *SCN9A* [33]. The time course and symmetry differentiate this from complex regional pain syndrome.

Ehlers Danlos Syndrome: Reviews of adults with Ehlers Danlos syndrome have documented that the majority of patients report spontaneous pain as part of their symptom complex. However, recent studies have also documented that these same patients demonstrate a decrease in their intradermal epithelial nerve fiber density (IENFD) consistent with a diagnosis of small fiber peripheral neuropathy [34].

A number of other genetically determined conditions are additional, rare causes of small fiber neuropathy in children and young adults. These include Wilson's disease [35, 36], Fabry's disease [37], Pompe disease [38], and familial amyloidosis [39]. Quantitative pupillary responses have been shown to correlate with the severity of the *PHOX2B* mutation in CCHS [40].

Acquired

One of the most frequent causes of small fiber neuropathy is glucose intolerance (less severe degrees of glucose intolerance, frank diabetes mellitus or metabolic syndrome). There are individuals who develop small fiber peripheral neuropathy with glucose intolerance demonstrated by a 2 hour post prandial (or 2 hour GTT) test who have normal hemoglobin A1c levels and no other identifiable cause of small fiber dysfunction [41]. In adults, a full metabolic syndrome which includes hyperlipidemia and obesity as well as diabetes mellitus appears to be more likely to cause isolated small fiber peripheral neuropathies [3]. The frequency of these disorders of glucose tolerance causing small fiber peripheral neuropathy has not been clearly identified in children; however, it has been documented that autonomic dysfunction is an early complication of diabetes mellitus in children and young adults [42].

Autoimmune autonomic ganglionopathy (AAG), with or without antibodies to the α3 subunit of the acetylcholine receptor, is an acquired disorder characterized by various combinations of neuropathic pain, orthostatic intolerance, gastrointestinal dysmotility and photophobia [43]. In addition to abnormalities on QSWEAT, TST, IENFD and HUT, a characteristic abnormality has been described on pupillometry [44]. With normal pupillary function, the iris remains constricted as long as a bright light is directed toward the eye. In AAG, the pupillary constriction fatigues if a prolonged (e.g., 2 second) light stimulus is directed toward the eye. Pupillometry demonstrates "escape" or redilation of the iris while the light is still directed toward the pupil.

Other acquired causes of small fiber peripheral neuropathy in children include thyroid dysfunction, celiac disease [45], Sjögren's disease [46, 47], systemic lupus erythematosus [48], nutritional factors including elevated pyridoxal phosphate or mercury or deficiencies in vitamins B1 or B12 [49], HIV/hepatitis C infections

[50], autoimmune impact of self-directed antibodies such as anti-Hu antibodies [51], and rare instances of chronic inflammatory demyelinating polyradiculoneuropathy (CIDP) which are selectively directed toward antigens on small nerve fibers [52]. Adults with restless leg syndrome [53] and fibromyalgia [54] have been shown to have reduced intraepidermal nerve fiber density on skin biopsy.

Children with chronic neuropathic pain have been demonstrated to have small fiber dysfunction. A recent series of 41 children and adolescents with disabling, chronic generalized pain of undetermined cause were evaluated by Oaklander and Klein [55]. More than half (59%) had definite and 17% had probable small fiber polyneuropathy (SFPN) by objective measures. 30% of skin biopsies for intraepidermal nerve fiber density, 100% of peripheral nerve biopsies, and 53% of autonomic function tests were diagnostic for SFPN. QSART was abnormal in 82%, HUT tests were abnormal in 75%, VR was abnormal in 42% and HR_{DB} abnormal in 27% of these children and adolescents with chronic generalized debilitating pain. An autoimmune etiology was felt likely as 61% had a history of a preceding infection, 52% had a family history of autoimmunity, 33% had prior personal history of autoimmune disease and two more were diagnosed with autoimmune systemic disease during the ongoing evaluation (Sjögren's syndrome and diabetes mellitus). Standard motor and sensory nerve conduction studies and needle electromyography were noncontributory when performed.

A number of potentially neurotoxic medications, useful for treatment of other types of disease in children and young adults, are well-documented to cause small fiber peripheral neuropathy. These include chemotherapeutic agents (particularly platinum-based compounds), the antiretroviral agents used to treat HIV infection [50], statins [56], TNF inhibitor medications [57] and metronidazole [58]. There is a single case report of an acquired acute onset small fiber neuropathy temporally associated with vaccination in an adult [59].

Conclusions

While small fiber neuropathies occur less frequently in children than adults, their presence can be associated with significant pain and functional limitation. The inability of infants and younger children to describe their symptoms and cooperate with focused sensory examinations makes availability of specialized diagnostic testing for small nerve fiber function more important. There are a number of types of sensory and autonomic testing, outlined in this chapter, which are tolerable by most children and relatively non-invasive. However, normal values for these tests are not always available in the same young age group where they are most valuable. The implementation of some of the novel techniques for evaluation of small fiber function, such as corneal confocal microscopy, will require collaboration with investigators across disciplines.

References

1. Kuntz NL, Patwari PP. Laboratory evaluation of pediatric autonomic disorders. Semin Pediatr Neurol. 2013;20(1):35–43.
2. Kuntz NL, Fealey RD. Pain can obscure autonomic dysfunction in acute, acquired small fiber neuropathies in children. Clin Auton Res. 2008;18(5):264.
3. Hivagyunuab A, Gibbons CH. Diagnosis and treatment of pain in small fiber neuropathy. Curr Pain Headache Rep. 2011;14(3):193–200.
4. Van Barneveld S, van der Palen J, van Putten MH. Evaluation of the finger wrinkling test: a pilot study. Clin Auton Res. 2010;20(4):249–53.
5. Freeman R, Chase KP, Risk MR. Quantitative sensory testing cannot differentiate simulated sensory loss from sensory neuropathy. Neurology. 2003;60:465–70.
6. Blackmore D, Siddizi ZA. Pinprick testing in small fiber neuropathy: accuracy and pitfalls. J Clin Neuromuscul Dis. 2016;17(4):181–6.
7. Lagerburg V, Bakkers M, Bouwhuis A, Hoeijmakers JGJ, Smit AM, Van Den Berg SJM, Hordijk-de Boer I, Broouwer-van Der Lee MDG, Kranendonk D, Reujlen JPH, Faber CG, Merkies ISJ. Contact heat-evoked potentials: normal values and use in small fiber neuropathy. Muscle Nerve. 2015;51:743–9.
8. Vallbo AB, Hagbarth KE, Wallin BG. Microneurography: how the technique developed and its role in the investigation of the sympathetic nervous system. J Appl Physiol. 2004;96(4):1262–9.
9. Singer W, Sletten DM, Opfer-Gehrking TL, et al. Postural tachycardia in children and adolescents—what is abnormal? J Pediatr. 2012;160(2):222–6.
10. Low PA, Sleeten DM. Laboatory evaluation ofautonomic failure. In: Low PA, Enarroch EE, editors. Clinical autonomic disorders. 3rd ed. Philadelphia, PA: Lippincott-Raven; 2008. p. 130–60.
11. Staino A, Santoro L, De Marco R, et al. Autonomic dysfunction in children with Hirschsprung's disease. Dig Dis Sci. 1999;44(5):960–5.
12. Novak P. Electrochemical skin conductance correlates with skin nerve fiber density. Front Aging Neurosci. 2016;8:199.
13. Longin E, Dimitriadis C, Shazi S, et al. Autonomic nervous system function in infants and adolescents: impact of autonomic tests on heart rate variability. Pediatr Cardiol. 2009;30:311–24.
14. Longin E, Schaible T, Lenz T, Konig S. Short term heart rate variability in healthy neonates: Normative data and physiologic observations. Early Hum Dev. 2005;81(8):883–671.
15. Daluwatte C, Miles JH, Christ SE, Beversdorf DQ, Takahashi TN, Yao G. Age-dependent pupillary light reflex parameters in children. Conf Proc IEEE Eng Med Biol Soc. 2012;2012:3776–9.
16. Kuntz NL, Fealey RE. Utility of diagnostic thermoregulatory sweat test in children. Neurology. 2010;76(9 Supp4):A575.
17. Shahani BT, Halperin JJ, Boulu P, Cohen J. Sympathetic skin response—a method of assessing unmyelinated axon dysfunction in peripheral neuropathies. J Neurol Neurosurg Psychiatry. 1984;47(5):536–42.
18. Pereon Y, Laplaud D, Nguyen TT, Radafy E. A new application for the sympathetic skin response: the evaluation of auditory thresholds in cochlear implant patients. Clin Neurophysiol. 2001;112(2):314–8.
19. Provitera V, Gibbons CH, Wendelschafer-Crabb G, Donadio V, Viktale DF, Stancanelli A, Caporaso G, Liguori R, Wang N, Santoro L, Kennedy WR, Nolano M. A multicenter, multinational age- and gender-adjusted normative dataset for immunofluorescent Intraepidermal nerve fiber density at the distal leg. Eur J Neurol. 2016;23(2):333–8.
20. McArthur JC, Stocks EA, Auer BS, Cornblath DR, Griffin JW. Epidermal nerve fiber density: normative reference range and diagnostic efficiency. Arch Neurol. 1998;55:1513–20.
21. Liu Y, Billiet J, Ebenezer GJ, Pan B, Hauer P, Wei J, Polydefkis M. Factors influencing sweat gland innervation in diabetes. Neurology. 2015;84(16):1652–9.
22. Chen X, Graham J, Dabbah MA, Petropoulos IN, Panirakis G, Asghar O, Alam U, Marshall A, Fadavi H, Ferdousi M, Azmi S, Tavakoli M, Efron N, Jeziorska M, Malik RA. Small nerve fiber quantification in the diagnosis of diabetic sensorimotor polyneuropathy: comparing corneal confocal microscopy with intraepidermal nerve fiber density. Diabetes Care. 2015;38:1138–44.

23. Bucher F, Schneider C, Blau T, Cursiefen C, Fink GR, Lehmann HC, Heindl LM. Small fiber neuropathy is associated with corneal nerve and dendritic cell alterations: an in vivo confocal microscopy study. Cornea. 2015;34(9):1114–9.
24. Birnbaum J, Duncan T, Owoyemi K, Wang KC, Carrino J, Chhabra A. Use of novel high-resolution magnetic reonance neurography protocol to detect abnormal dorsal root ganglia in Sjogren patients with neuropathic pain: case series of 10 patients and review of literature. Medicine (Baltimore). 2014;93(3):121–34.
25. Ebadi H, Siddiqui H, Ebadi S, Ngo M, Breiner A, Bril V. Peripheral nerve ultrasound in small fiber peripheral neuropathy. Ultrasound Med Biol. 2015;41(11):2820–6.
26. Houlden H, Reilly MM, Smith S. Pupil abnormalities in 131 cases of genetically defined inherited peripheral neuropathy. Eye. 2009;23(4):966–74.
27. Nicholson GA. Hereditary sensory neuropathy type Ia. In: Pagon RA, Adam MP, Ardinger HH, et al., editors. Gene reviews; 2015. http://www.ncbi.hlm.nih.gov/books/NBK1390/.
28. Kurth I. Hereditary sensory and autonomic neuropathy type II. In: Pagon RA, Adam MP, Ardinger HH, et al., editors. Gene reviews; 2015. http://www.ncbi.hlm.nih.gov/books/NBK1390/.
29. Shohat M, Hubshman MW. Familial dysautonomia. In: Pagon RA, Adam MP, Ardinger HH, et al., editors. Gene reviews; 2014. http://www.ncbi.hlm.nih.gov/books/NBK1390/.
30. Indo Y. Congenital insensitivity to pain with anhidrosis. In: Pagon RA, Adam MP, Ardinger HH, et al., editors. Gene reviews; 2014. http://www.ncbi.hlm.nih.gov/books/NBK1390/.
31. Cox JJ, Reimann F, Nicholas AK, Thornton G, Roberts E, Springell K, Karbani G, Jafri H, Mannan J, Raashid Y, Al-Gazali L, Hamamy H, Valente EM, Gorman S, Williams R, McHale DP, Wood JN, Gribble FM, Woods CG. An SCN9A channelopathy causes congenital inability to experience pain. Nature. 2006;444:894–8.
32. Emery EC, Habib AM, Nicholas AK CJJ, Gribble FM, Woods GG, Reimann F. Novel SCN9A mutations underlying extreme pain phenotypes: unexpected electrophysiological and clinical phenotype correlations. J Neurosci. 2015;35(20):7674–81.
33. Norris-Cook RH. Pediatric erythromelalgia: a retrospective review of 32 cases evaluated at Mayo Clinic over a 37 year period. J Am Acad Dermatol. 2012;66(3):416–23.
34. Cazzato D, Castori M, Lombardir R, Caravello F, Dalla Bella E, Petrucci A, Grammatico P, Dordoni C, Colombi M, Lauria G. Small fiber neuropathy is a common feature of Ehlers-Danlos Syndromes. Neurology. 2016;216(87):155–9.
35. Sturniolo GC, Lazzarini D, Bartolo O, Berton M, Leonardi A, Fregona IA, Parrozzani R, Midena E. Small fiber peripheral neuropathy in Wilson's Disease: An in vivo documentation by corneal confocal microscopy. Invest Ophthalmol Vis Sci. 2015;56(2):1390–5.
36. Soni D, Shukla G, Sing S, Goyal V, Behari M. Cardiovascular and sudomotor autonomic dysfunction in Wilson's disease—limited correlation with clinical severity. Auton Neurosci. 2009;151:154–8.
37. Schiffman R, Ries M. Fabry disease: a disorder of childhood onset. Pediatr Neurol. 2016;64:10–20.
38. Hobson-Webb LD, Austin SL, Jain S, Case LE, Greene K, Kishman PS. Small fiber neuropathy in Pompe Disease: first reported cases and prospective screening of a clinic cohort. Am J Case Rep. 2015;16:196–201.
39. Hafner J, Ghaoui R, Coyle L, Burke D, Ng K. Axonal excitability in primary amyloidosis neuropathy. Muscle Nerve. 2015;51(3):443–5.
40. Patwari PP, Stewart TM, Rand CM, Carroll MS, Kuntz NL, Kenny AS, Brogadir CD, Weese-Mayer DE. Pupillometry in Congenital Central Hypoventilation Syndrome (CCHS): Quantitative evidence of autonomic nervous system dysregulation. Pediatr Res. 2012;71(3):280–5.
41. Farhad K, Traub R, Ruzhansky KM, Brannagan RH III. Causes of neuropathy in patients referred as "idiopathic neuropathy". Muscle Nerve. 2016;53(6):856–61.
42. Vinik AI, Maser RE, Mitchell BD, Freeman R. Diabetic autonomic neuropathy. Diabetes Care. 2003;26(5):1553–79.
43. Dale RC, Lang B, Brilot F, Polfrit Y, Smith GH, Wong M. Treatment responsive pandysautonomia in an adolescent with ganglionic a3-AChR antibodies. Eur J Paediatr Neurol. 2012;16(4):296–8.

44. Muppidi S, Schribner M, Giibbons C, Adams-Huet B, Spaeth EB, Vernino SA. Unique manifestation of pupillary fatigue in autoimmune autonomic ganglionopathy. Arch Neurol. 2012;69(5):644–8.
45. Brannagan TH III, Hays AP, Chin SS, Sander HW, Chin RL, Magda P, Green PH, Latov N. Small-fiber neuropathy/neuronopathy associated with celiac disease: skin biopsy findings. Arch Neurol. 2005;62:1574–8.
46. Pereira PR, Viala K, Maisonbe T, aroche J, Mathian A, Hie M, Amoura Z, Aubart FC. Sjogren sensory neuronopathy (Sjogren ganglionopathy): Long term outcome and treatment response in series of 13 cases. Med (Balt). 2016;95(19):e3632–7.
47. Chai J, Herrmann DN, Stanton M, Barbano RL, Logigian EL. Painful small-fiber neuropathy in Sjogren syndrome. Neurology. 2005;65:925–7.
48. Goransson LG, Tjensvoll AB, Herigstad A, Mellgren SI, Omdal R. Small-diameter nerve fiber neuropathy in systemic lupus erythematosus. Arch Neurol. 2006;63:401–14.
49. Latov N, Vo ML, Chin RL, Carey BT, Langsdrf JA, Feuer NT. Abnormal Nutritional Factors in Patients Evaluated at a Neuropathy Center. J Clin Neuromuscul Dis. 2016;178(4):212–4.
50. Gonzalez-Duarte A, Robinson-Papp J, Simpson DM. Diagnosis and management of HIV-associated Neuropathy. Neurol Clin. 2008;26:821–32.
51. Camdessanche JP, Antoine JC, Honnorat J, Vial C, Petiot P, Convers P, Michel D. Paraneoplastic peripheral neuropathy associated with anti-Hu antibodies. A clinical and electrophysiological study of 20 patients. Brain. 2002;125:166–75.
52. Schneider C, Bucher F, Cursiefen C, Fink GR, Heindl LM, Lehmann HC. Corneal confocal microscopy detects small fiber damage in chronic inflammatory demyelinating polyneuropathy (CIDP). J Peripher Nerv Syst. 2014;19(4):322–7.
53. Polydefkis M, Allen RP, Hauer P, Earley CJ, Griffin JW, McArthur JC. Subclinical sensory neuropathy in late-onset restless legs syndrome. Neurology. 2000;55:1115–21.
54. Doppler K, Rittner HL, Deckart M, Sommer C. Reduced dermal nerve fiber diameter in skin biopsies of patients with fibromyalgia. Pain. 2015;156:2319–25.
55. Oaklander AL, Klein MM. Evidence of small-fiber polyneuropathy in unexplained, Juvenile-Onset, widespread pain syndrome. Pediatrics. 2013;131(4):1091–100.
56. Novak P, Pimentel DA, Sundar B, Moonis M, Qin L, Novak V. Association of Statins with Sensory and Autonomic Ganglionopathy. Front Aging Neurosci. 2015;7:Article 191.
57. Birnbaum J. Sensory neuronopathy associated with tumor necrosis factor inhibitor treatment. Neurol Clin Pract. 2014;4(6):516–8.
58. Tan CH, Chen YF, Chen CC, Chao CC, Liou HH, Hsieh ST. Painful neuropathy due to skin denervation after metronidazole-induced neurotoxicity. J Neurol Neurosurg Psychiatry. 2010;82(4):462–5.
59. Kafaie J, Kim M, Krause E. Small fiber neuropathy following vaccination. J Clin Neuromuscul Dis. 2016;18(1):37–40.

Chapter 20
Mononeuropathies

Ioannis Karakis

Introduction

Suspected mononeuropathies are the second most common reason for referral to the pediatric EMG laboratory. In a large series of 2100 pediatric studies performed in a single tertiary center over 11 years, polyneuropathy evaluation was consistently the leading indication, ranging from 29% to 35% of the requested studies per year, while mononeuropathy evaluations constituted 13–26% of requests per year. Similarly, polyneuropathy and, less frequently, mononeuropathy were the prevailing abnormal diagnoses, ranging together from 40 to 74% of the abnormal studies per year. Overall, peroneal (24%) and ulnar (22%) lesions constituted approximately half of all diagnosed mononeuropathies, followed by median (17%), facial (9%), sciatic (9%), radial (8%), tibial (4%), femoral (2%), and sural (2%) neuropathies [1] (Fig. 20.1).

Mononeuropathies are seen in childhood as well as in adulthood, but as with other disease categories, the presentation and distribution of specific mononeuropathies is often different in children compared to adults. Akin to every other field in neurology, evaluation of a child presenting with mononeuropathy starts with a detailed history and a meticulous clinical examination. Traumatic, compressive and entrapment etiologies are most frequently elicited on history. The clinical examination may confirm single nerve involvement, and exclude alternative musculoskeletal or neurological (e.g., radiculopathy or plexopathy) mimickers. When multiple mononeuropathies are suspected, a quest for additional historical symptoms or clinical signs for a multisystemic disease (e.g., hereditary neuropathy with liability to pressure palsies, vasculitis, sarcoidosis, amyloidosis, leprosy, etc.) should be performed. A summary of the clinical signs and differential diagnosis of the upper and lower extremity mononeuropathies is provided in (Tables 20.1 and 20.2).

I. Karakis, MD, PhD, MSc, FAAN, FAANEM, FAES
Department of Neurology, Emory University School of Medicine, Atlanta, GA, USA
e-mail: ioannis.karakis@emory.edu

© Springer International Publishing AG 2017

H.J. McMillan, P.B. Kang (eds.), *Pediatric Electromyography*,
DOI 10.1007/978-3-319-61361-1_20

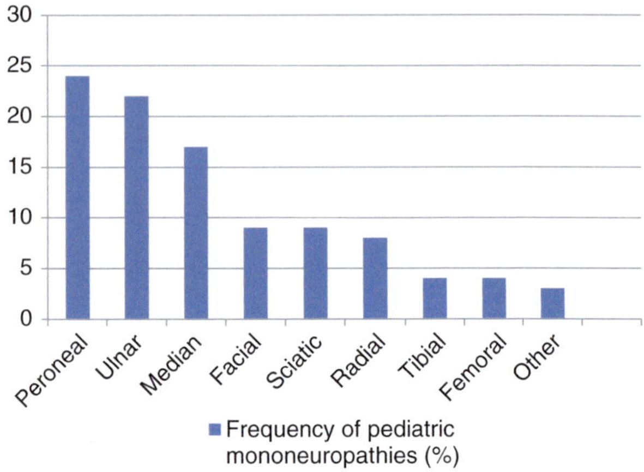

Fig. 20.1 Frequency of pediatric mononeuropathies (%)

The electrodiagnostic approach to potential mononeuropathies aims to 1) confirm the presence of a mononeuropathy, 2) exclude alternative monomelic (e.g., radiculopathy or plexopathy) or polymelic (e.g., mononeuritis multiplex or polyneuropathy) diagnoses, 3) localize the injury site, 4) assess the chronicity of the lesion, 5) evaluate for nerve continuity, and 6) clarify underlying pathophysiological mechanisms (demyelination vs. axonal vs. mixed) that may provide prognostic information. During electrodiagnostic testing, the examiner should remember that normative values vary significantly with age for the first five years of life, and that side-to-side comparisons are often helpful when potential abnormalities arise, given that older children and adolescents often have values that are perceptibly robust compared to what would be expected. A summary of the electrodiagnostic findings and electrodiagnostic differential diagnosis of the most common upper and lower extremity mononeuropathies is provided in Tables 20.3 and 20.4.

Prognosis is heavily dependent on the underlying etiology and the associated pathophysiological mechanism. With the advent of sophisticated imaging modalities, such as MR neurography and ultrasound as useful adjuncts to the clinical and electrodiagnostic examination, surgical exploration is saved nowadays for unclarified cases without recovery portending significant disability. Overall, neurapraxic lesions (i.e., segmental demyelination) are associated with auspicious recovery potential, while axonotmetic (i.e., axonal damage with intact epineurium) and especially neurotmetic (i.e., loss of any nerve continuity) lesions carry a grimmer prognosis, unless surgical repair is attempted in a timely fashion [2]. Physical therapy to prevent joint contractures and occupational therapy to improve function, use of splints and analgesia are also important during recuperation [3].

The following chapter reviews the electrodiagnostic approach for potential pediatric mononeuropathies. Additional information on the neuromuscular aspect of mononeuropathies in children is available in other textbooks [4, 5].

Table 20.1 Clinical diagnosis of focal neuropathies in the upper extremity

Nerve	Common lesion site	Typical causes	Weakness	Numbness	Deep tendon reflexes	Differential diagnosis
Median	Wrist	Mucopolysaccharidosis	Thumb abduction, extension and flexion	Palmar surface of first 3.5 digits	Present	Proximal median neuropathy, middle trunk/lateral cord (for sensory symptoms) or lower trunk/medial cord brachial plexopathy (for motor symptoms), C6–C7 sensory radiculopathy or C8–T1 motor radiculopathy
Ulnar	Elbow	Elbow fracture	Finger abduction and adduction, finger flexion of distal last two digits	Palmar and dorsal surface of last 1.5 digits and dorsum of the medial hand	Present	Lower trunk/medial cord brachial plexopathy, C8–T1 radiculopathy
Radial	Spiral groove	Humeral fracture	Finger and wrist extension, elbow flexion with semipronated hand	Dorsal surface of lateral hand and proximal phalanges of first 3.5 digits	Absent brachioradialis	Middle trunk/posterior cord brachial plexopathy, C6–C7 radiculopathy

(continued)

Table 20.1 (continued)

Nerve	Common lesion site	Typical causes	Weakness	Numbness	Deep tendon reflexes	Differential diagnosis
Axillary	Quadrilateral space	Shoulder dislocation	Shoulder abduction and external rotation	Lateral shoulder	Present	Upper trunk/posterior cord plexopathy, C5–C6 radiculopathy
Long thoracic	Scalene muscle	Parsonage Turner syndrome	Scapular winging w anterior shoulder flexion	None	Present	C5–C7 radiculopathy
Suprascapular	Suprascapular notch	Scapular fracture	Shoulder abduction and external rotation	None	Present	C5–C6 radiculopathy
Spinal Accessory	Sternocleidomastoid triangle	Lymph node biopsy	Head deviation to contralateral side and shoulder elevation. Scapular winging with shoulder abduction	None	Present	C3–C4 radiculopathy
Musculocutaneous	Biceps heads	Humeral fracture	Elbow flexion with hand supinated, hand supination with elbow flexed, partial shoulder anterior flexion	Lateral forearm	Absent biceps	Upper trunk/lateral cord brachial plexopathy, C5–C6 radiculopathy
Phrenic	Mediastinum	Mediastinal surgery	Diaphragmatic weakness	None	Present	C3–C5 radiculopathy

Table 20.2 Clinical diagnosis of focal neuropathies in the lower extremity

Nerve	Common lesion site	Typical causes	Weakness	Numbness	Deep tendon reflexes	Differential diagnosis
Peroneal	Fibular head	Leg crossing after weight loss	Foot dorsiflexion and eversion	Dorsum of the foot	Present	Peroneal division of sciatic nerve, lumbosacral plexopathy, L5 radiculopathy, conus medullaris/cauda equina syndrome
Tibial	Popliteal fossa and ankle	Knee and ankle fractures	Toes plantarflexion and abduction (distal) Additionally, foot plantarflexion and inversion (proximal)	Plantar surface of the foot	Absent ankle jerk (proximal)	Tibial division of sciatic nerve, lumbosacral plexopathy, S1 radiculopathy, conus medullaris/cauda equina syndrome
Sciatic	Pelvis and thigh	Injection trauma	Foot dorsi- and plantarflexion, foot inversion and eversion, knee flexion	Dorsum and plantar surface of the foot, lateral and posterior foreleg	Absent ankle jerk	Lumbosacral plexopathy, L5–S1 radiculopathy, conus medullaris/cauda equina syndrome
Femoral	Pelvis and thigh	Psoas hematoma	Knee extension (distal) and also hip flexion (proximal)	Anterior thigh and medial foreleg	Absent knee jerk	Lumbar plexopathy, L2–L4 radiculopathy, cauda equina syndrome
Obturator	Obturator foramen	Hip fracture	Hip adduction	Medial thigh	Present	Lumbar plexopathy, L2–L4 radiculopathy, cauda equina syndrome
Pudendal	Alcock's canal	Cycling	Perineal muscles	Penis or labia majora	Present	S2–S4 radiculopathies, sacral plexopathy, conus medullaris/ cauda equina syndrome

(continued)

Nerve	Common lesion site	Typical causes	Weakness	Numbness	Deep tendon reflexes	Differential diagnosis
Lateral Femoral Cutaneous	Inguinal ligament	Obesity	None	Lateral thigh	Present	Lumbar plexopathy, L2–L3 radiculopathy
Posterior Femoral Cutaneous	Buttock	Trauma	None	Posterior thigh	Present	Sacral plexopathy, S1–S3 radiculopathy, conus medullaris/cauda equina syndrome
Sural	Calf	Nerve biopsy	None	Posterior foreleg and lateral foot	Present	Lumbosacral plexopathy, S1 radiculopathy, conus medullaris/cauda equina syndrome
Saphenous	Thigh or knee	Knee surgery	None	Medial foreleg and foot	Present	Lumbosacral plexopathy, L4 radiculopathy, cauda equina syndrome
Superior gluteal	Pelvis	Hip fracture and surgery	Hip abduction and internal rotation	None	Present	Lumbosacral plexopathy, L4–S1 radiculopathy, conus medullaris/cauda equina syndrome
Inferior gluteal	Pelvis	Hip fracture and surgery	Hip extension	None	Present	Lumbosacral plexopathy, L5–S2 radiculopathy, conus medullaris/cauda equina syndrome
Iliohypogastric, ilioinguinal and genitofemoral	Retroperitoneal space and inguinal ligament	Hernioraphy	Lower lateral abdominal muscles and cremaster muscle weakness	Lower abdomen and upper anterior and medial thigh	Present	T12–L2 radiculopathies

Table 20.3 Electrophysiologic differential diagnosis of the most common focal neuropathies in the upper extremity

Nerve/muscle	Median neuropathy at the wrist	Ulnar neuropathy at the elbow	Radial neuropathy at the spiral groove	Lower trunk/ medial cord brachial plexopathy	Middle trunk/ posterior cord brachial plexopathy	C6–C7 radiculopathy	C8–T1 radiculopathy
Median SNAP digit II	Abnormal	Normal	Normal	Normal	Abnormal in middle trunk and normal in posterior cord	Normal	Normal
Ulnar SNAP digit V	Normal	Abnormal	Normal	Abnormal	Normal	Normal	Normal
Radial SNAP snuffbox	Normal	Normal	Abnormal	Normal	Abnormal	Normal	Normal
Medial antebrachial cutaneous	Normal	Normal	Normal	Abnormal	Normal	Normal	Normal
Median CMAP to abductor pollicis brevis	Abnormal	Normal	Normal	Abnormal	Normal	Normal	Abnormal
Ulnar CMAP to abductor digiti minimi	Normal	Abnormal	Normal	Abnormal	Normal	Normal	Abnormal
Radial CMAP to extensor indicis proprius	Normal	Normal	Abnormal	Abnormal in lower trunk and normal in medial cord	Abnormal in posterior cord and mostly normal in middle trunk	Normal	Abnormal
Abductor pollicis brevis EMG	Abnormal	Normal	Normal	Abnormal	Normal	Normal	Abnormal

(continued)

Table 20.3 (continued)

Nerve/muscle	Median neuropathy at the wrist	Ulnar neuropathy at the elbow	Radial neuropathy at the spiral groove	Lower trunk/ medial cord brachial plexopathy	Middle trunk/ posterior cord brachial plexopathy	C6–C7 radiculopathy	C8–T1 radiculopathy
First dorsal interosseous EMG	Normal	Abnormal	Normal	Abnormal	Normal	Normal	Abnormal
Extensor indicis proprius EMG	Normal	Normal	Abnormal	Abnormal in lower trunk and normal in medial cord	Abnormal in posterior cord and mostly normal in middle trunk	Mostly normal	Abnormal
Triceps EMG	Normal	Normal	Normal	Mostly normal	Abnormal	Abnormal	Mostly normal
Deltoid EMG	Normal	Normal	Normal	Normal	Abnormal in posterior cord and normal in middle trunk	Normal	Normal
Lateral antebracheal cutaneous SNAP	Normal	Normal	Normal	Abnormal	Normal	Normal	Normal
Infraspinatus EMG	Normal	Normal	Normal	Normal	Normal	Normal	Normal
Deltoid EMG	Normal	Normal	Normal	Normal	Normal	Normal	Abnormal
Biceps EMG	Normal	Normal	Normal	Normal	Normal	Abnormal	Abnormal

In purely demyelinating or hyperacute axonal lesions, NCS recorded from stimulation distal to the lesion would be preserved and needle examination of affected muscles would only show reduced recruitment

Certain studies (e.g., LAC or MAC) may be technically challenging or age dependent and should be interpreted with caution and/or using the unaffected, contralateral side (where available) for comparison

Table 20.4 Electrophysiologic differential diagnosis of the most common focal neuropathies in the lower extremity

Nerve/Muscle	Peroneal neuropathy at fibular head	Tibial neuropathy at popliteal fossa	Sciatic neuropathy at pelvis	Lumbosacral plexopathy	L5 radiculopathy	S1 radiculopathy
Superficial peroneal SNAP	Abnormal	Normal	Abnormal	Abnormal	Normal	Normal
Sural SNAP	Normal	Abnormal	Abnormal	Abnormal	Normal	Normal
Peroneal CMAP to tibialis anterior/extensor digitorum brevis	Abnormal	Normal	Abnormal	Abnormal	Abnormal	Normal
Tibial CMAP to abductor hallucis	Normal	Abnormal	Abnormal	Abnormal	Normal	Abnormal
Tibialis anterior/peroneus longus EMG	Abnormal	Normal	Abnormal	Abnormal	Abnormal	Normal
Tibialis posterior/Flexor digitorum longus EMG	Normal	Abnormal	Abnormal	Abnormal	Abnormal	Normal
Medial gastrocnemius EMG	Normal	Abnormal	Abnormal	Abnormal	Normal	Abnormal
Short head biceps femoris EMG	Normal	Normal	Abnormal	Abnormal	Normal	Abnormal
Gluteus medius/tensor fascia latae EMG	Normal	Normal	Normal	Abnormal	Abnormal	Normal
L5 paraspinals EMG	Normal	Normal	Normal	Normal	Abnormal	Normal
S1 paraspinals EMG	Normal	Normal	Normal	Normal	Normal	Abnormal

	Femoral neuropathy	Lumbar plexopathy	L2–L4 radiculopathy
Saphenous SNAP	Abnormal	Abnormal	Normal
Femoral CMAP to rectus femoris	Abnormal	Abnormal	Abnormal
Tibialis anterior EMG	Normal	Abnormal	Abnormal
Vastus lateralis EMG	Abnormal	Abnormal	Abnormal

Table 20.3 (continued)

	Femoral neuropathy	Lumbar plexopathy	L2–L4 radiculopathy
Adductor longus EMG	Normal	Abnormal	Abnormal
L2–L4 paraspinals	Normal	Normal	Abnormal

Incipient mononeuropathies may affect the sensory fibers of mixed nerve first, before affecting the motor fibers. Moreover, peak latency of NCS may be first affected prior to amplitude drop

In purely demyelinating or hyperacute axonal lesions, NCS recorded from stimulation distal to the lesion would be preserved and needle examination of affected muscles would only show reduced recruitment

In fascicular involvement (e.g., peroneal division sciatic neuropathy at the pelvis or deep peroneal neuropathy at the fibular head), not all abnormalities depicted above are expected

Given the dual innervation of most muscles (e.g., paraspinals), subtle abnormalities may be seen beyond the classical distribution, but they are typically less prominent. For the same reason, amplitude drop may be seen in severe single radiculopathies

Clinical syndromes often do not respect strict anatomic boundaries (e.g., radiculoplexus neuropathy) and therefore, a combination of listed findings may be seen

Certain studies (e.g., femoral CMAP and saphenous SNAP) may be technically challenging or age dependent and should be interpreted with caution and with contralateral comparison

Upper Extremity Mononeuropathies

Median Nerve

Anatomy

The median nerve is formed from the union of portions of the lateral and medial cord in the brachial plexus. The lateral cord is derived from the C5–C6 nerve root fibers from the upper trunk and C7 nerve root fibers from the middle trunk and serves predominantly sensory and proximal motor functions. The medial cord is derived from C8–T1 nerve root fibers through the lower trunk and serves exclusively motor functions. The nerve does not innervate any muscles in the upper arm, which can present challenges for precise localization in proximal medial neuropathies. In the forearm the nerve innervates the pronator teres (C6–C7), flexor carpi radialis (C6–C7), palmaris longus (C7–T1), and flexor digitorum superficialis (C7–C8). In the forearm the anterior interosseous nerve branches off the main stem of the median nerve, providing exclusively motor innervation to the lateral head of the flexor digitorum profundus (C7–C8), flexor pollicis longus (C7–C8), and pronator quadratus (C7–C8). The remainder of the median nerve enters the wrist through the carpal tunnel, with the palmar cutaneous nerve branching off proximal to the carpal tunnel. It then provides sensation to the palmar surface of the first three digits and half of the fourth digit along with the dorsum of their distal phalanges, as well as motor input to the first two lumbricals (C8–T1), the abductor pollicis brevis (C8–T1), the opponens pollicis (C8–T1), and the superficial head of the flexor pollicis brevis (C8–T1).

Etiology

Traumatic causes, typically from elbow fractures, lacerations or medical procedures, are the leading culprits for proximal medial neuropathies. Entrapment from the fibromuscular bands such as lacertum fibrosus, the ligament of Struthers, bicipital aponeurosis, hypertrophied heads of pronator teres muscle and the sublimis bridge of the flexor digitorum superficialis, as well as compression from soft tissue or bone tumors have also been reported [6]. Additionally, the anterior interosseous branch can be selectively affected from idiopathic brachial plexitis [7]. Distal median neuropathies (a.k.a. carpal tunnel syndrome) are rare in children. Metabolic (e.g., mucopolysaccharidoses), genetic (e.g., familial carpal tunnel syndrome or hereditary neuropathy with liability to pressure palsies) and mechanical (e.g., sport trauma, arthritis, tenosynovitis, macrodactyly, hemophilia, tumors) disorders constitute the main etiologies for carpal tunnel syndrome in children [8–10].

Clinical Evaluation

In infants and young children or in older children with cognitive difficulties related to inborn errors of metabolism, sensory complaints are hard to tease out. When present, they conform to the palmar surface of the first three and a half digits, and in proximal cases, also to the thenar eminence. Subtle symptoms such as clumsiness, nocturnal waking, and nibbling of the fingers should be noted. Examination will typically reveal atrophy and weakness in the thenar eminence ("simian hand"), and in proximal lesions, also of the median-innervated finger flexors ("benediction hand") [4]. Tinel's and/or Phalen's signs may be present, though notoriously fraught by variable sensitivity and specificity, especially in childhood [10]. In anterior interosseous neuropathies, the inability to make a round "O" with the thumb and index finger is a classic sign (Table 20.1).

Electrophysiologic Evaluation

Nerve conduction studies should include SNAP recording either from one of the median-innervated digits (typically the second, though in infants the middle finger is sometimes used), CMAP recording from the thenar eminence, and needle examination of distal and proximal median innervated muscles. In mild carpal tunnel syndrome cases, the only abnormalities detected may be sensory findings, starting with peak latency prolongation, or median to ulnar or median to radial comparison studies. In more severe cases, amplitude reduction of the median sensory study and similar abnormalities in the median motor studies are present. In young children, normal values for distal latencies cannot be used due to the difficulty of standardizing distances between the stimulating and the recording electrodes, thus nerve conduction velocities are important values to calculate, when applicable. For proximal median neuropathies, sensory and motor median amplitudes may be reduced with stimulation above the area of compression, in conjunction with normal distal latencies and reduced conduction velocity at the forearm. In contrast, nerve conduction studies are typically normal in pure anterior interosseous neuropathies. Needle examination can be very helpful in localizing the lesion. In demyelinating lesions affecting the motor fibers, only reduced recruitment is seen, while in cases involving axonal damage, signs of denervation and/or reinnervation should be observed. The possibility of congenital thenar hypoplasia should be remembered. For this benign diagnosis, electrophysiologic testing only shows a reduced CMAP in the abductor pollicis brevis with normal sensory NCS and needle exam [11]. When sensory symptoms predominate, the differential diagnosis also includes a middle trunk brachial plexopathy and C6–C7 radiculopathy. When motor complaints dominate the clinical picture, the differential diagnosis of median neuropathy also includes a medial cord/lower trunk plexopathy (e.g., thoracic outlet syndrome) and C8–T1 radiculopathy (Table 20.3). Thus, testing of the ulnar and radial SNAPs, as well the ulnar CMAP recording abductor digiti minimi is important, in addition to needle examination of non-median C6–C7 (e.g., triceps) and C8–T1 (e.g., first dorsal interosseous) muscles. Finally, NCS and needle EMG results should be evaluated with caution when a Martin-Gruber anastomosis is present, both in distal (e.g., positive dip in median CMAP studies with proximal stimulation along with artificially increased conduction velocity at the forearm), as well as in proximal (e.g., abnormalities may be detected in aberrantly innervated distal ulnar muscles) median neuropathies. The clinical and electrodiagnostic findings may require further investigations to pinpoint the underlying cause (e.g., imaging, metabolic or genetic screening, etc.).

Treatment and Prognosis

Management and prognosis rely heavily on the nature and degree of the underlying insult. Demyelinating lesions and axonal lesions with preserved continuity carry a better prognosis. In such cases, conservative measures with avoidance of aggravating activities, orthoses and steroid injections are typically recommended first. In more severe cases, surgical decompression and repair may be required [10]. In the setting of mucopolysaccharidoses, surgical release of carpal tunnel syndrome has been documented to be beneficial [12, 13].

Ulnar Nerve

Anatomy

The ulnar nerve is derived from nerve fibers of the C8 and T1 roots descending down the brachial plexus through the lower trunk and medial cord. Similar to the median nerve, it does not innervate muscles in the upper arm, rendering precise localization of proximal lesions challenging. After traveling through the epicondylar groove and subsequently the cubital tunnel, it enters the forearm, where it innervates the flexor carpi ulnaris (C8–T1) and the medial head of the flexor digitorum profundus (C8–T1). In a minority of people, anastomotic ulnar fibers destined for various ulnar innervated intrinsic hand muscles travel down the humerus within the median nerve, before crossing over the ulnar nerve above the wrist (Martin-Gruber anastomosis). Prior to reaching the palm, it provides cutaneous innervation in the dorsum of the medial hand and the last one and a half digits through the dorsal ulnar cutaneous branch. At the wrist, the nerve passes through Guyon's canal, where it diverges into a superficial and a deep palmar branch. The former branch is predominantly sensory, providing sensation to the last one and a half digits, aside from motor input to the palmaris brevis muscle (C8–T1). The latter is exclusively motor, innervating the hypothenar muscles (abductor digiti minimi, opponens digiti minimi and flexor digiti minimi) and then loops around the palm innervating the third and fourth lumbricals, as well as all the interossei, before terminating at the thenar eminence (adductor pollicis and deep head of flexor pollicis brevis) (all C8–T1).

Etiology

In contrast to the adult population where it ranks second to median neuropathy, ulnar neuropathy is the most common upper extremity mononeuropathy in childhood and adolescence [1]. The most common causes include trauma (elbow fractures or dislocations, lacerations, repetitive elbow movements), entrapment (cubital tunnel syndrome), compression (chair arm rests or bicycle handles, compartment syndrome and hematoma) and neural tumors [4, 14].

Clinical Evaluation

When present, sensory complaints localize to the fifth digit. In proximal ulnar neuropathies, sensation at the dorsum of the medial side of the hand is also affected. Weakness and atrophy universally involves the ulnar-innervated intrinsic hand muscles, though to variable degrees depending on the location of the lesion. In advanced cases, hand clawing may develop. For proximal ulnar neuropathies, there is also weakness in medial wrist flexion and flexion of the last phalanges of the last two digits, leading to less prominent hand clawing. There may be an inability to hold a piece of paper between the first and second digits without needing to flex the last phalanx of the thumb (Froment sign) or an inability to hold the last two digits together (Wartenberg sign). A Tinel's sign at the cubital tunnel may be present in compressive cases in that region (Table 20.1).

Electrophysiologic Evaluation

Nerve conduction studies of the ulnar SNAP to digit V and the dorsal ulnar cutaneous nerve should be performed, as well as motor nerve conduction studies of the FDI and the ADM; some younger children and most older children will tolerate all of this testing well, while a few who are anxious and cannot be easily soothed may end up with studies restricted to a digit V SNAP and motor study recording ADM. In distal ulnar neuropathies at Guyon's canal, the dorsal ulnar cutaneous SNAP and occasionally the digit V SNAP are spared (pure motor distal ulnar neuropathy). In other cases, an abnormal digit V SNAP may be the only evidence of a distal ulnar neuropathy restricted to the superficial branch (pure sensory distal ulnar neuropathy). When the motor branches are affected, the FDI CMAP is typically abnormal, whereas the ADM CMAP may be spared, depending on how distal the lesion is. In proximal ulnar neuropathies, there is usually conduction slowing with or without conduction block across the elbow, that can be further substantiated with inching studies. Proper and stable positioning of the elbow in a flexed position is paramount to avoid erroneous results, thus such meticulous testing may not be practical to perform in an anxious child. Distal sensory and motor potentials may be spared in purely demyelinating or hyperacute lesions, but are usually affected in axonal and mixed lesions. It is important to remember that an amplitude drop at the forearm may be due to a Martin-Gruber anastomosis rather than a true conduction block. When the question of a Martin-Gruber anastomosis arises, stimulation of the median nerve at the antecubital fossa while recording from the aberrantly innervated distal ulnar muscles can resolve the question.

Needle examination should include at least one proximal and one distal ulnar innervated muscle, in addition to non-ulnar innervated C8–T1 muscles. The differential diagnosis of an ulnar neuropathy typically includes a medial cord/lower trunk brachial plexopathy and a C8–T1 radiculopathy (Table 20.3). When the electromyographer is faced with an anxious child who may not tolerate examination of more than a handful of muscles, clinical information such as the location of a fracture or other traumatic lesion helps prioritize which muscles are most important to examine.

In the largest study of 49 children and adolescents published to date [15], sensory loss at digit V was the most common complaint (89%). The predominant localization was at the elbow (55%), followed by the forearm (23%) and humerus (14%). In ulnar neuropathies localized at the elbow, slowing was seen in about half of the cases, while conduction block was seen in a quarter. In all cases, diminished ulnar SNAP was the most common abnormality (71%), dorsal ulnar cutaneous SNAP was reduced in 55% and first dorsal interosseous CMAP was reduced half of the time. There was high correlation between ulnar SNAP median axon loss estimate with median axon loss estimate in the dorsal ulnar cutaneous SNAP and ADM and FDI CMAPs. Neurogenic changes were seen in the ADM and FDI in almost 79% and 77% of the cases, as opposed to the FCU in 25% and the FDP IV in 35% of the cases. In proximal localizations, intrinsic hand muscles were more affected than proximal ulnar muscles in 52% of cases. Pathophysiology was demyelinating in 27%, axonal in 59% and mixed in 14%. There is therefore frequent axonal and fascicular injury in pediatric ulnar neuropathy, similar to adults [16]. In proximal axonal lesions, sensory and motor fibers to distal muscles are predominantly affected, whereas in demyelinating lesions, slowing occurs twice as commonly as conduction block.

Treatment and Prognosis

Treatment varies from splinting and avoidance of aggravating factors in mild compressive cases, to decompression in severe entrapment cases and grafting when the nerve has been transected. Simple decompression is very effective, while neurolysis often leads to improvement [17]. As with other nerve injuries, recovery tends to be better with atraumatic or mildly traumatic insults to the ulnar nerve [14].

Radial Nerve

Anatomy

The radial nerve is one of the two terminal branches of the posterior cord of the brachial plexus, carrying nerve fibers from the C5–C8 nerve roots. In contrast to the median and ulnar nerves, it provides branches along its course and innervates muscles in the humerus. Proximal to the spiral groove, the posterior cutaneous nerve of the arm, motor branches to the triceps (C6–C8) and the anconeus (C6–C8), and the posterior cutaneous nerve of the forearm all branch off. Distal to spiral groove and before entering the elbow, it innervates the brachioradialis (C5–C6) and extensor carpi radialis longus (C5–C6). It then bifurcates into the superficial radial nerve that will provide sensation to the dorsum of the lateral hand and the first three and a half digits, and the predominantly motor posterior interosseous nerve. The latter enters the forearm through the arcade of Frohse of the supinator muscle (C6–C7) and, in addition to that muscle, it innervates sequentially the extensor carpi radialis brevis (C5–C7), the extensor digitorum communis (C7–C8), the extensor digiti minimi (C7–C8), the extensor carpi ulnaris (C7–C8), the abductor pollicis longus (C7–C8), the extensor pollicis brevis (C7–C8) and the extensor indicis proprius (EIP) (C7–C8).

Etiology

Radial mononeuropathies are the second most common upper extremity mononeuropathy in children. Once again, traumatic causes (fractures, injections, lacerations) predominate followed by compression (perioperative positioning, compartment syndrome and hematoma) and neural tumors [4, 18, 19].

Clinical Evaluation

The cardinal feature of a radial neuropathy is difficulty extending the fingers with or without concomitant wrist drop. In posterior interosseous lesions, there is partial preservation of wrist extension, typically with radial deviation, accounting for sparing of the extensor carpi radialis longus. In such occasions, sensation in the dorsum of the hand is unaffected. More proximal severe lesions are associated with sensory deficits in the dorsum of the hand along with complete wrist drop/finger drop. Concomitant brachioradialis weakness suggests a lesion at the spiral groove, while concomitant triceps weakness suggests a lesion at the axilla. Examination of other major nerves of the upper extremity to exclude a brachial plexopathy or cervical radiculopathy should be performed carefully while the affected wrist is passively hyperextended; other nerves may artifactually appear to be affected when examined with the affected wrist in a dropped position. A Tinel's sign at a site of blunt traumatic injury may be present (Table 20.1).

Electrophysiologic Evaluation

In addition to routine nerve conduction studies in the ulnar and median nerves, the radial sensory response and the radial motor response to EIP with stimulation up to the axilla should be evaluated. Needle EMG should include posterior interosseous nerve muscles (e.g., finger or wrist extensors) in addition to muscles innervated by branches that originate below (e.g., brachioradialis) and above (e.g., triceps) the spiral groove. In a posterior interosseous neuropathy, the superficial sensory response remains intact, but the radial motor response to the EIP is impaired, with sparing of radial-innervated muscles above the elbow. In more proximal lesions with at least partial axonal involvement, the superficial sensory response and motor response are both affected, commonly with a superimposed conduction block observed with stimulation below and above the injury site. Needle examination for lesions at or below the spiral groove in the upper arm spares the triceps, but affects the brachioradialis. For more proximal lesions, a posterior cord brachial plexopathy should be excluded by sampling axillary nerve muscles (e.g., deltoid or teres minor) and a middle trunk/C6–7 radiculopathy must be excluded by testing non-radial C6–C7 innervated muscles (e.g., flexor carpi radialis) (Table 20.3).

In the largest pediatric study published to-date, radial neuropathy localized to the proximal main radial nerve in 13%, distal main radial nerve trunk in 56% and posterior interosseous nerve in 31% of affected children in the cohort [18].

Treatment and Prognosis

Treatment depends on the etiology, severity, pathophysiology and chronicity and ranges from conservative measures to surgical exploration and repair. Prognosis in children with radial mononeuropathies is also dependent on the aforementioned factors. In the previously published series, radial neuropathy generally had a favorable prognosis in both neonates [20] and children [21]. Typically the convalescent period lasted 6–12 weeks for demyelinating lesions and up to 17 months for axonal injuries [18].

Other Upper Extremity Nerves

Axillary Nerve

Along with the radial nerve, the axillary nerve is the second terminal branch of the posterior cord of the brachial plexus. It runs in close proximity to the humeral head and provides sensory innervation to the lateral shoulder and motor innervation to the deltoid (C5–C6) and teres minor (C5–C6) muscles. Thus, injury of this nerve results in a patch of numbness at the lateral shoulder along with weakness in shoulder abduction and external rotation (Table 20.1). In children this nerve is usually injured in the setting of shoulder joint trauma [22]. Neurodiagnostic evaluation typically focuses on the affected muscles and muscles that may help exclude mimickers (e.g., upper trunk plexopathy or C5–C6 radiculopathy) (Table 20.3).

Long Thoracic Nerve

The long thoracic nerve originates from the C5–C7 cervical nerve roots prior to their merging into the brachial plexus. It innervates the anterior serratus muscle (C5–C7), participating in shoulder blade stabilization. Therefore, injury to that nerve manifests with scapular winging that becomes more evident during anterior flexion of the arm (Table 20.3). Most cases in children are traumatic in origin, [21, 23] but it can also represent a form fruste of brachial neuritis. Needle examination of the serratus anterior should be performed with caution due to the risk of pneumothorax, and should not be attempted at all in an anxious or uncooperative child. It should be remembered that scapular winging may occur in some myopathies such as facioscapulohumeral muscular dystrophy, and that this muscular dystrophy may be initially asymmetric and can also be associated with a normal serum creatine kinase level.

Musculocutaneous Nerve

The musculocutaneous nerve is derived from the lateral cord of the brachial plexus. After providing innervation to the coracobrachialis, brachialis and biceps (all innervated at C5–C6), it continues in the lateral forearm as a sensory nerve. Its damage results in weakness of arm and elbow flexion, hand supination in a flexed elbow position, numbness in the lateral forearm and a reduced biceps jerk. (Table 20.1) In the pediatric population, most causes are traumatic, [21, 24] though it can also be affected in cases of brachial plexitis. Electrophysiologic testing includes nerve conduction studies of bilateral lateral antebrachial cutaneous responses and needle examination of the biceps. The possibility of a C5–C6 radiculopathy, upper trunk or lateral cord plexopathy needs to be clinically and electrodiagnostically excluded (Table 20.3).

Suprascapular Nerve

The suprascapular nerve is composed of C5–C6 nerve fibers that branch off the upper trunk of the brachial plexus to innervate the supraspinatus and infraspinatus muscles. When injured, this nerve results in shoulder abduction and external rotation weakness (Table 20.1). Suprascapular neuropathies are usually of traumatic etiology and can occur proximally, at the level of the suprascapular notch, [25] leading to needle EMG abnormalities in both supra-and infraspinatus muscles (both C5–C6), or more distally, at the level of the spinoglenoid notch, [26] leading to needle EMG abnormalities only at the infraspinatus muscle. It can also be the initial manifestation of brachial plexitis (Parsonage-Turner syndrome). Caution should be exerted with testing of that muscle to avoid misinterpretation of the results due to the presence of the overlying trapezius muscle. Differential diagnosis includes an upper trunk plexopathy or C5–C6 radiculopathy (Table 20.3).

Accessory Nerve

The spinal root of the accessory nerve is derived from anterior horn cells at C3–C4 and enters the skull through the foramen magnum. After it unites with the cranial root that arises from the medulla, they both exit the skull through the jugular foramen and innervate first the sternocleidomastoid muscle and subsequently the trapezius muscle (both C3–C4). Damage to that nerve causes inability to turn the head to the contralateral side, and inability with ipsilateral shoulder shrug, along with scapular winging upon arm abduction. (Table 20.1) As in adults, traumatic lesions from medical procedures at the neck (e.g., lymph node biopsy, radical resection) constitute the prevailing culprits [27, 28]. NCS can be obtained by stimulating Erb's point and recording from the upper portion of the trapezius and should be always compared with the contralateral side; however, stimulation of Erb's point is often painful and should only be attempted in children who are cooperative and not upset. Needle examination should include sampling of the sternocleidomastoid and trapezius muscles, along with other muscles that can cause scapular instability (Table 20.3).

Phrenic Nerve

The phrenic nerve is formed from the ventral rami of the C3–C5 nerve roots. It follows a long route down the neck and the thorax before innervating the diaphragm (C3–C5) and providing sensory input to the pleura, pericardium and diaphragmatic peritoneum. It can be damaged from any lesion along that protracted course, proximally in the anterior horn cells, as an incipient sign of brachial plexitis or as part of more widespread acquired [29] or inherited polyneuropathy [30]. Unilateral lesions are usually asymptomatic. In some cases, clinical examination may reveal mild dyspnea, particularly upon recumbency, accessory respiratory muscle use, and paradoxical movement of the abdominal wall with inspiration (Table 20.1). NCS can be obtained by stimulating Erb's point and recording from the lower part of the ribcage and should be always compared with the contralateral side; as noted above, stimulation of Erb's point is often painful and should be performed selectively in children. Needle examination of the diaphragm is possible but caution should be exerted to avoid pneumothorax. A "sniff" test under fluoroscopy can confirm the presence of a phrenic nerve lesion, and imaging along the course of the nerve may provide additional information about the cause.

Lower Extremity Mononeuropathies

Sciatic Nerve

Anatomy

The sciatic nerve is formed from the anterior rami of the L4–S2 nerve roots through the lumbosacral plexus. It passes beneath the gluteus maximus muscle and emerges from the pelvis through the sciatic notch, underneath the piriformis muscle, along with the inferior gluteal artery, its major blood supplier. As it descends in the posterior thigh it provides innervation to the semitendinosus (L4–S2), semimembranosus (L4–S2), adductor magnus and the long and short head of the biceps femoris (L4–S2). All these muscles, aside from the short head of the biceps femoris, are innervated by the tibial division of the sciatic nerve. The peroneal division lies more laterally and superficially, has limited supportive tissue and is more taut, rendering it more susceptible to compression and/or traction injury [31]. Thus, an injury to the sciatic nerve may at times mimic a peroneal neuropathy, making it important to examine a number of relevant muscles during needle EMG to help confirm the location of the lesion. The two divisions of the sciatic nerve separate just above the popliteal fossa into the tibial and the common peroneal nerve, with the exception of 10% of individuals, where this segregation can occur more proximally in the thigh.

Etiology

The most common injury to the sciatic nerve is related to trauma from pelvic, hip or femoral fractures, penetrating injuries including intramuscular injections to the gluteus maximus, crush injuries and lacerations. Compression from prolonged immobilization, lithotomy position for perineal surgical exploration, fibroids, endometriosis, and calcifications constitutes an additional pathogenetic mechanism. Individuals with hereditary neuropathy with liability to pressure palsies (HNPP) are also at risk of sciatic nerve injury with relatively minor trauma. Traction during delivery or orthopedic procedures has also been described. Ischemic insult to the nerve has been reported with umbilical artery catheterization, iliac artery aneurysms and arteriovenous malformations, congenital vascular anomalies and meningococcemia. Neoplastic (neurofibroma, neuroblastoma, perineurioma, rhabdomyoma, bone and lymphoproliferative tumors) as well as postviral etiologies can occur [4, 21, 32, 33]. Piriformis syndrome has been reported in children but is quite rare [34]. Occasionally, no cause is identified [35].

Clinical Evaluation

Patients with sciatic injury present with weakness in foot/toe dorsiflexion and foot eversion (peroneal division), as well as foot/toe plantar flexion and foot inversion (tibial division). However, predominant impairment of the peroneal division is a frequent occurrence, mimicking at first glance a peroneal neuropathy. Thus, it is important to seek subtle signs of tibial nerve involvement. Additionally, for proximal lesions the hamstrings are affected leading to knee flexion weakness. It is paramount to confirm sparing of hip abduction and extension to exclude concomitant involvement of the gluteii muscles that would be seen in more proximal lesions that may mimic sciatic neuropathy, such as lumbosacral plexopathies and radiculopathies. Sensory examination should reveal deficits, including painful dysesthesias, in both the dorsal and plantar surfaces of the foot (Table 20.2).

Electrophysiologic Evaluation

Electrophysiologic evaluation should include testing of both peroneal and tibial motor responses, as well as superficial peroneal and sural sensory responses, which are all typically affected. Common peroneal F waves, tibial F waves, and tibial H reflexes are also classically impaired, though these late responses may not always be practical to obtain in young children, especially H reflexes. Needle examination reveals abnormalities both in peroneal and tibial innervated muscles. Ideally, a broad selection of muscles in both territories should be examined, but children may sometimes tolerate only a handful of needle examinations; thus, the bare minimum would be examination of at least one muscle, preferably two, from each branch. The hamstrings should be affected, at times more prominently in the short head of the biceps femoris that receives peroneal fibers. Sampling of that muscle is important on rare occasions where the peroneal division is exclusively affected within the sciatic nerve. In that case, the tibial motor responses and sural sensory response will be largely or completely spared and the peroneal motor response would be universally reduced without conduction block or slowing across the fibular head [31]. Occasionally the adductors may reveal neurogenic changes due to the dual innervation of adductor magnus from sciatic and obturator nerves [31]. Quadriceps, tensor fascia latae and gluteii muscles should be spared, unless the culprit is a lumbosacral plexopathy or polyradiculopathies, with additional involvement of the respective paraspinal muscles in the last case scenario (Table 20.4).

In the largest study of 51 pediatric patients with sciatic neuropathies published to date, abnormalities in motor conduction studies were seen in 44/53 (83%) of the cases in the peroneal nerve, as opposed to 35/51 (67%) of the cases in the tibial nerve. Abnormalities in sensory conduction studies were recorded in 34/43 (79%) of the cases in the sural nerve and in 15/25 (60%) of the cases in the superficial peroneal nerve. Needle EMG was abnormal in peroneal innervated muscles in all subjects, in tibial nerve innervated muscles in 43/51 (84%), and in the hamstrings in 18/29 (62%) [32].

Treatment and Prognosis

Prognosis for recovery is variable and depends on the etiology, pathophysiology and severity of the injury [32, 33].

Common Peroneal Nerve

Anatomy

The peroneal (also known as the fibular) nerve is one of the two terminal branches of the sciatic nerve, deriving its innervation from the anterior rami of the L4, L5, and to a lesser extent, the S1 nerve roots. Along its course within the sciatic nerve, the peroneal fibers are situated more laterally and superficially, rendering them more susceptible to injury compared to their tibial counterparts. After providing a branch to the short head of the biceps femoris (L5–S1) at the thigh, the peroneal division diverges from the tibial division just above the popliteal fossa. The common peroneal nerve then wraps around the fibular head, separating into the deep peroneal and the superficial peroneal nerves. The deep peroneal nerve innervates muscles in the anterior compartment of the foreleg [tibialis anterior (L4–L5), extensor digitorum longus (L4–L5), extensor hallucis longus (L4–S1), peroneus tertius (L4–S1)], as well as the extensor digitorum brevis (L5–S1) intrinsic foot muscles. The deep peroneal nerve also carries sensory input from the web space between the first two toes. The superficial peroneal nerve supplies the lateral compartment of the foreleg [peroneus longus and brevis (L5–S1)], providing sensation to the lateral calf and the dorsum of the foot. In 10–15% of the population, an accessory branch branches off the superficial peroneal nerve and participates in the innervation of the extensor digitorum brevis after passing behind the lateral malleolus.

Etiology

The majority of the cases are due to injury of the nerve fibers at the fibular head. The most common etiologies include compression (e.g., from habitual leg crossing, orthopedic appliances, synovial or intraneural ganglion cysts, compartment syndrome), entrapment (e.g., myofascial bands), trauma (e.g., lacerations, fibular head fractures), neoplasms (e.g., schwannoma, perineuroma, osteochondroma, etc.), systemic disease (e.g., vasculitis, diabetes, leprosy or HNPP) and abrupt weight loss [35]. Some cases are idiopathic. In neonates, peroneal neuropathy has been associated with stretch injury from breech presentation, intrauterine compression, umbilical artery catheterization and compartment syndrome from iatrogenic local infiltration of intravenous fluids and/or medications [4, 21, 36].

Clinical Evaluation

The hallmark of a peroneal neuropathy is weakness in foot dorsiflexion and eversion. That is in contrast to a sciatic neuropathy, where foot inversion and plantar flexion, as well as knee flexion, would be at least partially affected, and an L5 radiculopathy, where foot inversion, hip internal rotation and hip abduction would be also affected. Examination of the other major nerves of the lower extremity should be performed carefully upon passive hyperextension of the dropped foot. Numbness and pain may be reported by older children on the dorsum of the foot. A Tinel's sign at the most common site of insult, the fibular head, may be present (Table 20.2).

Electrophysiologic Evaluation

Nerve conduction studies should include evaluation of the superficial peroneal and sural sensory responses, the peroneal (recording from both the extensor digitorum brevis and the tibialis anterior muscles) and the tibial motor responses. The peroneal responses are typically impaired, while the tibial are spared. That can be corroborated with testing of respective late responses when tolerated by the child, in which case the peroneal F responses may be affected, while the tibial F and H responses remain normal (H reflexes are often not well-tolerated in young children). The needle examination would ideally include at least a deep peroneal-innervated muscle, one superficial peroneal-innervated muscle, a tibial-innervated muscle (e.g., gastrocnemius) but especially one non-peroneal muscle innervated by the L5 nerve root (e.g., tibialis posterior, the short head of the biceps femoris, tensor fascia latae, gluteus medius, and L5 paraspinals). However, examination of a complete list of muscles is often not practical in a young child. Thus, it is crucial to obtain a brief history and physical examination to determine what muscles would have the highest diagnostic value, and examine them in order of priority, in case the examination needs to be terminated prematurely. In a peroneal neuropathy at the fibular head, the peroneal muscles classically demonstrate variable degrees of neurogenic changes, while the others remain unaffected. If the peroneal injury is more proximal, the short head of the biceps femoris is also affected. The differential electrodiagnosis of a peroneal neuropathy includes a peroneal division predominant sciatic neuropathy, a lumbosacral plexopathy and an L5 radiculopathy [4] (Table 20.4).

As in adults, [37] there are diverse clinical and electrophysiologic presentations of common peroneal neuropathies in children, accounting for variable involvement of the deep and superficial peroneal fascicles: 1) common peroneal neuropathies with axonal loss; 2) common peroneal neuropathies with conduction block; 3) common peroneal neuropathies with mixed axonal loss and conduction block; and 4) isolated deep peroneal neuropathy [36, 38, 39]. In a large study of 53 children and adolescents with common peroneal neuropathy tested in a tertiary center, conduction block at the fibular head was present in 35% of cases and deep peroneal axonal loss in 77%, while superficial peroneal axonal loss was identified in 45%. The pathophysiology was predominantly axonal in 72%, mostly demyelinating in 6%, and mixed in 22%. Given though that the mean disease duration was >6 months in 2/3 of these cases and that the subjects were ascertained at a tertiary care pediatric hospital, it is possible that mild demyelinating lesions were under-represented in this cohort. Predominantly demyelinating lesions at the fibular head demonstrated sparing of the superficial peroneal sensory nerve, while predominantly axonal lesions showed a moderate correlation between superficial and deep peroneal axonal loss [36].

Treatment and Prognosis

Prognosis of peroneal neuropathies is variable and is largely dependent on the underlying etiology and the pathophysiology of the acquired damage. Prompt reversal of the igniting cause and the presence of a demyelinating lesion carry better prognoses, while significant axonal damage resulting in absent or low extensor digitorum brevis motor responses are associated with poor prognosis [38]. In cases where surgical repair is indicated, that should be attempted within 3–4 months of acute nerve injury. When improvement is not achieved, tendon transfers may help re-establish foot dorsiflexion [4].

Tibial Nerve

Anatomy

The tibial nerve is derived from the anterior divisions of the L5–S2 nerve roots. It travels down the pelvis and the thigh as an individual division within the sciatic nerve along with the peroneal division. At the distal thigh the tibial division bifurcates from the sciatic nerve. It first passes through the popliteal fossa, where the sural nerve arises, with additional input from a communicating branch from the peroneal nerve. The tibial nerve then passes through the two heads of the gastrocnemius muscles and supplies innervation to the gastrocnemii (L5–S2), soleus (S1–S2), tibialis posterior (L5–S1), flexor digitorum longus (L5–S1), and flexor hallucis longus (S1–S2) muscles of the calf. As it passes through the tarsal tunnel behind the medial malleolus the medial calcaneal nerve branches off to supply sensation to part of the sole, then the terminal tibial nerve divides into medial and lateral plantar nerves that innervate most of the intrinsic foot muscles (S1–S2) and sensation to part of the sole [5].

Etiology

Tibial neuropathies in children are exceedingly rare [40–43]. Traumatic and entrapment causes have been reported, both in the popliteal fossa as well as the ankle (tarsal tunnel syndrome) [43].

Clinical Evaluation

In proximal tibial neuropathies, there is weakness and atrophy in plantar flexion of the toes and the foot, along with weakness in foot inversion and toe abduction. Painful dysesthesias in the back of the calf and the lateral and bottom (sole) surfaces of the foot may be reported by children who can describe their symptoms in detail. The ankle jerk on the affected side may be diminished or lost. In distal tibial neuropathies, calf muscle strength, calf sensation, and the ankle jerk are typically spared. There is weakness of the intrinsic foot muscles aside from the extensor digitorum brevis and pain at the medial and/or lateral plantar surface. A Tinel's sign may be present at the tarsal tunnel (Table 20.2).

Electrophysiologic Evaluation

Electrophysiologic evaluation should include testing of both peroneal and tibial motor responses, as well as superficial peroneal and sural sensory responses. Additionally, for distal tibial neuropathies, evaluation of the medial and lateral plantar sensory responses is indicated. Contralateral testing should be performed to exclude a more generalized process, such as a length dependent peripheral neuropathy, and to evaluate for side to side asymmetries. Common peroneal (F) and tibial (F and H) late responses can also be tested when tolerated; H reflexes should only be attempted in awake older children and adolescents who are tolerating the study quite well. Needle examination should include sampling of both peroneal and tibial innervated muscles of the calf. For distal tibial neuropathies, evaluation of the medial and lateral plantar nerve muscles should be performed when tolerated, as well as the extensor digitorum brevis for comparison, given the frequent mild abnormalities seen in intrinsic foot muscles of normal patients, presumably from compression due to wearing shoes. Needle examination of intrinsic foot muscles can be quite uncomfortable, and should only be attempted in awake pediatric patients who are older and are tolerating the study well up until that point.

In a proximal tibial neuropathy, the tibial CMAP is often abnormal. Depending on the level and intensity of the damage, the sural response may be also affected. The peroneal CMAP and SNAP should be spared. When examined, tibial F and H responses are typically prolonged or absent while the peroneal F responses are present. Needle EMG abnormalities are confined to tibial-innervated muscles. The differential electrodiagnosis of a proximal tibial neuropathy is depicted in Table 20.4.

In a distal tibial neuropathy such as tarsal tunnel syndrome, distal latency/conduction velocity and often amplitudes of medial and/or lateral plantar potentials are impaired with normal sensory responses in more proximal nerves. The tibial CMAP recorded from the AH may also be affected. Similarly, tibial-innervated intrinsic foot muscles manifest abnormalities that are not seen in the extensor digitorum brevis in the foot or any of the calf muscles.

Treatment and Prognosis

As with the other mononeuropathies, identification and reversal of the predisposing factor is of paramount importance and is closely linked to final outcome.

Femoral Nerve

Anatomy

The femoral nerve arises from the anterior rami of the L2-L4 nerve roots. The psoas is innervated by the spinal nerve, while the iliacus (L2-L3) is the first muscle innervated by the femoral nerve. The femoral nerve then enters the thigh beneath the inguinal ligament through the femoral triangle providing innervation to the pectineus, sartorius and quadriceps muscles (L2-L4). Two sensory branches, the anterior femoral cutaneous nerve and the saphenous nerve, provide cutaneous innervation to the anteromedial thigh and the medial foreleg and foot respectively. The lateral femoral cutaneous nerve arises from the L2-L3 nerve roots but branches off proximal to the formation of the femoral nerve and thus is not technically a branch of the femoral nerve. It innervates sensation to the lateral aspect of the thigh.

Etiology

Most insults occur either at the retroperitoneal pelvic space or at the inguinal ligament. Pediatric femoral neuropathies have been reported in the context of perioperative trauma (e.g., femoral catheterization, [44] reduction of hip dysplasia, [45] hernia repair [46]), retroperitoneal [47] or intraneural hematomas, [48] tumors (e.g., neurofibroma, [49] perineurioma [50]) or without identifiable cause [35]. Meralgia paresthetica is caused by injury to the lateral femoral cutaneous nerve, which as noted above is not technically part of the femoral nerve but arises from the same nerve roots. Meralgia paresthetica is characterized by numbness, paresthesias, and pain over the lateral thigh, and is caused by various compressive injuries in the inguinal area, including those caused by tight clothing.

Clinical Evaluation

The patient usually presents with inability to flex the hip and extend the knee, noticed primarily upon walking upstairs. When reportable, sensory abnormalities localize at the anterior thigh and medial foreleg and foot. When sensory loss is restricted to the anterolateral thigh and no weakness is evident, the possibility of meralgia paresthetica should be considered. When the motor branches of the femoral nerve are affected, the knee jerk is dropped on the affected side. The adductors should be spared unless a lumbar radiculopathy or plexopathy is the culprit (Table 20.2).

Electrophysiologic Evaluation

In addition to routine NCS of the affected lower extremity, evaluation of the femoral CMAP recording from the quadriceps and the saphenous SNAP is desirable, though it may be difficult to obtain these responses, especially in young children. Both nerves can be technically challenging to study and are not routinely evaluated; therefore, any abnormalities should be compared to the contralateral unaffected extremity. Needle EMG should reveal abnormalities in some or all femoral innervated muscles, depending on the level of the injury, sparing the adductors and the lumbar paraspinals (Table 20.4). EMG will typically be normal in cases of meralgia paresthetica as the lateral femoral cutaneous nerve cannot easily be evaluated directly, but neurophysiological studies are often still warranted to exclude injury to the femoral nerve or other lumbosacral structures.

Treatment and Prognosis

In cases of complete nerve disruption, exploration and nerve repair should be considered [51]. In partial injuries, conservative management with analgesia, physical therapy and clinico-electrophysiologic monitoring is recommended first, [5] unless other surgical indications exist (e.g., progressive compressive lesion or hemodynamic instability from retroperitoneal hematoma). Meralgia paresthetica often responds to conservative measures, including wearing looser clothing.

Other Lower Extremity Nerves

Pediatric focal mononeuropathies have also been rarely reported in the obturator [52], pudendal, lateral femoral cutaneous [53–57], posterior femoral cutaneous, sural [58], saphenous [59], superior and inferior gluteal, iliohypogastric, ilioinguinal and genitofemoral nerves. Their clinical evaluation is depicted in (Table 20.2). Electrodiagnostic testing should aim to confirm the clinical diagnosis by stimulating and recording from the affected nerve and sampling affected muscles, and by investigating the pertinent differential diagnosis by testing nerves and muscles that share similar anatomical pathways more proximally. Unfortunately, electrophysiologic evaluation of many of these nerves is either technically challenging or impossible due to their small caliber and location in proximity to adipose tissue, and therefore an accurate diagnosis is frequently dependent exclusively on clinical (history, exam and diagnostic nerve blocks) or radiological (US, MR neurography) grounds.

References

1. Karakis I, Liew W, Darras BT, Jones HR, Kang PB. Referral and diagnostic trends in pediatric electromyography in the molecular era. Muscle Nerve. 2014;50(2):244–9.
2. Sunderland S. Nerves and nerve injuries. Edinburgh: E. & S. Livingstone; 1968.
3. Fuller G. Focal peripheral neuropathies. J Neurol Neurosurg Psychiatry. 2003;74(Suppl 2):ii20–i4.
4. Ryan MM, Jones HR. In: Darras BT, Jones HR, Ryan MM, De Vivo DC, editors. Mononeuropathies. 2nd ed. San Diego: Academic Press; 2015.
5. Stewart J. Focal peripheral neuropathies. New York: Elsevier; 1987.
6. Deymeer F, Jones HR Jr. Pediatric median mononeuropathies: a clinical and electromyographic study. Muscle Nerve. 1994;17(7):755–62.
7. Nakano KK, Lundergran C, Okihiro MM. Anterior interosseous nerve syndromes. Diagnostic methods and alternative treatments. Arch Neurol. 1977;34(8):477–80.
8. Davis L, Vedanarayanan VV. Carpal tunnel syndrome in children. Pediatr Neurol. 2014;50(1):57–9.
9. Van Meir N, De Smet L. Carpal tunnel syndrome in children. Acta Orthop Belg. 2003;69(5):387–95.
10. Batdorf NJ, Cantwell SR, Moran SL. Idiopathic carpal tunnel syndrome in children and adolescents. J Hand Surg [Am]. 2015;40(4):773–7.
11. Sonel B, Senbil N, Yavus Gurer YK, Evcik D. Cavanagh's syndrome (congenital thenar hypoplasia). J Child Neurol. 2002;17(1):51–4.
12. Van Heest AE, House J, Krivit W, Walker K. Surgical treatment of carpal tunnel syndrome and trigger digits in children with mucopolysaccharide storage disorders. J Hand Surg [Am]. 1998;23(2):236–43.
13. Haddad FS, Jones DH, Vellodi A, Kane N, Pitt MC. Carpal tunnel syndrome in the mucopolysaccharidoses and mucolipidoses. J Bone Joint Surg. 1997;79(4):576–82.

14. Felice KJ, Royden Jones H Jr. Pediatric ulnar mononeuropathy: report of 21 electromyography-documented cases and review of the literature. J Child Neurol. 1996;11(2):116–20.
15. Karakis I, Liew W, Szelag Fournier H, Jones HR, Darras BT, Kang PB. American Association of neuromuscular and electrodiagnostic. Medicine. 2016.
16. Stewart JD. The variable clinical manifestations of ulnar neuropathies at the elbow. J Neurol Neurosurg Psychiatry. 1987;50(3):252–8.
17. Baysefer A, Izci Y, Akay KM, Kayali H, Timurkaynak E. Surgical outcomes of ulnar nerve lesions in children. A retrospective clinical study. Pediatr Neurosurg. 2004;40(3):107–11.
18. Escolar DM, Jones HR Jr. Pediatric radial mononeuropathies: a clinical and electromyographic study of sixteen children with review of the literature. Muscle Nerve. 1996;19(7):876–83.
19. Monica JT, Waters PM, Bae DS. Radial nerve palsy in the newborn: a report of four cases and literature review. J Pediatr Orthop. 2008;28(4):460–2.
20. Alsubhi FS, Althunyan AM, Curtis CG, Clarke HM. Radial nerve palsy in the newborn: a case series. CMAJ. 2011;183(12):1367–70.
21. Jones HR Jr. Compressive neuropathy in childhood: a report of 14 cases. Muscle Nerve. 1986;9(8):720–3.
22. Tyagi A, Drake J, Midha R, Kestle J. Axillary nerve injuries in children. Pediatr Neurosurg. 2000;32(5):226–9.
23. Vastamaki M, Kauppila LI. Etiologic factors in isolated paralysis of the serratus anterior muscle: a report of 197 cases. J Shoulder Elb Surg. 1993;2(5):240–3.
24. Henry D, Bonthius DJ. Isolated musculocutaneous neuropathy in an adolescent baseball pitcher. J Child Neurol. 2011;26(12):1567–70.
25. Laulund T, Fedders O, Sogaard I, Kornum M. Suprascapular nerve compression syndrome. Surg Neurol. 1984;22(3):308–12.
26. Montagna P, Colonna S. Suprascapular neuropathy restricted to the infraspinatus muscle in volleyball players. Acta Neurol Scand. 1993;87(3):248–50.
27. Park SH, Esquenazi Y, Kline DG, Kim DH. Surgical outcomes of 156 spinal accessory nerve injuries caused by lymph node biopsy procedures. J Neurosurg Spine. 2015;23(4):518–25.
28. Grossman JA, Ruchelsman DE, Schwarzkopf R. Iatrogenic spinal accessory nerve injury in children. J Pediatr Surg. 2008;43(9):1732–5.
29. Ravishankar N. Respiratory paralysis in a child: the severe axonal variant of childhood Guillain-Barre syndrome. J Pediatr Neurosci. 2015;10(1):67–9.
30. Sevilla T, Jaijo T, Nauffal D, Collado D, Chumillas MJ, Vilchez JJ, et al. Vocal cord paresis and diaphragmatic dysfunction are severe and frequent symptoms of GDAP1-associated neuropathy. Brain J Neurol. 2008;131(Pt 11):3051–61.
31. Katirji B. Electrodiagnostic approach to the patient with suspected mononeuropathy of the lower extremity. Neurol Clin. 2002;20(2):479–501, vii.
32. Srinivasan J, Ryan MM, Escolar DM, Darras B, Jones HR. Pediatric sciatic neuropathies: a 30-year prospective study. Neurology. 2011;76(11):976–80.
33. Jones HR Jr, Gianturco LE, Gross PT, Buchhalter J. Sciatic neuropathies in childhood: a report of ten cases and review of the literature. J Child Neurol. 1988;3(3):193–9.
34. Bhattad SB, Gupta A, Suri D, Sharma D, Sinha A, Singh S. Piriformis syndrome in a young child—an unusual clinical entity. Indian J Pediatr. 2016;83(4):361–2.
35. Engstrom JW, Layzer RB, Olney RK, Edwards MB. Idiopathic, progressive mononeuropathy in young people. Arch Neurol. 1993;50(1):20–3.
36. Karakis I, Khoshnoodi, M., Liew, W., Nguyen E.S., Jones H.R., Darras B.T., Kang, P.B. Electrophysiologic features of peroneal neuropathy in childhood and adolescence. Muscle Nerve. 2016;55(5):693–7.
37. Wilbourn AJ. AAEE case report #12: common peroneal mononeuropathy at the fibular head. Muscle Nerve. 1986;9(9):825–36.
38. Jones HR Jr, Felice KJ, Gross PT. Pediatric peroneal mononeuropathy: a clinical and electromyographic study. Muscle Nerve. 1993;16(11):1167–73.
39. Kang PB, Preston DC, Raynor EM. Involvement of superficial peroneal sensory nerve in common peroneal neuropathy. Muscle Nerve. 2005;31(6):725–9.

40. Molloy AP, Lyons R, Bergin D, Kearns SR. Flexor digitorum accessorius causing tarsal tunnel syndrome in a paediatric patient: a case report and review of the literature. Foot Ankle Surg. 2015;21(2):e48–50.
41. Smuts I, Potgieter D, van der Westhuizen FH. Combined tarsal and carpal tunnel syndrome in mucolipidosis type III. A case study and review. Ann N Y Acad Sci. 2009;1151:77–84.
42. Brockmann K, Schneider-Sickert F, Kolenda H, Aden I, Hanefeld F. Tarsal tunnel syndrome in a 7-year-old boy. Eur J Pediatr. 2004;163(1):46–7.
43. Albrektsson B, Rydholm A, Rydholm U. The tarsal tunnel syndrome in children. J Bone Joint Surg. 1982;64(2):215–7.
44. Kachko L, Ben Ami S, Liberman A, Birk E, Kronenberg S. Duloxetine contributing to a successful multimodal treatment program for peripheral femoral neuropathy and comorbid 'reactive depression' in an adolescent. Pain Res Manag. 2011;16(6):457–9.
45. Murnaghan ML, Browne RH, Sucato DJ, Birch J. Femoral nerve palsy in Pavlik harness treatment for developmental dysplasia of the hip. J Bone Joint Surg Am. 2011;93(5):493–9.
46. van Hoff J, Shaywitz BA, Seashore JH, Collins WF. Femoral nerve injury following inguinal hernia repair. Pediatr Neurol. 1985;1(3):195–6.
47. Murray IR, Perks FJ, Beggs I, Moran M. Femoral nerve palsy secondary to traumatic iliacus haematoma—a young athlete's injury. BMJ Case Reports. 2010;2010 doi:10.1136/bcr.05.2010.3045.
48. Ehrmann L, Lechner K, Mamoli B, Novotny C, Kos K. Peripheral nerve lesions in haemophilia. J Neurol. 1981;225(3):175–82.
49. Shetty GM, Murari AS, Song HR, Lee SH, Yang JH. Neurofibromatous sensory neuropathy of the thigh in a 7-year-old boy. Arch Orthop Trauma Surg. 2008;128(10):1093–7.
50. McMillan HJ, Torres C, Michaud J, Ying Y, Boyd KU, Bourque PR. Diagnosis and outcome of childhood perineurioma. Childs Nerv Syst. 2016;
51. Kim DH, Kline DG. Surgical outcome for intra- and extrapelvic femoral nerve lesions. J Neurosurg. 1995;83(5):783–90.
52. Bradshaw C, McCrory P, Bell S, Brukner P. Obturator nerve entrapment. A cause of groin pain in athletes. Am J Sports Med. 1997;25(3):402–8.
53. Nishimura M, Kodama Y, Fukano R, Okamura J, Ogaki K, Sakaguchi Y, et al. Meralgia paresthetica as a presentation of acute appendicitis in a girl with acute lymphoblastic leukemia. J Pediatr Hematol Oncol. 2015;37(3):e182–3.
54. Fernandez-Mayoralas DM, Fernandez-Jaen A, Jareno NM, Perez BC, Fernandez PM, Sola AG. Meralgia paresthetica in the pediatric population: a propos of 2 cases. J Child Neurol. 2010;25(1):110–3.
55. Tejwani SG, Scaduto AA, Bowen RE. Transient meralgia paresthetica after pediatric posterior spine fusion. J Pediatr Orthop. 2006;26(4):530–3.
56. Edelson R, Stevens P. Meralgia paresthetica in children. J Bone Joint Surg Am. 1994;76(7):993–9.
57. Richer LP, Shevell MI, Stewart J, Poulin C. Pediatric meralgia paresthetica. Pediatr Neurol. 2002;26(4):321–3.
58. Reisin R, Pardal A, Ruggieri V, Gold L. Sural neuropathy due to external pressure: report of three cases. Neurology. 1994;44(12):2408–9.
59. Hattori H, Asagai Y, Yamamoto K. Sudden onset of saphenous neuropathy associated with hereditary multiple exostoses. J Orthop Sci. 2006;11(4):405–8.

Chapter 21
Neuromuscular Junction Disorders

Wendy K.M. Liew

Pediatric neuromuscular junction disorders are less common in children compared to adults, but both autoimmune and inherited subtypes of this disease category occur in the pediatric age group. Neuroanatomically, these can either be classified into presynaptic, synaptic or postsynaptic disorders. Symptoms occur when there is a disruption in the normal synthesis, storage, or release of acetylcholine, the microanatomy of the synapse, the acetylcholinesterase enzyme, or the function of the acetylcholine receptor complex. The specific clinical manifestations are dependent on the pathophysiology and severity of the disorder. The hallmarks of neuromuscular junction disorders are weakness and fatiguability, especially with extraocular muscles and bulbar muscles. However, due to the rarity of the condition and the overlap of the major symptoms with other neuromuscular or metabolic disorders, making the diagnosis can be quite challenging, from first conception of the possibility to confirmatory testing, especially as several of the classic diagnostic tests have limitations with regard to sensitivity. It is also frequently difficult to differentiate these disorders from one another, especially in children. Electrodiagnostic studies can be a valuable tool in not only detecting the presence of a disorder involving the neuromuscular junction, but also differentiating the type of neuromuscular disorders using a combination of nerve conduction studies, repetitive stimulation studies, exercise testing and needle EMG. Single fiber EMG and stimulated single fiber EMG are techniques that are also valuable in these evaluations. The results can then aid the pediatric neurologist in selecting the appropriate serologies or genetic tests to help confirm a definitive diagnosis in these patients.

With respect to etiology, neuromuscular junction disorders can be divided into autoimmune, metabolic, toxic and congenital syndromes. The most commonly encountered subtypes in children are the autoimmune and congenital syndromes.

W.K.M. Liew, M.B.Ch.B., M.R.C.P.C.H., F.A.M.S
SBCC Baby and Child Clinic, Neurology Centre, Singapore, Singapore
e-mail: wendyliewkm@gmail.com

© Springer International Publishing AG 2017

H.J. McMillan, P.B. Kang (eds.), *Pediatric Electromyography*,
DOI 10.1007/978-3-319-61361-1_21

Physiology of a Normal Neuromuscular Junction

The neuromuscular junction forms the nerve-muscle synapse and connects the motor nerve axon with the skeletal muscle. Though an individual motor neuron and its primary axon typically innervate multiple muscle fibers, the axon will divide into a number of terminal branches, each of which is connected to an individual muscle fiber by a neuromuscular junction (NMJ). At the end of each branch is a small swelling called the terminal bouton. The terminal bouton contains choline acetyltransferase (required for the synthesis of ACh), multiple vesicles of acetylcholine, and transmembrane voltage-gated calcium channels (VGCCs) that mediate the release of ACh into the synaptic cleft [1, 2].

Each synaptic vesicle in the terminal bouton contains approximately 10,000 molecules of ACh, which is defined as one quantum of ACh. The primary clusters of these vesicles congregate near the presynaptic membrane in close proximity to the voltage-gated calcium channels that mediate ACh release into the synaptic space. These vesicles are immediately available for release. An action potential that moves down the axon to the terminal bouton triggers an influx of calcium ions through the voltage-gated calcium channels. The calcium influx in turn triggers fusion of the synaptic vesicle membrane with the presynaptic membrane before the quantum of ACh is released into the synaptic space [1, 3, 4]. Larger quantities of vesicles (the "secondary" store) are located further away from the presynaptic membrane and are mobilized closer to the membrane as additional acetylcholine is needed. Lastly, there is a "reserve" store of more than 100,000 quanta of ACh and these are situated even more remotely, in the motor axon and cell body.

Upon release from the synaptic vesicles, ACh diffuses across the synaptic space to the postsynaptic membrane and binds with acetylcholine receptors (AChR), triggering an influx of cations, mostly sodium ions, through channels within these receptors. This leads to local depolarization that activates sodium channels located deeper in the junctional folds, resulting in a further influx of sodium ions that launches the muscle action potential, which spreads along the muscle fiber and is the immediate trigger for muscle fiber contraction. ACh is metabolized by acetylcholinesterase.

Neuromuscular transmission operates via an "all or none" mechanism. If the nerve impulse fails to induce an end plate potential above threshold, muscle fiber contraction will not occur. Such failure of neuromuscular transmission is known as "blocking" for individual muscle fibers and results in muscle weakness when a significant number of NMJs are "blocked".

Approach to a Child with a Neuromuscular Transmission Disorder

In any child suspected of having a neuromuscular junction disorder, the electrodiagnostic evaluation includes routine nerve conduction studies (NCS), low frequency repetitive motor nerve stimulation (RNS), needle electromyography (EMG) and in some cases, single-fiber electromyography (SFEMG), particularly a variant known as stimulated single-fiber electromyography (SSFEMG). For additional details regarding these techniques, please refer to Chap. 6 on repetitive nerve stimulation and Chap. 10 on single fiber EMG. There are practical considerations that are unique to the pediatric population. The repetitive stimulation studies cause more discomfort than standard nerve conduction studies, and young children may not be able to perform the exercise tasks of specific muscles that are required in some sophisticated repetitive nerve stimulation protocols. SFEMG and SSFEMG may also be associated with some discomfort, depending on the approach used. Both are more technically challenging in children compared to adults. Strategies to maximize the diagnostic yield while minimizing discomfort include performing low frequency repetitive stimulation at rest only, given evidence that post-exercise measurements may not often increase the diagnostic yield substantially, and using SSFEMG, which requires minimal cooperation from the child aside from lying reasonably still for a period of time. In the United States, specially trained child life specialists, when available, can help distract and soothe young children. Such approaches will often enable the examiner to perform an accurate and informative series of studies without sedation or general anesthesia. A suggested approach to the diagnostic evaluation of children with suspected disorders of neuromuscular transmission is listed in Table 21.1.

Table 21.1 A protocol for the evaluation of suspected disorders of neuromuscular transmission in children

1.	Routine sensory and motor nerve conduction studies
	• At least one upper and one lower extremity
	• It is preferable to focus on symptomatic extremities
2.	Repetitive nerve stimulation
	• Low frequency repetitive stimulation studies on at least 1 distal and 1 proximal site
	• In younger children with limited cooperation, focus on obtaining high-quality baseline studies at rest rather than being distracted by exercise testing, as the latter will usually lead to further declines in cooperation
	• If baseline studies do not yield a clear decrement, a cooperative child or adolescent should perform voluntary exercise for 1 min, which will be followed by repetitive nerve stimulations at 1–4 min post exercise to seek signs of decremental responses
	• If a decrement is present on either baseline or exercise testing, a cooperative child should perform voluntary exercise for 10 seconds, followed by repetitive nerve stimulation to evaluate for postexercise facilitation
3.	Needle electromyography
	• Routine needle EMG in distal and proximal muscles, focusing on symptomatic muscles
	• A myopathic pattern will suggest either a presynaptic disorder of the neuromuscular junction or the alternative diagnosis of myopathy, depending the context of other findings in the study
4.	Stimulated single-fiber EMG (SSFEMG)
	• Stimulated single fiber EMG is preferred over traditional single fiber EMG studies in children since considerable cooperation, namely sustained muscle contraction, is required for the latter to be carried out
	• SSFEMG may be used as a secondary evaluation when the studies above do not yield sufficient diagnostic information, however some electromyographers prefer to use SSFEMG as a primary screen

Single Fiber EMG

SFEMG is the most sensitive test in detecting defects in the neuromuscular junction [5, 6]. A variant of this procedure, stimulated single-fiber EMG (SSFEMG), is much easier to perform in children compared to the traditional SFEMG approach. Details of this technique may be found in Chap. 10.

Congenital Myasthenic Syndromes

Congenital myasthenic syndromes are a heterogeneous group of disorders that classically present at birth, but may also present later in childhood [7–10]. These syndromes are typically classified according to the neuroanatomical localization of the defect: presynaptic, synaptic, and post synaptic. Infants usually present with various combinations of generalized hypotonia, weakness, respiratory distress, episodic apnea, and feeding difficulties. Symptoms are often exacerbated by crying and feeding, with improvement after sleeping. Respiratory symptoms may be intermittent, in some cases presenting as brief resolved unexplained events (BRUEs), previously known as acute life threatening events (ALTEs). Older children will classically present with a combination of fatiguable or fluctuating ptosis, ophthalmoplegia, and motor difficulties caused by muscle weakness. Prenatal symptoms may include reduced fetal movements and polyhydramnios due to dysphagia; the former may result in arthrogryposis that is apparent at birth. The range of clinical presentations is broad, from severe, life-threatening disease at birth to mild symptoms with onset later in childhood. The differential diagnosis for the presentations at both ends of the spectrum is broad and there are no easily detected serum biomarkers, in contrast to the antibody tests available for autoimmune disorders of the neuromuscular junction, often leading to difficulties in pinpointing the diagnosis. Distinctive clinical and electrophysiologic features may help the clinician distinguish between the different syndromes, as noted below.

Congenital myasthenic syndromes are caused by mutations in genes that are expressed at the neuromuscular junction. Such mutations disrupt the normal signaling that occurs between the motor axon and the muscle fiber. Mutations in *CHRNE* are responsible for more than half of the cases. Mutations in *RAPSN*, *CHAT*, *COLQ*, and *DOK7* account for many of the others. As in other categories of inherited disorders associated with multiple genetic loci, there remain cohorts of patients who do not have mutations identified in the known causative genes. Table 21.2 shows a classification of known causative genes based on the neuroanatomical site of defect, and Table 21.3 correlates electrophysiologic and clinical findings with specific subtypes. Postsynaptic CMSs are more frequent than the presynaptic or synaptic CMSs, in large part due to the high incidence of *CHRNE* mutations. The inheritance of congenital myasthenic syndrome is usually autosomal recessive. Less commonly, these diseases may also be inherited in an autosomal dominant pattern, typically a result of de novo spontaneous mutations.

Table 21.2 Genes associated with congenital myasthenic syndrome

Presynaptic
• *CHAT*
Synaptic
• *COLQ*
• *LAMB2*
Postsynaptic
• *CHRNA*, *CHRNB*, *CHRND*, and *CHRNE*
• *CHRNG* (this subunit is expressed exclusively *in utero*)
• *RAPSN*
• *DOK7*
• *MUSK*
• *SCN4A*
• *AGRIN*
• *GFPT1*
• *PLEC1*

Presynaptic Congenital Myasthenic Syndrome

The hallmarks of presynaptic congenital myasthenic syndrome include episodic apnea resulting from respiratory distress and bulbar weakness. These episodes may be triggered by fever or intercurrent illness. Neonatal, infantile and juvenile forms have been described, primarily associated with mutations in *CHAT* [11–13].

Low frequency repetitive nerve stimulation at 3 Hz typically results in a significant decremental response (greater than 10%) (Fig. 21.1), though some patients may not manifest this classic electrophysiologic abnormality. A mild incremental response has also been reported in a small group of patients [12, 14].

Lambert Eaton-like congenital myasthenic syndrome is distinct from Lambert Eaton myasthenic syndrome in that the former is genetic in origin, albeit without identified mutations to date, while the latter is autoimmune in origin, as in adults. Both are extremely rare in childhood. The classical nerve conduction findings in both include a low compound muscle action potential at rest, with an incremental increase after high frequency repetitive stimulation or voluntary exertion [15, 16]. The genetic etiology of Lambert Eaton-like congenital myasthenic syndrome presumably affects the presynaptic region, though this will only be confirmed structurally when genetic mutations are confirmed for this disorder.

Synaptic Congenital Myasthenic Syndrome

Endplate acetylcholinesterase deficiency of the motor plate and abnormal laminin β2 chain can each cause synaptic congenital myasthenic syndrome, with the former being more common.

Table 21.3 Electrophysiologic features of congenital myasthenic syndromes

Microanatomy	Subtype	Low frequency repetitive nerve stimulation	High frequency repetitive nerve stimulation	SFEMG findings	Distinctive clinical features	Treatment
Presynaptic	Choline acetyltransferase deficiency	Decrement in weak muscles, or after prolonged stimulation in muscles that are not weak	No facilitation	Increased jitter, blocking	Episodic apnea	Pyridostigmine
	Lambert-Eaton- like CMS	Decrement	Incremental increase	Increased jitter, blocking	Low amplitude CMAP	Pyridostigmine 3,4-DAP Guanidine
Synaptic	Endplate ACE deficiency	Decrement, no improvement with acetylcholinesterase	Decrement	Increased jitter, blocking		Ephedrine, Albuterol
	Laminin β2 chain	Decrement	Decrement	Increased jitter, blocking	Cholinesterase inhibitors ineffective, may worsen symptoms	Ephedrine
Postsynaptic	Acetylcholine receptor deficiency without kinetic abnormality	Decrement	May have partial improvement of decrement, with facilitation	Increased jitter, blocking		Pyridostigmine 3,4-DAP
	Slow channel CMS	Decrement, no improvement with acetylcholinesterase	Decrement, worse at higher frequency	Increased jitter, blocking		Quinidine sulfate Fluoxetine
	Fast channel CMS	Decrement	No decrement	Increased jitter, blocking		Pyridostigmine
	Rapsyn deficiency	Decrement can be variable	Decrement may be present after exertion	Increased jitter, blocking		Pyridostigmine 3,4-DAP
	DOK-7 deficiency	Decrement	Decrement	Increased jitter, blocking		3,4-DAP
	Plectin deficiency				Myopathic features on EMG	

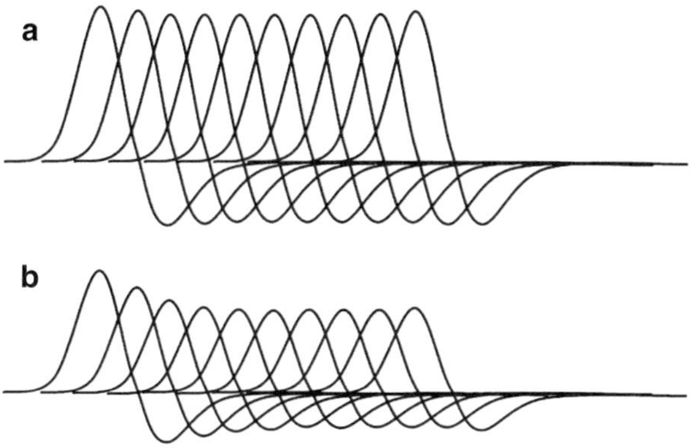

Fig. 21.1 At 3 Hz repetitive stimulation, presynaptic neuromuscular diseases may show either (**a**) no decrement or (**b**) a decrement of greater than 10% of the compound motor action potential amplitude by the fourth stimulation

Recessive mutations in *COLQ* cause defects in a subunit of acetylcholinesterase, leading to endplate acetylcholinesterase deficiency [17, 18]. Acetylcholinesterase hydrolyses acetylcholine after its action at the cholinergic synapse. Defective acetylcholinesterase is unable to bind to acetylcholine and its receptor, leading to prolonged exposure of the receptor to acetylcholine. This prolonged exposure results in several damaging consequences at the neuromuscular junction, including desensitization of the ACh receptor to acetylcholine [19].

In laminin β2 chain congenital myasthenic syndrome caused by mutations in *LAMB2* [20], the pathophysiology has been postulated to be an abnormal formation of the neuromuscular junction.

Low frequency repetitive nerve stimulation at 3 Hz usually demonstrates a decremental response in the compound muscle action potential, with confirmation of the diagnosis by the identification of mutations in *COLQ* and *LAMB2*.

Postsynaptic Congenital Myasthenic Syndrome

Mutations in the genes encoding the α, β, δ and ε subunits of the acetylcholine receptor and various proteins that interact with the acetylcholine receptor lead to postsynaptic defects of the neuromuscular junction. The other proteins include rapsyn, tyrosine kinase 7 and muscle-specific tyrosine kinase. Within this subgroup, there is significant heterogeneity and overlap in clinical presentations and electrophysiologic findings [7, 11, 21].

Mutations of genes causing defects in acetylcholine receptors can be classified into two subtypes: those that reduce the expression of AChR without altering its kinetic properties, and those that do alter its kinetic properties. The latter may be further subdivided into slow channel mutations and fast channel mutations. Slow channel mutations increase the synaptic response to acetylcholine while fast channel mutations decrease the synaptic response to acetylcholine [22]. More recently, it has been found that certain novel subtypes of postsynaptic congenital myasthenic syndrome do not fall into any of these three categories, including those associated with mutations in *SCN4A* (which encodes a sodium channel) [23], *AGRIN* (whose protein product aggregates ACh receptors) [24], *CHRNG* (which is associated with Escobar syndrome, recently confirmed to be caused by neuromuscular junction defects, but without ongoing postnatal weakness or fatigability as *CHRNG* is only expressed in the fetal form of the ACh receptor) [25, 26]; and *PLEC1* (which is associated with concomitant muscular dystrophy and epidermolysis bullosa) [27, 28].

For those patients with postsynaptic disorders who have ACh receptor deficiency without altered ACh receptor kinetics, the most common mutations occur in *CHRNE*, which encodes the ε subunit of the acetylcholine receptor; mutations have also been reported in such a context for *CHRNB*, *CHRND*, *RAPSN*, *DOK7*, *MUSK*, and *GFPT1*. The clinical phenotype of this subgroup includes hypotonia, ptosis, ophthalmoplegia, fatiguable weakness, dysphagia, and respiratory difficulties. Skeletal deformities such as arthrogryposis and/or scoliosis are usually present [7, 11, 21]. The inheritance pattern is autosomal recessive. The primary electrophysiologic finding is a decremental response on low frequency repetitive stimulation, thus there is a not a distinct electrophysiologic signature for this subgroup.

Slow-channel CMS is an autosomal dominant disorder that is associated with mutations in *CHRNA*, *CHRNB*, *CHRND*, and *CHRNE*, and may present at any age [22, 29, 30]. Patients present with ptosis, ophthalmoplegia, neck weakness, and distal muscle weakness. The weakness tends to affect the upper limbs more than the lower limbs, and may be asymmetric after exertion [29, 31]. An electrophysiologic hallmark of slow-channel syndromes is a repetitive CMAP after single stimulation. Thus, the sweep speed should be adjusted after performing standard motor nerve conduction studies in children suspected of this diagnosis to seek cryptic second CMAPs that on first glance may not appear on the screen. In nerve conduction studies, there is a decremental response to both low and high frequency repetitive stimulation, with a greater decremental response to high frequency repetitive stimulation. Conventional needle EMG may show a myopathic pattern [11, 32]. As slow-channel CMS has distinct electrophysiologic findings, patients with a suggestive pattern of weakness along with a dominant pattern of inheritance should have the complete electrophysiologic evaluation that is described, when feasible.

Fast-channel CMS is an autosomal recessive condition that is associated with mutations in *CHRNA*, *CHRND*, and *CHRNE*, and presents in infancy. Clinical signs include ptosis, ophthalmoplegia, dysphagia, and muscle weakness [21, 31]. Repetitive stimulation studies demonstrate a decremental response, which improves with volitional muscle contractions [22, 31]. When it is feasible to stimulate voluntary contractions in patients under examination, it is worth re-checking repetitive stimulation studies after volitional movement in an attempt to find signs of fast-channel CMS.

Myasthenia Gravis

Myasthenia gravis is an acquired autoimmune disorder, in contrast to the inherited congenital myasthenic syndromes. Autoimmune myasthenia gravis is caused by autoantibodies directed against different proteins at the motor end plate, most commonly the acetylcholine receptor (AChR). Other autoantibodies that have been associated with myasthenia gravis are IgG autoantibodies to muscle-specific kinase (MuSK), striated muscle protein, or low density lipoprotein receptor-related protein [33–35]. These autoantibodies disrupt the neuromuscular junction via various mechanisms. One mechanism is binding of the antibody to the acetylcholine receptor, decreasing the number of functional acetylcholine receptors and disrupting the normal function of the postsynaptic neuromuscular transmission by causing an accelerated degradation of the AChR. Another mechanism is blocking of the binding sites of the AChR by the antibody. A third is via deposition of complement. Some cases of myasthenia gravis are associated with antecedent infections, but many cases are not associated with a clear infectious trigger for the autoimmune reaction. In rare cases, drugs such as penicillamine may trigger autoimmune myasthenia gravis.

The child with myasthenia gravis may present with either primary ocular or generalized symptoms. Differences in clinical phenotypes have been described between Western and Eastern countries, with the former having a predisposition to generalized subtype. Patients in East Asia most often experience the primary ocular subtype, and onset is usually prepubertal. The hallmarks of myasthenia gravis are fatiguability and fluctuating symptoms. Symptoms are often worse at the end of the day or after exertion, with milder symptoms at the beginning of the day or after naps. Onset most frequently occurs in the elementary (primary) school years and during adolescence; however, onset has been reported as early as 15 months.

Classical clinical symptoms include ocular findings such as fatiguable ptosis, ophthalmoplegia, generalized weakness and bulbar weakness. Ocular symptoms are present in approximately 90% of children with myasthenia gravis. Ptosis, strabismus, and ophthalmoplegia may be unilateral or bilateral. There may also be differing severity between the eyes. It is important for the clinician to recognize myasthenic crisis, which is a life-threatening condition that occurs in children as well as adults, resulting from weakness of the bulbar and respiratory muscles. Mentation of the patient is preserved. A patient with myasthenic crisis requires admission to the intensive care unit as respiratory support with mechanical intubation may be needed on short notice. An increased incidence of co-morbid autoimmune disorders such as thyroid disorders, rheumatoid arthritis, diabetes and lupus, are seen in both the patients and their first-degree family members.

The diagnosis of autoimmune myasthenia gravis remains a clinical one, but it is most convincing when abnormalities are found on at least one of the following confirmatory diagnostic tests: autoantibody titers, edrophonium test, ice pack test, low frequency repetitive stimulation, or stimulated single fiber EMG [33]. The edrophonium test and the ice pack test are not as sensitive or specific as the serological and electrophysiologic studies. Single fiber EMG is usually reserved for selected patients where previous investigations have been negative or equivocal, but in some centers this test modality is used successfully as the primary screen for children. Muscle biopsy may reveal small accumulations of lymphoid cells but these are not specific for myasthenia gravis. Electron microscopy demonstrates a simplification of the postsynaptic membrane, with a reduction in AChR at the neuromuscular junction. Immunostaining may demonstrate IgG deposits and complements deposition at the motor end plates. These specialized tests are generally not indicated in majority of the cases, and muscle biopsy is not a good clinical diagnostic test for myasthenia gravis.

The aim of therapy for autoimmune myasthenic gravis is to improve neuromuscular transmission. This is achieved by increasing the amount of active acetylcholine with acetylcholinesterase inhibitors and/or immunomodulation via corticosteroids, intravenous immunoglobulins, plasmapheresis, azathioprine, and/or mycophenolate [36, 37]. More recently rituximab has been used in some children with therapeutic effect [38]. The three standard immunomodulatory treatments that are available in the pediatric population are corticosteroids, plasmapheresis and immunoglobulin [39–41]. Long-term corticosteroid therapy is associated with significant side effects such as weight gain, short stature and bone demineralization. A study comparing the efficacy of plasmapheresis and intravenous immunoglobulin in children has shown that both appear to be comparable in terms of efficacy and are reasonable alternatives to corticosteroids not only in the acute setting, but also as maintenance therapy, with children showing more consistent responses to plasmapheresis [33, 42]. In children with generalized myasthenia gravis who are not responding to a combination of acetylcholinesterase inhibitors and immunomodulatory therapy, the current literature supports thymectomy. Thymectomy performed within 12 months of symptom onset appears to be associated with more favorable outcomes [43, 44]. The role of thymectomy in patients with anti-MuSK myasthenia gravis and ocular myasthenia gravis is not well defined. There have been controversies regarding the timing of thymectomy in younger children due to the role of thymus in the development of immune system, however, isolated reports have documented good outcomes without apparent negative consequences for the immune system in children as young as 17 months [45].

On standard nerve conduction studies, motor and sensory nerve responses are usually normal in myasthenia gravis. Repetitive nerve stimulation studies will often demonstrate one or more of the following characteristic features: (1) decrement in CMAP amplitude of at least 10% by the fourth stimulation on low frequency stimulations, with partial or complete recovery by the tenth stimulation; (2) post-exercise facilitation/recovery after brief maximal muscle contraction for 10 seconds; and/or (3) exaggerated decrement after 1 minute of muscle contraction. Repetitive stimulation is usually applied to at least one distal and one proximal motor nerve. Ideally, nerves innervating clinically affected muscles should be tested. Abnormal repetitive stimulation studies confirm the presence of a disorder of the neuromuscular junction, but such findings are not specific to myasthenia gravis. The sensitivity of repetitive stimulation studies is approximately 80% for generalized myasthenia gravis and approximately 50% for ocular myasthenia gravis, for children [33] as well as adults. This sensitivity is reduced when the studies are performed on distal or strong muscles.

Single fiber electromyography (SFEMG) and, in children particularly, stimulated single fiber electromyography (SSFEMG) is the most sensitive electrophysiologic test for the detection of deficient neuromuscular transmission, but this test modality does not differentiate between different types of neuromuscular junction disorders, and may also be abnormal in other types of neuromuscular disorders entirely. The primary abnormalities seen in SFEMG are increased jitter and blocking, which become more apparent with higher stimulation frequencies; the latter finding is suggestive of a post-synaptic defect. In the proper clinical context, such findings are consistent but not specific for a postsynaptic defect of the neuromuscular junction [46]. Sensitivity of SFEMG is greater than 95% in both generalized and ocular myasthenia gravis, especially when facial muscles are tested.

Infantile Botulism

Infantile botulism is classically recognized by the acute presentation of hypotonia and descending weakness in infants, usually in the first 6 months of life. More than 60% of reported botulism cases are infantile, accounting for approximately 75 cases per year in the United States [47].

Clostridium botulinum is an obligatory anaerobic, gram positive, spore forming rod. Spores of *Clostridium botulinum* are found in soil, agricultural products, household dust and certain foods, especially honey [48]. In the United States, spores and thus infant botulism are endemic in the mid-Atlantic region, parts of Utah, and parts of California. The spores are generally harmless to older children and adults; however, in infants, the spores have the ability to multiply and produce botulinum toxin in the gut due to the immature gut flora at that age. These toxins target and inactivate proteins that are involved in the release of synaptic vesicles in the presynaptic terminal, resulting in a disturbance of neuromuscular transmission. Most *C. botulinum* strains produce one of seven known botulinum toxin types (A–G) [49]. Infantile botulism typically results from strains that produce botulinum types A and B. It has been postulated that different botulinum subtypes cause neuromuscular paralysis of different durations, resulting in a range of recovery times [47, 50].

The first symptom is typically decreased stooling frequency or frank constipation [51]. Pupillary light reflexes, extraocular and bulbar muscles are often affected early, the latter manifesting with a hypophonic cry and poor suck. This is followed by a progressive, descending weakness, frequently resulting in respiratory failure from the weak bulbar and respiratory muscles. The length of time between the presentation of the first symptom and time of most marked weakness is variable and can range from less than 24 hours to greater than a week.

Examination typically shows dilated pupils with sluggish pupillary light reflexes. There may be ptosis, ophthalmoplegia, facial weakness with drooling and a reduced gag reflex. Affected infants are hypotonic and weak, especially at the neck flexor muscles. Tendon reflexes may be normal, reduced or absent. Consciousness is usually not affected unless the infant is in respiratory failure.

Botulism should be included in the differential diagnosis, along with sepsis and metabolic disorders, in any infant presenting with feeding difficulties, hypotonia, weakness and respiratory difficulties. Early recognition, timely supportive care with mechanical ventilation if indicated, and treatment often result in full recovery and an excellent prognosis.

Definitive confirmation is obtained via detection of the organism or toxin in stool specimens, however receiving results often takes days, or sometimes even weeks depending on the laboratory running the test. Given the distinctive clinical features, electrophysiology will often help confirm the diagnosis, which will help with prognosis and also decision-making regarding whether to order the botulism immune globulin treatment, which is quite expensive but cost-effective when administered early in the course, based on the resulting shortening of critical care and hospital stays [52].

In routine nerve conduction studies, infants frequently have reduced CMAP amplitudes. Sensory nerve action potentials, distal latencies and conduction velocities are usually normal.

Low frequency repetitive nerve stimulation studies at 2–3 Hz produce a modest decremental response, although responses can be variable, and a decrement may be difficult to detect with confidence when the baseline CMAP has a significantly reduced amplitude. The characteristic finding in infantile botulism is an incremental facilitation of CMAP amplitudes at high frequency repetitive nerve stimulation rates of 20–50 Hz. Post-exercise exhaustion is usually absent in botulism, and is difficult to test in infants anyway. Such high stimulation rates are uncomfortable and distressing for the infants, thus some form of sedation or anesthesia is needed, which is relatively accessible in a critical care setting. EMG may demonstrate low amplitude, polyphasic motor units, with fibrillations, and positive sharp wave potentials [53]. It is important to perform accurate repetitive stimulation studies whenever possible as the other findings are suggestive of a myopathic pattern, and the repetitive stimulation studies may be the sole finding to point towards a disorder of the neuromuscular junction rather than a myopathy in these cases.

Single-fiber EMG demonstrates increased jitter and blocking which improves as the stimulation frequency increases. This finding is consistent with a presynaptic defect.

Organophosphate Poisoning

Organophosphates, which are commonly used in agricultural settings as pesticides, are sometimes accidentally ingested. Some of the substances in this category have been banned as chemical weapons, indicating how potent they are. Organophosphates block cholinesterases, including acetylcholinesterase, thus leading to overstimulation of the motor endplate and a disorder of neuromuscular transmission. The clinical presentation is characterized by prominent cholinergic symptoms, accompanied by muscle weakness that may be profound. Atropine is the most easily accessible antidote in most circumstances.

The electrophysiology of organophosphate poisoning is more complex than for other disorders of the neuromuscular junction. On single stimulation, repetitive CMAPs may be seen [54], as in slow channel congenital myasthenic syndromes. Low frequency repetitive stimulation does not typically induce a decrement in the CMAP amplitude, whereas high frequency repetitive stimulation induces a decrement-increment response [54]. There are only rare case reports of organophosphate poisoning in children. One report noted a delayed onset of a radiculopathy with absent F waves that recovered later in the course [55], suggestive of a phenomenon called organophosphate-induced delayed polyneuropathy that was been documented in greater detail in adults [56]. However, as this is a single pediatric case and some of the details were disputed [57], it is not clear how generalizable these electrophysiologic findings are for children with organophosphate poisoning.

References

1. Reichardt LF, Kelly RB. A molecular description of nerve terminal function. Annu Rev Biochem. 1983;52:871–926.
2. Rutecki PA. Neuronal excitability: voltage-dependent currents and synaptic transmission. J Clin Neurophysiol. 1992;9(2):195–211.
3. Engel AG. The neuromuscular junction. Handb Clin Neurol. 2008;91:103–48.
4. Elmqvist D. Neuromuscular transmission with special reference to Myasthenia Gravis. Acta Physiol Scand Suppl. 1965;Suppl 249:1–34.
5. Pitt M. Paediatric electromyography in the modern world: a personal view. Dev Med Child Neurol. 2011;53(2):120–4.
6. Single fiber EMG reference values: a collaborative effort. Ad Hoc Committee of the AAEM special interest group on single fiber EMG. Muscle Nerve. 1992;15(2):151–61.
7. Kinali M, Beeson D, Pitt MC, Jungbluth H, Simonds AK, Aloysius A, et al. Congenital myasthenic syndromes in childhood: diagnostic and management challenges. J Neuroimmunol. 2008;201–202:6–12.
8. Engel AG. Congenital myasthenic syndromes in 2012. Curr Neurol Neurosci Rep. 2012;12(1):92–101.
9. Nogajski JH, Kiernan MC, Ouvrier RA, Andrews PI. Congenital myasthenic syndromes. J Clin Neurosci. 2009;16(1):1–11.
10. Engel AG. The therapy of congenital myasthenic syndromes. Neurotherapeutics. 2007;4(2):252–7.
11. Lorenzoni PJ, Scola RH, Kay CS, Werneck LC. Congenital myasthenic syndrome: a brief review. Pediatr Neurol. 2012;46(3):141–8.
12. Ohno K, Tsujino A, Brengman JM, Harper CM, Bajzer Z, Udd B, et al. Choline acetyltransferase mutations cause myasthenic syndrome associated with episodic apnea in humans. Proc Natl Acad Sci U S A. 2001;98(4):2017–22.
13. Mallory LA, Shaw JG, Burgess SL, Estrella E, Nurko S, Burpee TM, et al. Congenital myasthenic syndrome with episodic apnea. Pediatr Neurol. 2009;41(1):42–5.
14. Maselli RA, Chen D, Mo D, Bowe C, Fenton G, Wollmann RL. Choline acetyltransferase mutations in myasthenic syndrome due to deficient acetylcholine resynthesis. Muscle Nerve. 2003;27(2):180–7.
15. Bady B, Chauplannaz G, Carrier H. Congenital Lambert-Eaton myasthenic syndrome. J Neurol Neurosurg Psychiatry. 1987;50(4):476–8.
16. Hajjar M, Markowitz J, Darras BT, Kissel JT, Srinivasan J, Jones HR. Lambert-Eaton syndrome, an unrecognized treatable pediatric neuromuscular disorder: three patients and literature review. Pediatr Neurol. 2014;50(1):11–7.
17. Donger C, Krejci E, Serradell AP, Eymard B, Bon S, Nicole S, et al. Mutation in the human acetylcholinesterase-associated collagen gene, COLQ, is responsible for congenital myasthenic syndrome with end-plate acetylcholinesterase deficiency (Type Ic). Am J Hum Genet. 1998;63(4):967–75.
18. Ohno K, Brengman J, Tsujino A, Engel AG. Human endplate acetylcholinesterase deficiency caused by mutations in the collagen-like tail subunit (ColQ) of the asymmetric enzyme. Proc Natl Acad Sci U S A. 1998;95(16):9654–9.

19. Katz B, Thesleff S. A study of the desensitization produced by acetylcholine at the motor end-plate. J Physiol. 1957;138(1):63–80.
20. Maselli RA, Ng JJ, Anderson JA, Cagney O, Arredondo J, Williams C, et al. Mutations in LAMB2 causing a severe form of synaptic congenital myasthenic syndrome. J Med Genet. 2009;46(3):203–8.
21. Barisic N, Chaouch A, Muller JS, Lochmuller H. Genetic heterogeneity and pathophysiological mechanisms in congenital myasthenic syndromes. Eur J Paediatr Neurol. 2011;15(3):189–96.
22. Engel AG, Shen XM, Selcen D, Sine SM. What have we learned from the congenital myasthenic syndromes. J Mol Neurosci. 2010;40(1–2):143–53.
23. Tsujino A, Maertens C, Ohno K, Shen XM, Fukuda T, Harper CM, et al. Myasthenic syndrome caused by mutation of the SCN4A sodium channel. Proc Natl Acad Sci U S A. 2003;100(12):7377–82.
24. Huze C, Bauche S, Richard P, Chevessier F, Goillot E, Gaudon K, et al. Identification of an agrin mutation that causes congenital myasthenia and affects synapse function. Am J Hum Genet. 2009;85(2):155–67.
25. Hoffmann K, Muller JS, Stricker S, Megarbane A, Rajab A, Lindner TH, et al. Escobar syndrome is a prenatal myasthenia caused by disruption of the acetylcholine receptor fetal gamma subunit. Am J Hum Genet. 2006;79(2):303–12.
26. Oskoui M, Jacobson L, Chung WK, Haddad J, Vincent A, Kaufmann P, et al. Fetal acetylcholine receptor inactivation syndrome and maternal myasthenia gravis. Neurology. 2008;71(24):2010–2.
27. Forrest K, Mellerio JE, Robb S, Dopping-Hepenstal PJ, McGrath JA, Liu L, et al. Congenital muscular dystrophy, myasthenic symptoms and epidermolysis bullosa simplex (EBS) associated with mutations in the PLEC1 gene encoding plectin. Neuromuscul Disord. 2010;20(11):709–11.
28. Selcen D, Juel VC, Hobson-Webb LD, Smith EC, Stickler DE, Bite AV, et al. Myasthenic syndrome caused by plectinopathy. Neurology. 2011;76(4):327–36.
29. Chaouch A, Muller JS, Guergueltcheva V, Dusl M, Schara U, Rakocevic-Stojanovic V, et al. A retrospective clinical study of the treatment of slow-channel congenital myasthenic syndrome. J Neurol. 2012;259(3):474–81.
30. Spillane J, Beeson DJ, Kullmann DM. Myasthenia and related disorders of the neuromuscular junction. J Neurol Neurosurg Psychiatry. 2010;81(8):850–7.
31. Engel AG, Ohno K, Sine SM. Congenital myasthenic syndromes: progress over the past decade. Muscle Nerve. 2003;27(1):4–25.
32. Lorenzoni PJ, Kay CS, Arruda WO, Scola RH, Werneck LC. Neurophysiological study in slow-channel congenital myasthenic syndrome: case report. Arq Neuropsiquiatr. 2006;64(2A):318–21.
33. Liew WK, Powell CA, Sloan SR, Shamberger RC, Weldon CB, Darras BT, et al. Comparison of plasmapheresis and intravenous immunoglobulin as maintenance therapies for juvenile myasthenia gravis. JAMA Neurol. 2014;71(5):575–80.
34. Lindstrom JM, Seybold ME, Lennon VA, Whittingham S, Duane DD. Antibody to acetylcholine receptor in myasthenia gravis: prevalence, clinical correlates, and diagnostic value. 1975. Neurology. 1998;51(4):933; and 6 pages following
35. Chiang LM, Darras BT, Kang PB. Juvenile myasthenia gravis. Muscle Nerve. 2009;39(4):423–31.
36. McMillan HJ, Darras BT, Kang PB. Autoimmune neuromuscular disorders in childhood. Curr Treat Options Neurol. 2011;13(6):590–607.
37. Engel AG. Morphologic and immunopathologic findings in myasthenia gravis and in congenital myasthenic syndromes. J Neurol Neurosurg Psychiatry. 1980;43(7):577–89.
38. Koul R, Al Futaisi A, Abdwani R. Rituximab in severe seronegative juvenile myasthenia gravis: review of the literature. Pediatr Neurol. 2012;47(3):209–12.
39. Zinman L, Ng E, Bril V. IV immunoglobulin in patients with myasthenia gravis: a randomized controlled trial. Neurology. 2007;68(11):837–41.

40. Snead OC 3rd, Benton JW, Dwyer D, Morley BJ, Kemp GE, Bradley RJ, et al. Juvenile myasthenia gravis. Neurology. 1980;30(7 Pt 1):732–9.
41. Mandawat A, Mandawat A, Kaminski HJ, Shaker ZA, Alawi AA, Alshekhlee A. Outcome of plasmapheresis in myasthenia gravis: delayed therapy is not favorable. Muscle Nerve. 2011;43(4):578–84.
42. Millichap JG, Dodge PR. Diagnosis and treatment of myasthenia gravis in infancy, childhood, and adolescence: a study of 51 patients. Neurology. 1960;10:1007–14.
43. Adams C, Theodorescu D, Murphy EG, Shandling B. Thymectomy in juvenile myasthenia gravis. J Child Neurol. 1990;5(3):215–8.
44. Gronseth GS, Barohn RJ. Practice parameter: thymectomy for autoimmune myasthenia gravis (an evidence-based review): report of the quality standards subcommittee of the American Academy of Neurology. Neurology. 2000;55(1):7–15.
45. Tracy MM, McRae W, Millichap JG. Graded response to thymectomy in children with myasthenia gravis. J Child Neurol. 2009;24(4):454–9.
46. Stalberg E. Clinical electrophysiology in myasthenia gravis. J Neurol Neurosurg Psychiatry. 1980;43(7):622–33.
47. Fox CK, Keet CA, Strober JB. Recent advances in infant botulism. Pediatr Neurol. 2005;32(3):149–54.
48. Spika JS, Shaffer N, Hargrett-Bean N, Collin S, MacDonald KL, Blake PA. Risk factors for infant botulism in the United States. Am J Dis Child. 1989;143(7):828–32.
49. Barash JR, Tang TW, Arnon SS. First case of infant botulism caused by Clostridium baratii type F in California. J Clin Microbiol. 2005;43(8):4280–2.
50. Eleopra R, Tugnoli V, Rossetto O, De Grandis D, Montecucco C. Different time courses of recovery after poisoning with botulinum neurotoxin serotypes A and E in humans. Neurosci Lett. 1998;256(3):135–8.
51. Mitchell WG, Tseng-Ong L. Catastrophic presentation of infant botulism may obscure or delay diagnosis. Pediatrics. 2005;116(3):e436–8.
52. Arnon SS, Schechter R, Maslanka SE, Jewell NP, Hatheway CL. Human botulism immune globulin for the treatment of infant botulism. N Engl J Med. 2006;354(5):462–71.
53. Cornblath DR, Sladky JT, Sumner AJ. Clinical electrophysiology of infantile botulism. Muscle Nerve. 1983;6(6):448–52.
54. Singh G, Mahajan R, Whig J. The importance of electrodiagnostic studies in acute organophosphate poisoning. J Neurol Sci. 1998;157(2):191–200.
55. Aiuto LA, Pavlakis SG, Boxer RA. Life-threatening organophosphate-induced delayed polyneuropathy in a child after accidental chlorpyrifos ingestion. J Pediatr. 1993;122(4):658–60.
56. Jokanovic M, Kosanovic M, Brkic D, Vukomanovic P. Organophosphate induced delayed polyneuropathy in man: an overview. Clin Neurol Neurosurg. 2011;113(1):7–10.
57. Gutmann L, Bodensteiner JB. Organophosphate-induced delayed polyneuropathy. J Pediatr. 1993;123(5):837.

Chapter 22
Myopathies and Myotonic Disorders

Jiri Vajsar, Hernan D. Gonorazky, and James J. Dowling

Myopathies are a clinically and genetically heterogeneous group of disorders with a wide spectrum of symptom onset and severity as well as a range of morbidity and mortality. In childhood, myopathies are most commonly due to genetic mutations, with acquired disease being a less frequent cause [1]. Currently, with the evolution of molecular diagnostics and the application of next generation sequencing technology, along with the use of muscle MRI/ultrasound and muscle biopsy, the role of electromyography (EMG) in myopathies has diminished, but retains significant utility when the differential diagnosis also includes neuromuscular diseases that are not primarily myopathic, disorders of the neuromuscular junction, as well as myotonic disorders [2, 3]. The clinical history and physical examination are crucial to orient the electrophysiologic (EDX) study. The age of onset, pattern of inheritance, distribution of muscle weakness, presence of axial or limb contractures, presence of ophthalmoplegia, myopathic facies, cardiomyopathy or accompanying dermatological lesions are some of the features to have in mind when deciding to pursue EDX and for determining the specifics of the EDX study.

Clinically, myopathies present as pure motor syndromes (with the exception of congenital myotonic dystrophy (cDM1) and some congenital muscular dystrophies, which can have prominent central nervous system (CNS) involvement). Depending on the age of onset, they can be classified as congenital, most frequently presenting as neonatal hypotonia (i.e., congenital myopathies, congenital muscular dystrophies, congenital myotonic dystrophy type 1) or have an onset later in childhood. Beyond infancy the child will usually have a history of gross motor developmental delay and/or difficulties walking, frequent tripping and falls. The distribution is usually symmetric except for diseases such as facioscapulohumeral muscular dystrophy (FSHD) and Pompe disease, among others. Although myopathies are usually described to have a proximal distribution of weakness, a predominant distal

J. Vajsar, M.D., M.Sc., F.R.C.P.C. (✉) • H.D. Gonorazky, M.D. • J.J. Dowling, M.D., Ph.D.
Hospital for Sick Children, University of Toronto, Toronto, ON, Canada
e-mail: jiri.vajsar@sickkids.ca

© Springer International Publishing AG 2017

H.J. McMillan, P.B. Kang (eds.), *Pediatric Electromyography*,
DOI 10.1007/978-3-319-61361-1_22

involvement can be present in disorders such as myotonic dystrophy type 1 (DM1) or myofibrillar myopathies and in some cases of congenital myopathies [4, 5]. The presentation of bulbar symptoms with myopathic facies should direct the diagnosis towards congenital myopathies or cDM1. The involvement of extraocular muscles is an important clue, since they are compromised in a small group of diseases, such as centronuclear myopathies, recessive forms of *RYR1*-related myopathy, mitochondrial disorders, and neuromuscular junction disorders (NMJ) [2]. A history of rhabdomyolysis, defined as an acute muscle breakdown, with myalgia, pigmenturia, elevated serum creatine kinase (CK) triggered by exercise, heat or medications should alert the clinician to a primary genetic cause for myopathy, especially if there are recurrent episodes [6]. The complications after administration of volatile anaesthetic gases and/or depolarizing muscle relaxants, such as succinylcholine, related to symptoms such as muscle rigidity, hyperthermia, elevated CK and multisystemic failure is a classical history of malignant hyperthermia, which is usually related to mutations in the gene *RYR1*, though malignant hyperthermia or similar syndromes have been associated in a minor proportion with other genes [7–9]. It is also important to determine if symptoms such as fatigue, weakness or muscle cramps are associated with exercise, or fasting. These should suggest a primary metabolic disorder or potentially a NMJ disorder, though many patients with myopathies and dystrophies also complain of easy fatigability and/or myalgias [6].

With markedly elevated serum CK (>5 × upper limit of normal) the diagnosis of metabolic, autoimmune or dystrophic muscle disease should be suspected (Fig. 22.1). However, there is no direct correlation between CK levels and the severity of EMG findings. One will usually see an increase in CK when there is inflammation or necrosis of the myofibers and as these disorders may ultimately lead to the detachment of myofibers from the neuromuscular junction, the needle EMG

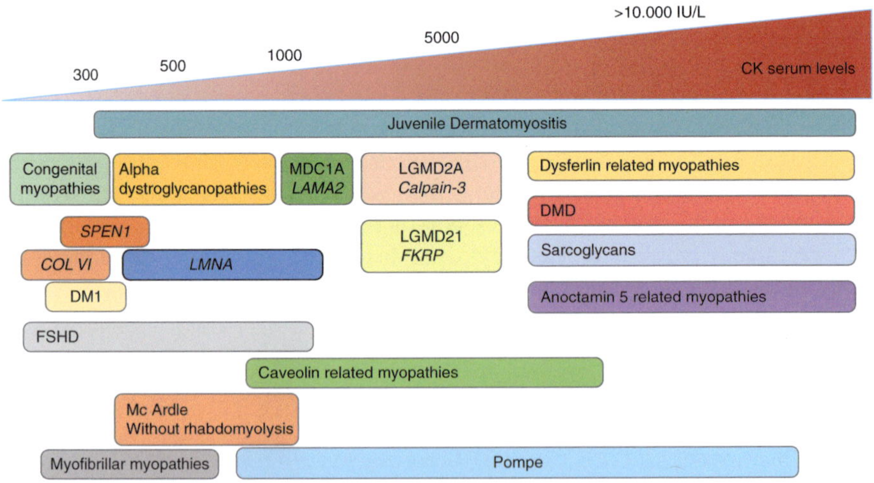

Fig. 22.1 CK serum levels on most muscle disorders in paediatric population. (serum CK expressed in IU/L)

often shows the presence of fibrillations and positive sharp waves (PSW) [10]. Importantly, normal CK levels do not rule out muscle disease. Disorders of the neuromuscular junction (e.g., botulism) and some forms of congenital myopathies may be associated with fibrillation potentials, positive sharp waves, and "myopathic" appearing motor unit potentials (MUAP), often in the context of a normal CK level [11–13]. While mild serum CK elevation (2–5 × upper limit of normal) can reflect muscle disorders, this can also be seen with motor neuronopathies (e.g., spinal muscular atrophy) or polyneuropathies (Charcot-Marie-Tooth disease) due to the secondary loss of muscle that occurs with motor nerve atrophy [14]. For patients in whom there is a high clinical suspicion of Duchenne muscular dystrophy (DMD), FSHD, or DM1, the best practice is to request genetic testing as the first step toward obtaining a definitive diagnosis [15–17]. For other suspected genetic muscle diseases, the decision to pursue genetic testing first or instead a muscle biopsy is an evolving one. Particularly as the cost for genetic testing continues to drop, it is rapidly becoming the first choice test for all or most childhood muscle diseases with a suspected genetic cause.

Electrophysiologic Evaluation

EDX evaluation for muscle disorders in the pediatric population can be challenging and is usually used to differentiate between primary muscle disorders and mimics such as NMJ diseases. The EMG diagnostic yield for neurogenic diseases and NMJ disorders is high in young children. A recent large retrospective study of myopathies (age range 6 months to 18 years) showed that EMG is similarly highly sensitive for detecting abnormalities in documented myopathies (91% sensitive), but less specific in terms of distinct diagnoses (67%) [18]. However, different cohorts, particularly those that include infants being evaluated for neonatal hypotonia, have shown that the yield for diagnosis of myopathy with only EMG may be low, with a high frequency of false-negative results. The reason for such a low diagnostic yield is unclear. Possible explanations include technical issues, patchy distribution of myopathic findings, the lower number of muscles often sampled in infants and young children versus adults, and the difficulty of distinguishing between expected small MUAPs in infants versus MUAPs that are truly myopathic [10, 19, 20].

The usual protocol for myopathy should include one sensory and one motor nerve conduction study with an accompanying F response in one upper and one lower limb. For needle EMG, it is ideal to study at least two distal and two proximal muscles in the upper and lower extremities and at least one paraspinal muscle or the genioglossus. However, in practice the number of muscles studied in children is generally fewer, depending on circumstances such as the tolerance of the individual child. The use of sedatives like propofol can improve the quality and tolerability of some aspects of the study, however this must be balanced with the loss of active patient recruitment and reduced or absent visualization of MUAPs in a sedated or

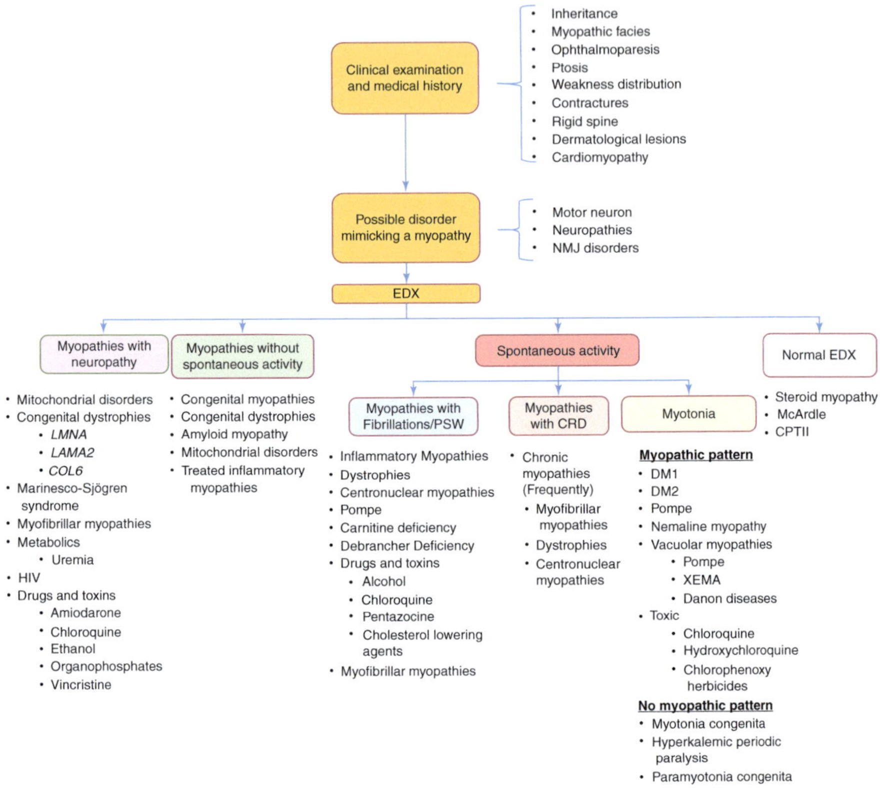

Fig. 22.2 Diagnostic algorithm by most prevalent electrophysiological findings in muscle disorders

anesthetised patient [21]. Thus, it is generally recommended to perform the majority of studies in children without sedation or general anesthesia, as explained in greater detail in Chap. 3.

One has to keep in mind that there can be a transient mild elevation of CK after an EMG study. Therefore, measuring the CK right after the EMG is not recommended if it is possible to have blood drawn for the test another day, though the elevation typically doesn't exceed 1.5× of baseline. Another precaution is to avoid performing a muscle biopsy in a muscle where a needle EMG was recently performed since the needle can generate a mild inflammation at the site of the recording.

EDX findings can be divided into 6 different groups that can assist with generating a differential diagnosis (Fig. 22.2).

1. Combined myopathies with neuropathies
2. Myopathic pattern with no spontaneous activity
3. Myopathic pattern with predominant fibrillation discharges
4. Myopathic pattern with myotonia
5. Myopathic pattern with complex repetitive discharges
6. Myopathies with normal EDX

Nerve Conduction Studies

Nerve conduction studies should be normal in myopathies, except in cases with severe muscle wasting where decreased compound muscle action potential (CMAP) amplitude may be observed. In the setting where there is a low CMAP amplitude and normal sensory nerve action potential (SNAP) amplitudes, one should also consider a disorder of neuromuscular transmission (especially presynaptic NMJ disorders such as Lambert-Eaton syndrome) as well as disorders of motor neurons and/or motor nerves. Lambert-Eaton myasthenic syndrome (LEMS) is rare in the paediatric population but it has been reported in a handful of cases associated with paraneoplastic or autoimmune disorders [22–25]. Testing should include a single supramaximal stimulation delivered before and after short (10-second) exercise. Presynaptic NMJ disorders such as LEMS will classically demonstrate a dramatic post-exercise facilitation, namely a > 60–100% increase in CMAP amplitude above baseline values [26, 27]. When such a diagnosis is under consideration, it is helpful to perform a repetitive nerve stimulation study (RNS) (see Chap. 6) with a proper protocol that includes the evaluation of the presynaptic NMJ disorders (see Chap. 21).

The existence of both a neuropathy and myopathy should suggest a more limited differential diagnosis that includes mitochondrial disorders, congenital muscular dystrophies such as those associated with mutations in *LAMA2* (which can produce a demyelinating peripheral neuropathy), and more rarely *LMNA* (which rarely is also associated with a type 2 form of Charcot-Marie-Tooth disease) and *COL6* (where some cases of subclinical neuropathy have been observed), rare cases of glycogenosis type 3, Marinesco-Sjögren syndrome, myofibrillar myopathies, or injuries due to toxins (Fig. 22.2) [28–32].

Insertional Activity

Increased insertional activity in myopathies results from of muscle fiber irritability. Fiber necrosis, inflammation and/or fiber splitting can produce a "functional denervation" which is a partial detachment of a segment of the myofiber from its motor endplate. This represents the muscle-fiber equivalent of what is seen in denervation. In advanced stages of the disease with severe fatty replacement of the muscle, the insertional activity may appear more normal. However, increased insertional activity in isolation without other abnormalities is of unclear significance, and care should be taken not to base a neurophysiologic diagnosis entirely on increased insertional activity alone.

Spontaneous Activity

Fibrillation potentials and positive sharp waves (PSW) are the usual findings in neurogenic processes producing denervation. However, for the reason noted above, they can be frequently present in different muscle disorders and thus should not be relied on to distinguish between neurogenic and myopathic diseases.

Fibrillation potentials are usually up to 2 ms in duration and less than 100 μV in amplitude, with bi or triphasic morphology and an initial positive deflection. They have a regular frequency and the sound is usually described as "raindrops on a tin roof". Positive sharp waves (PSWs) are biphasic waves with an initial sharp positive deflection followed by a slow negative wave. The amplitude can be from 50 μV up to 1 mV. As with fibrillation potentials, they are regular in frequency and the sounds emanating from loudspeakers are described as dull pops, given their longer durations. The frequency of fibrillation potentials or PSWs is usually between 0.5 and 10 Hz and rarely up to 30 Hz. In muscle disorders, they result from segmental necrosis of the myofiber splitting in at least two fragments, one of which is separated from the motor plate. Therefore in those myopathies where the inflammation and necrosis is a typical finding in the muscle biopsy (inflammatory myopathies, dystrophies), it is common to observe fibrillation potentials and PSWs at the time of the EMG (Fig. 22.3a).

Another common finding is the presence of complex repetitive discharges (CRDs) due to irritability of the fibers (Fig. 22.3b). They are caused by ephaptic activation of a group of myofibers that will provoke an abrupt onset and abrupt end of the electrophysiological phenomenon. They have uniform frequency (5–100 Hz), morphology and amplitude and are stable in configuration. They are also known as

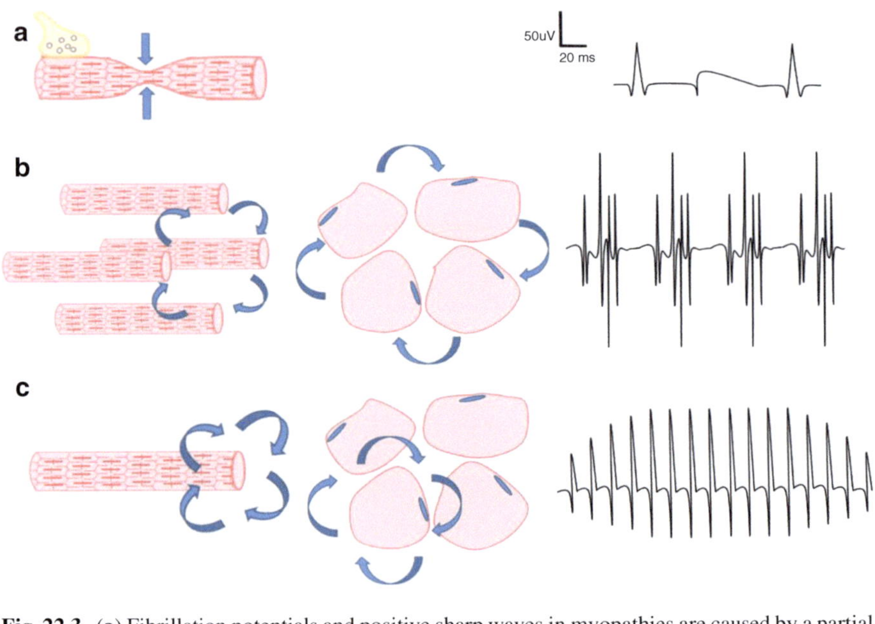

Fig. 22.3 (**a**) Fibrillation potentials and positive sharp waves in myopathies are caused by a partial detachment of the nerve terminal from the motor endplate due to segmental necrosis of the myofiber, producing a "denervated" healthy fragment. On EMG, they are biphasic or triphasic with an initial positive wave and a regular rhythm with a frequency up to 30 Hz. (**b**) Complex repetitive discharges are secondary to ephaptic firing of a group of myofibers. The MUAPs are regular and stable with an acute onset and stop. (**c**) Myotonia is caused by spontaneous rhythmic firing of one fiber. It has a characteristic waxing and waning morphology in amplitude and frequency and it produces a typical sound on the loudspeakers reminiscent of a "dive bomber" or "motorcycle"

pseudomyotonic discharges given their resemblance to myotonic discharges, however, we avoid the use of this term due to potential confusion that can result. Unlike myotonic discharges, CRDs do not have a waxing and waning configuration. The sounds produced by CRDs have been likened to machine or machine gun noises. This finding can be seen in both myopathic and neurogenic disorders and usually indicates a long standing process with associated atrophy of large groups of muscle fibers that are in close proximity to one another. CRDs by themselves do not indicate a specific diagnosis or class of diagnoses.

A third common finding in myopathies is myotonia (Fig. 22.3c). It is important to differentiate between those disorders that produce clinical and electrophysiological myotonia (i.e., DM1, myotonia congenita and some forms of periodic paralysis) with the ones that produce only electrophysiological myotonia (i.e., some centronuclear myopathies and metabolic disorders such as Pompe disease) [33] (Fig. 22.2).

Finally, cramps can be associated with underlying metabolic myopathies such as glycogen storage disorders (e.g., McArdle disease) or disorders of fatty acid oxidation (e.g., carnitine palmitoyltransferase II deficiency). Cramps in these cases result from sustained contraction or impaired relaxation resulting from energy failure and/or ion channel dysfunction. Whereas physiological cramping will be associated with high frequency firing of one or more MUAPs (20–150 Hz), patients with metabolic myopathy or channelopathies may demonstrate electrical silence during needle EMG. Hence, as this specific muscle symptom does not actually correspond to an electrophysiologic cramp, some have advocated that it be referred to as a contracture [10].

Voluntary Contraction

The motor unit potential in myopathies is characterized by a smaller morphology and early recruitment due to a dropout of muscle fibers from a motor unit, hence the need to recruit more motor units to generate a specific amount of muscle force. In general the recruitment pattern is appropriate for the firing frequency or activation (defined as the ability of a motor unit to increase the firing rate), but increased for the amount of force being generated. In general, the ratio is 1:5; that means, at a firing rate of 5 Hz only one motor unit should be recruited, at 30 Hz there should be at least 6 different motor units on the screen (Fig. 22.4a). In myopathies, since there are fewer contractile myofibers per motor unit, to generate a given amount of force, it requires a higher amount of active motor units. So, with a slight contraction of the muscle, there will be an inappropriately high number of firing MUAPs, corresponding to a higher number of active motor units (Fig. 22.4b). Traditionally, this finding could only be assessed by the neurophysiologist performing the study who can feel the amount of force generated by a muscle. Accordingly, with the loss of fibers for each motor unit, the amplitudes and durations of the MUAPs will be small, with frequent polyphasia and unstable morphologies (Fig. 22.5), due to loss of synchronicity of activation of the myofibers within a motor unit [34].

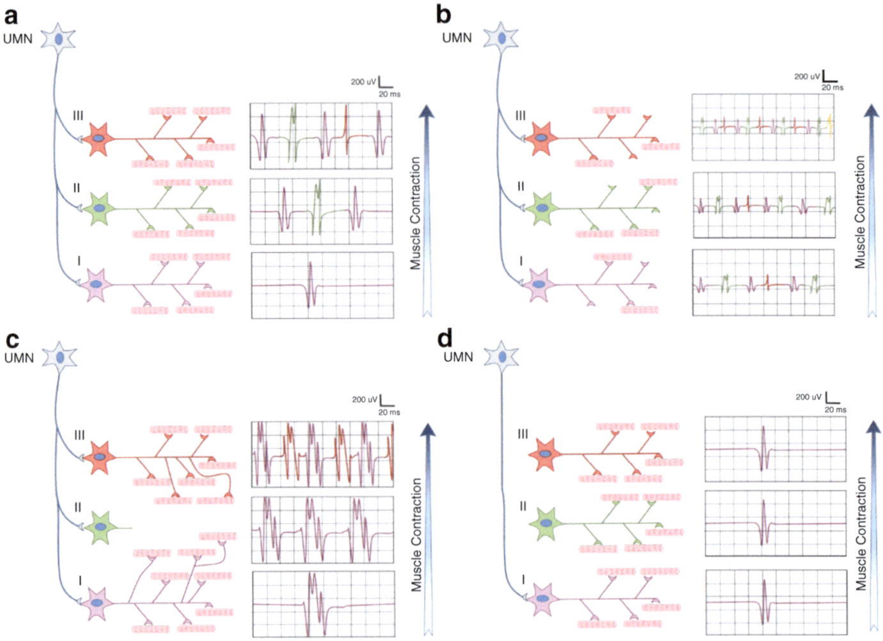

Fig. 22.4 Recruitment pattern. (**a**) Normal Motor Unit (MU) recruitment. The ratio of firing frequency (*activation*) to the number of different muscle action potentials (MUAPs) (*recruitment)* is approximately 5:1. When the firing rate of the first MUAP (I) is 10 Hz, a second MU is recruited (II). By 15 Hz, a third MU starts firing (III), and so forth. (**b**) Myopathic MU recruitment pattern. The loss of myofibers causes that under a mild muscle contraction there is an inappropriate higher number of activated MU, seen in the screen by different MUAPs at early stages of muscle activation. This is defined as early recruitment. However, the firing ratio is still appropriate at 5:1 producing an interference pattern but with reduced amplitude secondary to small MUs. (**c**) Neuropathic MU recruitment pattern. Since there is a loss of MU (II) the recruitment is reduced and the remaining MU are forced to fire at a higher frequency. At maximal contraction at approximately 30 Hz there are only 2 MU activated. This produces an abnormal ratio of 15:1. Also observe the nerve sprouting by MU I and III to reinnervate the muscle fibers of MU II. This produces a polyphasic, long duration, high amplitude MUAP. (**d**) Central MU recruitment pattern. Central involvement will produce an abnormal activation. The recruitment ratio will still be normal at 5:1, however there is an impaired ability to increase the firing rate. (UMN, upper motor unit)

Although the findings in minimal voluntary contraction in the setting of a muscle disease is what is traditionally termed a “myopathic pattern”, small MUAPs may also be found in neuromuscular junction disorders such as botulism, or during early re-innervation after severe neurogenic process [12, 34]. However, the early recruitment pattern is present only in true myopathies [10], and thus assessment of recruitment pattern is often crucial to the interpretation of a study in which small motor units are observed.

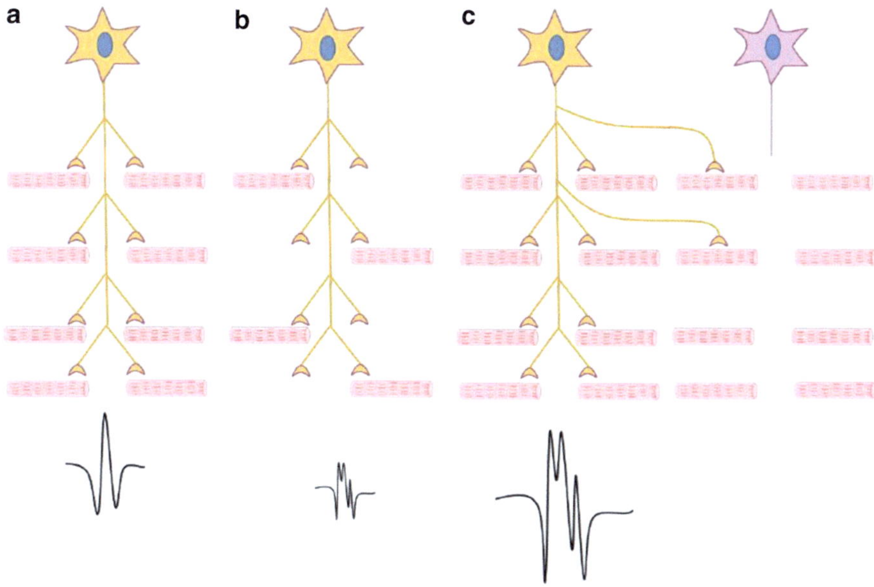

Fig. 22.5 Motor unit action potentials. (**a**) Normal MUAP. (**b**) Myopathic MUAP, due to the loss of myofibers the MUAPs are small and of short duration. Unstable and polyphasic potentials are secondary to malfunction of remaining myofibers. (**c**) Neuropathic MUAP. Nerve sprouting to denervated muscle fibers. This leads to a bigger MUAP of longer duration and polyphasic pattern due to lack of synchronicity with the newly incorporated myofibers

Clinical and Electrophysiological Description of Selected Muscle Disorders

As the overall goal of the present book is to describe EMG patterns specifically in the pediatric population, the childhood myopathies discussed below were selected as examples of electrodiagnostic patterns, and are not meant to comprise a comprehensive discussion of all muscle disorders.

Myopathic Pattern With Fibrillations

As mentioned earlier, fibrillation potentials in myopathies are mainly due to inflammation and necrosis of the myofibers. In children, this is mainly due to inflammatory myopathies and dystrophies.

Juvenile Dermatomyositis

While in adults there is a higher proportion of patients with polymyositis than dermatomyositis, in children the converse is true, with dermatomyositis being by far the most common inflammatory myopathy in childhood [35, 36]. Juvenile dermatomyositis is a chronic autoimmune disease characterized by limb girdle weakness, with involvement of neck flexors and extensors muscles and pathognomonic skin rashes. It is a multisystem disorder affecting primarily the muscle and skin due to a capillary vasculopathy. There is a predominance in females that ranges from 2:1 to 5:1 [21, 35, 37].

The diagnostic criteria include symmetrical limb girdle weakness, heliotrope dermatitis and/or Gottron's papules, increased CK (though it is important to note that some patients may have normal values), muscle biopsy consistent with diagnosis (the characteristic finding is the perimysial atrophy of muscle fibers) and an abnormal EMG [38]. In acute-subacute stages EMG shows prominent presence of fibrillation potentials and or positive sharp waves, with short small MUAPs and early recruitment. In long standing forms it is possible to find CRDs. These findings are more evident in proximal and paraspinal muscles. This last muscle group is the most sensitive and should be evaluated when there is no abnormal finding in other muscles [39]. In more chronic cases the MUAPs may have long durations and increased amplitudes, mimicking a neurogenic disorder. The NCVs are normal unless there is severe muscle atrophy in which case decreased CMAP amplitudes will be observed in conjunction with normal sensory responses.

Currently, EMG and muscle biopsy are not used as frequently for diagnosis of dermatomyositis as in the past, as they are considered invasive studies [40]. Muscle MRI has proven to be a useful method for the diagnosis of dermatomyositis and as a biomarker for treatment response, usually revealing increased T2 signals in affected muscles and subcutaneous tissues [41].

The main therapy is immunosuppressive medications such as corticosteroids, methotrexate or cyclosporine. In some patients who require prolonged corticosteroid use, a secondary proximal muscle weakness may develop, reflecting a steroid myopathy that is associated with selective type 2 fiber atrophy. EMG can be used in such cases to help differentiate among a relapse, refractory dermatomyositis, or a steroid myopathy since dermatomyositis is associated with increased spontaneous activity whereas steroid myopathy is not (see normal EDX group Fig. 22.2) [42].

Duchenne Muscular Dystrophy (DMD)

DMD is the most common form of muscular dystrophy in childhood [43]. Since it is an X-linked disorder it typically affects males, with heterozygous female carriers sometimes showing mild cardiac and muscle symptoms in adulthood; exceptionally, females will have more dramatic phenotypes such as in the setting of concomitant Turner syndrome, unfavorable X-linked inactivation, or relevant chromosomal translocation [44]. DMD most commonly results from an out-of-frame deletion or duplication within the *DMD* gene, or less commonly, a frameshift or nonsense mutation. Patients exhibit progressive proximal muscle weakness and contractures, eventually losing independent ambulation, developing cardiomyopathy and later death from cardiorespiratory complications [43]. The diagnosis is confirmed with genetic testing. When DNA testing is negative, muscle biopsy may be required to evaluate for the possibility of a mimicking disorder [45]. Typical muscle biopsy findings include absent dystrophin staining with characteristic dystrophic changes (e.g., split fibers, increased internalized nuclei, regenerating fibers, and replacement of muscle by fat and connective tissue). In some cases, it may be necessary to extract RNA to find direct evidence for cryptic splicing defects [46]. Published databases can also guide clinicians as to whether specific mutations are or are not known to be pathogenic, and clinical genetic test reports increasingly make use of such databases to reduce the reporting of the dreaded "variants of unknown significance". High serum CK levels (typically >20–150 × the upper limit of normal) should trigger the suspicion for this diagnosis, particularly when there is clinical onset after 1.5 years of age, toe-walking, pseudohypertrophy of the calves, and/or a positive Gowers sign [45]. EDX is rarely used in the diagnostic evaluation for Duchenne muscular dystrophy. In those rare instances when it is performed, nerve conduction studies will be normal, while needle EMG may reveal abnormal insertional activity, fibrillation potentials and PSW, with myopathic motor units and an early recruitment pattern, especially in proximal symptomatic muscles. With advancing disease, the CMAP amplitude will decrease, insertional activity will diminish, and the myopathic findings will become more apparent due to progressive muscle atrophy. In endstage muscle it may be difficult to find areas where motor units can be consistently recruited and evaluated.

Becker muscular dystrophy (BMD) also results from dystrophin mutations. However, unlike DMD, patients with BMD show some residual protein expression and activity, due to the association in most cases with in-frame deletions, duplications, and point mutations [43]. Consequently, patients have a milder symptomatology with a later onset compared to DMD.

DMD management requires a multidisciplinary approach. Corticosteroids have been used to slow disease progression, improving and preserving muscle strength and function, prolonging independent ambulation, and delaying the onset of complications such as scoliosis, respiratory decline and cardiomyopathy [45, 47]. Other therapies are emerging with the goal of improving the expression of dystrophin through novel molecular mechanisms. Such novel therapies include ones that transform an out-of-frame to an in-frame mutation via exon skipping induced by an antisense oligonucleotide that was recently provisionally approved by the US Food and Drug Administration; other novel therapies are in development [47–50].

Pompe Disease

Glycogen storage disease type II, also known as Pompe disease or acid maltase deficiency, is an autosomal recessive lysosomal glycogen storage disorder. It has two main phenotypes, an early onset form presenting during infancy and characterized by generalized hypotonia, weakness, macroglossia, cardiomegaly, hepatosplenomegaly, failure to thrive, and respiratory insufficiency [51]. The late onset form presents with progressive muscle weakness in both pediatric and adult populations that often mimics the phenotype of limb-girdle muscular dystrophy with frequent respiratory complications but usually without heart involvement [52]. The late onset patients are more difficult to recognize since the presentation can include a limb girdle muscular dystrophy pattern, an asymmetric scapular winging, ptosis, and/or asymptomatic hyperCKemia [53]. The muscle biopsy usually shows vacuoles positive for glycogen with PAS staining, but there are also atypical cases without glycogen accumulation [54, 55]. The serum CK is usually elevated, particularly in the infantile form of the disease (<10× upper limit of normal). Due to the phenotypic variability of this disease, particularly in the later onset form, EDX studies can provide important clues for the diagnosis. NCS are normal except in advanced cases with severe muscle atrophy. Needle EMG may demonstrate fibrillation potentials and PSW as well as myotonic discharges. This is seen in paraspinal muscles in half of the children and two-thirds of adults with this disease. The examination of this group of muscles is important since it may be the only site revealing abnormalities in the EDX [56]. It is important also to mention that this group of patients has electrophysiological myotonia but no clinical signs of it. The diagnosis is usually confirmed by analyzing the enzyme activity in the blood using a dried blood spot testing, followed by genetic testing [52]. The advent of enzyme replacement therapy (ERT) has changed the outcome of the infantile onset patients. Without ERT the early onset has a high mortality with death by the age of 1 year [51]. ERT has also improved symptomatology for patients with late onset Pompe [57].

Myopathic Pattern with no Spontaneous Activity

Congenital Muscular Dystrophies

The congenital muscular dystrophies (CMD) are a heterogeneous group of disorders. The diagnosis is usually made by the clinical exam, CK levels, which can range from normal to 6–10× high, brain MRI, and immunohistochemical staining in the muscle biopsy. An abnormal brain MRI may be seen in a subset of CMD patients, especially the dystroglycanopathies and merosinopathies. Muscle biopsy shows dystrophic features and may show abnormalities on immunohistochemical staining for merosin and or alpha-dystroglycan (aDG). It is the second most common reason for requests for EMG studies in floppy infants admitted to the NICU for suspected primary muscle disorders, after congenital myopathies [58]. The most common CMD subtype is MDC1A (primary merosin deficiency) [59]. The findings include generalized weakness, early contractures and respiratory insufficiency, high serum CK, diffuse white matter changes on brain MRI and deficient merosin on muscle biopsy [43, 59]. Partial merosin deficiency can be seen in some patients with *LAMA2* mutations and also in the alpha-dystroglycanopathies due to abnormalities in protein glycosylation of aDG. The findings include increased CK and frequent eye and brain malformations that range from abnormalities in the posterior fossa to lissencephaly. The most severe classic phenotypes are muscle-brain-eye disease, Walker-Warburg syndrome and Fukuyama CMD [60]. Other CMDs include the rigid spine syndrome due to mutations in *SEPN1* and the collagen VI related myopathies (Bethlem myopathy and Ullrich CMD). The latter is characterized by congenital hip dislocation, congenital torticollis, and joint hyperlaxity with development of early contractures and scoliosis and generalized muscle weakness [61].

Nerve conduction studies are usually normal except for patients with primary merosin deficiency. In this group there is a slowing in the conduction velocities of the motor nerves with normal amplitude and normal sensory studies [62]. Motor neuropathy is often associated with severe form of MDC1A. Also there has been a report of borderline low NCVs in a young patient with Ullrich CMD (due to mutations in *COL6*) [63]. EMG does not demonstrate the abnormal spontaneous activity that can be seen in other primary myopathies and more significantly in neuropathies. The typical "myopathic" potentials when demonstrated are usually present in more proximal muscles. One report describes brief repetitive decreasing discharges in distal muscles post-electrical stimulation. These were of high frequency (90–300 Hz) and short duration (median 61.5 ms) with the shape of single motor response. They were not elicited by muscle percussion and were different from myotonia due to the lack of the waxing and waning feature [63].

Congenital Myopathies

Congenital myopathies are a heterogeneous group of inherited muscle diseases that vary in age of onset, clinical features, morbidity and mortality. Although the classical description is of patients with onset in infancy, they can present in a wide range of ages. Signs that can help to establish the diagnosis include: lack of antigravity movements, ophthalmoplegia, ptosis, high arched palate, arthrogryposis, hip dysplasia, and lower facial muscle weakness with open tented mouth. The serum CK is typically within the normal range but can be slightly elevated. The diagnosis has been historically established by muscle biopsy, as the different types are classified according to pathological findings. As genetic testing has become more widely available there is a trend to classify them by gene, since numerous genes are now associated with multiple phenotypes and histopathological findings [2]. The different histological subtypes include:

Core myopathy. The muscle biopsy reveals areas lacking enzyme activity with oxidative stains such as SDH and NADH, hence, devoid of mitochondria. This category may further be subdivided into central core disease due to dominant mutations in the *RYR1* gene (90% of cases), minicore myopathy without ophthalmoplegia due to mutations in *SEPN1* and minicores with ophthalmoplegia due to recessive mutations in *RYR1* [64]. Other rare causes of core myopathy including mutations in *MYH7*, *ACTA1*, and *CCDC78*.

Congenital fiber-type disproportion. This term refers to the presence of significantly smaller type I fibers compared with type II without features suggestive of other subtypes of congenital myopathy. A pure CFTD is associated with mutations in *RYR1, SEPN1, ACTA1, TPM2* and *TPM3*. Clinically, CFTD overlaps with other types of congenital myopathies, but the phenotype is typically milder than the other subtypes [64].

Nemaline myopathy (NM) is diagnosed when the classic nemaline rods are observed on Gomori trichrome stain and on electron microscopy of a muscle biopsy specimen. Clinically, there is severe congenital NM, intermediate congenital NM, typical congenital NM, childhood/juvenile onset NM and adult-onset NM. There are at least 11 genes within this group. The most common are those in *NEB* causing a recessive disease and in *ACTA1* causing a dominantly inherited NM, typically due to de novo mutations. The characteristic features in this group include bulbar muscle involvement, a myopathic face (open mouth, tented lips, excessive drooling), and a high arched palate, with preservation of extraocular movements [64].

Centronuclear myopathy (including myotubular myopathy) can be caused by mutations in six genes identified to date (*MTM1, DNM2, BIN1, SPEG, TTN, and RYR1*). Muscle biopsy is characterized by centralized nuclei in at least 25% of the fibers with abnormal central oxidative aggregate staining with SDH and NADH. Certain genes are associated with particular features on muscle biopsy. With *DNM2* mutations there is often a "spoke on wheel" appearance with oxidative stains. *BIN1* mutations tend to present with clusters of central nuclei. Necklace fibers have been related to mutations in *MTM1* and correspond with internalised nuclei within a desmin positive stain ring [64].

EDX in congenital myopathies has a sensitivity of 36% in infants (<2 years of age) with a false negative rate of 25%. The presence of a "myopathic pattern" in a newborn is extremely low [20, 65]. The use of EMG in this age group has been largely replaced by muscle biopsy and genetic studies, but in some cases EMG may still yield useful diagnostic information. In patients >2 years of age there are no characteristics findings for most of the congenital myopathies. The NCS are normal with normal F-responses. The needle EMG will show MUAPs of small amplitude, short duration and polyphasic potentials with an early recruitment and no spontaneous activity [65]. Centronuclear myopathies can represent an exception since fibrillations, positive sharp waves, and more rarely complex repetitive discharges can be seen on needle EMG [13, 66]. The association of myopathic and myotonic findings have been reported in nemaline myopathy [33]. Abnormal repetitive nerve stimulation testing and other features of a NMJ disorder have been observed in cases of congenital myopathy, including those due to mutations in *DNM2, MTM1, RYR1, TPM2, TPM3* and *KLHL40* [67–72].

Myotonic Disorders

Clinical myotonia is a symptom and sign found in a subgroup of neuromuscular disorders. It is caused by muscle ion channel abnormalities and presents with stiffness or cramping in involved muscles. Myotonia may be detected clinically after

Table 22.1 Common genetic causes of myotonia

Diseases	Gene	Locus
Clinical myotonia and electrical myotonia		
Myotonic dystrophy type 1	*DMPK*	19q13.3
Myotonic dystrophy type 2 (proximal myotonic myopathy)	*ZNF9*	3q21.3
Myotonia congenita	*CLCN1*	7q34
Schwartz-Jampel syndrome	*HSPG2*	1p36.12
Clinical paramyotonia and electrical myotonia		
Hyperkalemic periodic paralysis	*SCN4A*	17q23
Paramyotonia congenita	*SCN4A*	17q23
Electrical myotonia without clinical myotonia		
Acid maltase deficiency	*GAA*	17q25.3

forced eye closure, leading to delay in eye opening or by making a fist followed by difficulty releasing the grip. Percussion myotonia can be elicited by tapping the thenar muscle, as well as the quadriceps, gastrocnemius or tongue. Myotonia usually decreases with repeated muscle contractions (positive "warm-up" phenomenon) in contrast to paramyotonia ("paradoxical myotonia") in which muscle relaxation becomes progressively delayed with repetitive contractions. This is an important clinical distinction that can help to differentiate these two types of myotonic disorders.

Historically, myotonias were classified accordingly to their clinical features and inheritance patterns. More recently, genetic testing has further defined the different types (Table 22.1).

Needle EMG in the detection of myotonia plays a very important role as electrical myotonia is quite often more easily detected than clinical myotonia. Myotonic potentials are recorded after insertion or movement of the EMG recording electrode in relaxed muscle or on percussion next to the needle. It presents as trains of rhythmic firing of grouped motor unit potentials in the form of positive waves or fibrillation potentials with waxing and waning frequency and amplitude with firing ranges of 20 to 80 Hz and amplitudes from 10 to 1000 μV [73]. Audio profile of the discharges has been characterized as that of dive bomber airplane, motorcycle, or chain saw engine [74].

Dystrophic Myotonias

The most common is myotonic dystrophy type 1 (DM1) and myotonic dystrophy type 2 (DM2) and they both share prominent clinical and electrical myotonia.

DM1 is an autosomal dominant disease caused by a CTG trinucleotide expansion in the untranslated region of the dystrophia myotonica-protein kinase (*DMPK*) gene on chromosome 19q13.3 [75–77]. Anticipation is characteristic in this disease with an increasing number of CTG repeats in subsequent generations, especially with maternal inheritance, with large CTG repeats of 1000–4000 typically occurring in the congenital form of DM1. Although cranial muscle weakness and wasting and predominantly distal muscles weakness and wasting are the main features of this disease along with myotonia, other systems can be involved leading to cognitive dysfunction, hypersomnia, dysphagia, cardiac arrhythmias, muscle pain, cataracts, respiratory insufficiency, insulin resistance and diabetes, and cancer [78, 79]. The childhood-onset form of DM1 can present as early as the neonatal period with muscle weakness and respiratory insufficiency and although these children improve with time, they have long term global developmental delays.

Needle EMG shows myotonic discharges most prominently in the distal muscles, usually with characteristic waxing and waning frequency. There are often myopathic motor unit potentials although they can be obscured by myotonic discharges. The characteristic clinical features with or without the help of EMG studies will point to myotonic dystrophy but the definite diagnosis and type is made through DNA testing. Of note, clinical and electrical myotonia are rarely evident at birth, and may not develop until later in childhood.

The management of DM1 involves ensuring adequate nutritional intake and monitoring for cataracts, cardiac arrhythmias and sleep disturbances (i.e., central or obstructive apneas) that can lead to day time fatigue. Developmental delay and later cognitive impairment are typical of children with cDM1. As such, modifications are typically required to their learning plan both due to learning problems and fine motor difficulties that can ensue. Genetic counseling should be offered to all families, especially as individuals with DM1 are usually able to reproduce and thus are at risk of transmitting the mutation to their offspring. Precautions are required during anesthesia. Mexiletine is helpful to reduce clinical myotonia and rehabilitation approaches are needed in cDM1 [80].

DM2 is an autosomal dominant disease caused by a CCTG repeat expansion in the *zinc finger protein 9* gene *(ZNF9)* on chromosome 3q21 [81–83]. There is no congenital form and the adult patients have both clinical and electrical myotonia, early cataracts and weakness which is more proximal than distal, and calves can be enlarged [84–86]. Proximal muscle pain is common and the patients can develop similar systemic involvement as in DM1 with memory loss, glucose intolerance, dysphagia, hypogonadism and cardiac arrhythmias but overall DM2 tends to be more benign than DM1 [84, 87]. EMG reveals myotonic discharges but they can be quite brief and less intense than in DM1 and associated myopathic potentials are more proximal than distal. Diagnosis is confirmed by DNA testing and there is no clear correlation between the number of CCTG repeats and the onset or severity of the disease.

Non-dystrophic Myotonias

Thomsen Myotonia Congenita

This is an autosomal dominant disease caused by mutations in the muscle chloride channel 1 *(CLCN1)* gene on chromosome 7q34. Clinically, there is transient muscle stiffness, mostly painless, without weakness. It begins in early childhood or infancy and the myotonia becomes more obvious after prolonged rest and there is a "warm up" effect (i.e., improvement with repeat exercise). Children may be described as clumsy in addition to being stiff and their muscles will show increased bulk, most likely due to sustained muscle contractions. Myotonia can be present on grip testing and muscle percussion. It may increase with strong emotions, pregnancy, hypothyroid disease, and depolarizing anesthetic agents [88–90]. Needle EMG examination shows myotonic discharges [88, 90]. Another useful finding is a transient reduction in the CMAP amplitude that can be observed with 3 Hz repetitive nerve stimulation or after brief isometric exercise (see Chap. 6).

Becker Myotonia Congenita

Autosomal recessive mutations in *CLCN1* gene cause Becker's myotonia congenita. Clinically, this disorder is associated with more severe myotonia than Thomsen's myotonia congenita. In severe cases of myotonia, the patients can have transient immobility after being startled, in particular after a few minutes of rest. EMG shows the same findings as in Thomsen's myotonia congenita. Management is similar for all of the myotonic chloride channelopathies and consists of symptomatic treatment of myotonia with mexiletine or other medications and physical therapy with stretching exercises in order to minimize possibly developing joint contractures [90]. Life span in both Thomsen and Becker myotonia congenita is normal.

Schwartz-Jampel Syndrome

Schwartz-Jampel syndrome is also known as chondrodystrophic myotonia and presents with severe myotonia, short stature, muscle hypertrophy, joint contractures, bone disease as well as ocular and facial abnormalities [91, 92]. It is caused by mutation in the *HSPG2* gene encoding perlecan, a heparin sulfate proteoglycan [93]. Clinically, there is no warm-up phenomenon for the myotonia. The needle EMG findings can resemble neuromyotonia or even complex repetitive discharges since it does not show the typical waxing and waning character that is typical of myotonic discharges.

Sodium Channelopathies

Paramyotonia Congenita

Paramyotonia congenita is an autosomal recessive disease caused by mutations in the α-subunit of the muscle sodium channel encoded by the *SCN4A* gene on chromosome 17q23 [94–96] and can clinically overlap with hyperkalemic periodic paralysis. Myotonia or weakness is exacerbated by cold or exercise and warming decreases the stiffness. It develops in infancy or childhood and the attacks of myotonia and weakness decrease by middle age. Needle EMG shows widespread myotonic discharges that are more pronounced in distal muscles and with exercise and cooling [97, 98].

Exercise or slow repetitive nerve stimulation can stimulate a drop in the CMAP amplitude [88, 99, 100]. Management includes cold exposure avoidance and symptomatic treatment of myotonia. Mexilitine can also provide symptomatic relief and improvement of clinical myotonia [101].

Myotonia Fluctuans and Myotonia Permanens

Myotonia fluctuans and permanens are autosomal dominant diseases due to *SCN4A* mutations. The latter is characterized by severe and continuous myotonia while the former is a mild disease and myotonia varies in severity from day to day.

Acetazolimide-responsive Myotonia

This is an autosomal dominant channelopathy due to *SCN4A* gene mutations which starts in childhood. Generalized myotonia that is often accompanied by muscle pain is triggered by potassium ingestion, fasting, and in some cases with cold and is relieved by acetazolimide therapy [102]. The myotonia paradoxically worsens with repeat activity. Needle EMG reveals myotonic discharges that are minimally responsive to cold temperatures [102].

Hyperkalemic Periodic Paralysis With Myotonia

This is an autosomal dominant sodium channelopathy due to mutations in *SCN4A* gene that can also present in infancy and childhood and clinically overlaps with paramyotonia congenita. Attacks of weakness typically begin in the morning before breakfast and resolve slowly within 15–90 minutes. Precipitants for the attacks are strenuous exercise, emotional stress, cold exposure, and ingestion of glucocorticosteroids, alcohol or potassium. The serum potassium level is normal between the episodes but increases during the episode. The myotonia is episodic and presents between attacks of weakness. Needle EMG examination may be normal between the attacks but in some kindreds it may reveal myotonia [103]. Prolonged exercise may reduce the CMAP amplitude in distal muscles [104]. Management involves avoidance of triggers. Oral glucose and insulin in severe cases may suppress impending attacks. Hydrochlorothiazide and carbonic anhydrase inhibitors may help prevent attacks [105–107].

Other Disorders that can be Associated With Myotonia

Other disorders may have associated myotonia, although usually not as a presenting feature. Electrical myotonia has been recorded in neuromuscular diseases such as polymyositis and inclusion body myositis, Pompe disease, myotubular or centronuclear myopathy, nemaline myopathy, caveolinopathy, malignant hyperthermia, hypothyroidism and severe denervation [73, 74, 108]. In some of these, complex repetitive discharges may be mistaken for electrical myotonia. Rarely, electrical myotonia can be caused by medications such as clofibrate, propranolol, penicilamine, cyclosporine and 2,4 dichlorophenoxyacetic acid [103].

Electromyography in Myotonic Disorders

Electrical myotonia is the most useful finding on EMG examination while NCS are often normal. Needle EMG can confirm the presence, severity and distribution of electrical myotonia and show additional myopathic features. Cold temperatures can prolong electrical myotonia bursts in myotonia congenita (Thomsen disease) and paramyotonia congenita while extremely cold temperatures may eliminate electrical myotonia and voluntary motor unit potentials in paramyotonia congenita [88, 97, 109]. Myotonic discharges are more easily evoked in DM1 than in DM2 [110]. There are additional several specialized tests that may assist in the diagnosis of disorders associated with myotonia: repetitive nerve stimulation, the short and long exercise tests and the provocative cold test.

Low frequency repetitive stimulation may trigger a CMAP decrement in paramyotonia congenita and Thomsen and Becker diseases [90, 99, 104].

The short exercise test entails brief exercise of the muscle in question for 10–30 seconds. Baseline CMAP amplitude is compared with post-exercise CMAP amplitude. The most precipitous decline is observed in paramyotonia congenita, particularly after cooling. Chloride channelopathies tend to have a decline in the first post-exercise CMAP and muscle cooling does not change this pattern [111]. DM1 will also show a decrease in CMAP while DM2 will not [112].

In the long exercise test as described by McManis et al. [104] the patient will maximally contract the adductor digiti minimi for 5 minutes with 3–4 seconds of rest every 15 seconds. In all forms of periodic paralysis, there is a decrease in the CMAP over time. The CMAP decrement in patients with hyperkalemic (and hypokalemic) paralysis differs from patients with paramyotonia congenita. In the former, the amplitude increases immediately after exercise and then declines slowly over the course of 15–30 minutes. In patients with paramyotonia congenita, there is a rapid decline in CMAP amplitude followed by a slow increase back to baseline over next hour. Myotonia congenita patients also may show decrements after exercise testing but this does not tend to be consistent.

Cold in the cooling test provokes weakness in patients with paramyotonia congenita. The CMAP amplitude drop in this disorder is greater than 75% after cooling the limb muscle for 15–30 minutes at 15 °C [113, 114].

Pharmacological Treatment

Antiarrhythmic Medications

Mexiletine Hydrochloride

Mexiletine hydrochloride is a class 1B anti-arrhythmic medication derived from lidocaine. It has been used in treatment of both non-dystrophic and dystrophic myotonias as well as both sodium and chloride channelopathies [115]. Mexiletine is believed to enhance fast inactivation of sodium channels and improvement in the chloride channelopathies probably results from nonspecific blockade of normal sodium channels [116, 117]. A randomized, double-blind, placebo controlled, cross over trial of mexiletine 200 mg three times daily in 59 adults (unpublished data) confirmed improvement in patient-reported stiffness, quality-of-life measures and quantitative measures of myotonia in non-dystrophic myotonias [118, 119]. Similarly, a double-blind, placebo controlled trial demonstrated mexiletine in a dose of 150–200 mg three times daily to be an effective antimyotonia therapy in DM1 patients [80, 120, 121]. Laryngospasm in an infant with *SCN4A* mutation was also relieved by mexiletine [122]. Baseline cardiac evaluation is recommended prior to initiating mexiletine, particularly in patients with cardiac or EKG abnormalities since there is an increased risk for arrhythmogenesis with this medication [123].

Tocainide is a class 1b antiarrhythmic agent, also derived from lidocaine. It has a similar effect on sodium channel function as mexiletine but it can cause more serious side effects [124]. Flecainide has been also used in patients with *SCN4A* mutations [125].

Antiepileptic Medications

Carbamazepine and phenytoin have sodium channel blocking properties, including the sodium channels found in skeletal muscle sarcolemma. The former has been preferred in children due to a lower side effect profile; they both have been reported to improve myotonia symptoms and signs [126, 127].

Antidepressant Medication

Imipramine, clomipramine and amitriptyline were previously used in the treatment of myotonia, but have been almost entirely supplanted by the above medications [128–130].

Acetazolimide

Acetazolamide is a carbonic anhydrase inhibitor and diuretic that increases the renal clearance of sodium and potassium and limits the entry of potassium in the muscle cells [131]. It increases chloride conductance through muscle voltage-gated chloride channels [132]. It has been used in most of the non-dystrophic myotonias and helps to prevent muscle weakness, pain and paralytic attacks [109, 131, 133].

Other Medications

Dantrolene has been observed to reduce hand myotonia in a child with Thomsen's myotonia congenita [134]. The use of nifedipine, a calcium channel blocker and antihypertensive medication, was associated with mild improvement in myotonic dystrophy patients [135].

References

1. Darin N, Tulinius M. Neuromuscular disorders in childhood: a descriptive epidemiological study from western Sweden. Neuromuscul Disord. 2000;10(1):1–9.
2. North KN, Wang CH, Clarke N, Jungbluth H, Vainzof M, Dowling JJ, Amburgey K, Quijano-Roy S, Beggs AH, Sewry C, Laing NG, Bonnemann CG, International Standard of Care Committee for Congenital. Approach to the diagnosis of congenital myopathies. Neuromuscul Disord. 2014;24(2):97–116.
3. Bonnemann CG, Wang CH, Quijano-Roy S, Deconinck N, Bertini E, Ferreiro A, Muntoni F, Sewry C, Beroud C, Mathews KD, Moore SA, Bellini J, Rutkowski A, North KN, Members of International Standard of Care Committee for Congenital Muscular. Diagnostic approach to the congenital muscular dystrophies. Neuromuscul Disord. 2014;24(4):289–311.
4. Shaibani A. Distal myopathies: case studies. Neurol Clin. 2016;34(3):547–64.
5. Dimachkie MM, Barohn RJ. Distal myopathies. Neurol Clin. 2014;32(3):817–42, x.
6. Chan EK, Kornberg AJ, Ryan MM. A diagnostic approach to recurrent myalgia and rhabdomyolysis in children. Arch Dis Child. 2015;100(8):793–7.
7. Rosenberg H, Pollock N, Schiemann A, Bulger T, Stowell K. Malignant hyperthermia: a review. Orphanet J Rare Dis. 2015;10:93.
8. Stamm DS, Aylsworth AS, Stajich JM, Kahler SG, Thorne LB, Speer MC, Powell CM. Native American myopathy: congenital myopathy with cleft palate, skeletal anomalies, and susceptibility to malignant hyperthermia. Am J Med Genet A. 2008;146A(14):1832–41.
9. Gurnaney H, Brown A, Litman RS. Malignant hyperthermia and muscular dystrophies. Anesth Analg. 2009;109(4):1043–8.
10. Preston DC, Shapiro BE. Electromyography and neuromuscular disorders clinical-electrophysiological correlations. London; New York: Elsevier Saunders; 2013. p. 1. online resource (xvii, 643 p.)
11. Chahin N, Selcen D, Engel AG. Sporadic late onset nemaline myopathy. Neurology. 2005;65(8):1158–64.
12. Witoonpanich R, Vichayanrat E, Tantisiriwit K, Rattanasiri S, Ingsathit A. Electrodiagnosis of botulism and clinico-electrophysiological correlation. Clin Neurophysiol. 2009;120(6):1135–8.
13. Fischer D, Herasse M, Bitoun M, Barragan-Campos HM, Chiras J, Laforet P, Fardeau M, Eymard B, Guicheney P, Romero NB. Characterization of the muscle involvement in dynamin 2-related centronuclear myopathy. Brain J Neurol. 2006;129(Pt 6):1463–9.
14. Rudnik-Schoneborn S, Lutzenrath S, Borkowska J, Karwanska A, Hausmanowa-Petrusewicz I, Zerres K. Analysis of creatine kinase activity in 504 patients with proximal spinal muscular atrophy types I-III from the point of view of progression and severity. Eur Neurol. 1998;39(3):154–62.

15. Tawil R, Kissel JT, Heatwole C, Pandya S, Gronseth G, Benatar M, D. Guideline Development, N. Implementation Subcommittee of the American Academy of, N. Practice Issues Review Panel of the American Association of, M. Electrodiagnostic. Evidence-based guideline summary: evaluation, diagnosis, and management of facioscapulohumeral muscular dystrophy: report of the guideline development, dissemination, and implementation subcommittee of the american academy of neurology and the practice issues review panel of the american association of neuromuscular & electrodiagnostic medicine. Neurology. 2015;85(4):357–64.
16. Falzarano MS, Scotton C, Passarelli C, Ferlini A. Duchenne muscular dystrophy: from diagnosis to therapy. Molecules. 2015;20(10):18168–84.
17. Bird TD. Myotonic dystrophy type 1. In: Pagon RA, Adam MP, Ardinger HH, Wallace SE, Amemiya A, Bean LJH, Bird TD, Fong CT, Mefford HC, Smith RJH, Stephens K, editors. Synonym: Steinert's Disease. Seattle (WA): GeneReviews(R); 2015.
18. Ghosh PS, Sorenson EJ. Diagnostic yield of electromyography in children with myopathic disorders. Pediatr Neurol. 2014;51(2):215–9.
19. David WS, Jones HR Jr. Electromyography and biopsy correlation with suggested protocol for evaluation of the floppy infant. Muscle Nerve. 1994;17(4):424–30.
20. Rabie M, Jossiphov J, Nevo Y. Electromyography (EMG) accuracy compared to muscle biopsy in childhood. J Child Neurol. 2007;22(7):803–8.
21. Symmons DP, Sills JA, Davis SM. The incidence of juvenile dermatomyositis: results from a nation-wide study. Br J Rheumatol. 1995;34(8):732–6.
22. Verbeek S, Vanakker O, Mercelis R, Lipka AF, Haerynck F, Dullaers M, Verloo P, Van Coster R, Verhelst H. Lambert-Eaton myasthenic syndrome in a 13-year-old girl with Xp11.22-p11.23 duplication. Eur J Paediatr Neurol. 2014;18(3):439–43.
23. Hoffman WH, Helman SW, Sekul E, Carroll JE, Vega RA. Lambert-Eaton Myasthenic syndrome in a child with an autoimmune phenotype. Am J Med Genet A. 2003;119A(1):77–80.
24. Tsao CY, Mendell JR, Friemer ML, Kissel JT. Lambert-Eaton myasthenic syndrome in children. J Child Neurol. 2002;17(1):74–6.
25. Morgan-Followell B, de Los Reyes E. Child neurology: diagnosis of Lambert-Eaton myasthenic syndrome in children. Neurology. 2013;80(21):e220–2.
26. A.Q.A.C.A.A.o.E. Medicine. Practice parameter for repetitive nerve stimulation and single fiber EMG evaluation of adults with suspected myasthenia gravis or Lambert-Eaton myasthenic syndrome: summary statement. Muscle Nerve. 2001;24(9):1236–8.
27. Chiou-Tan FY, Gilchrist JM. Repetitive nerve stimulation and single-fiber electromyography in the evaluation of patients with suspected myasthenia gravis or Lambert-Eaton myasthenic syndrome: review of recent literature. Muscle Nerve. 2015;52(3):455–62.
28. Konersman CG, Bordini BJ, Scharer G, Lawlor MW, Zangwill S, Southern JF, Amos L, Geddes GC, Kliegman R, Collins MP. BAG3 myofibrillar myopathy presenting with cardiomyopathy. Neuromuscul Disord. 2015;25(5):418–22.
29. Di Muzio A, De Angelis MV, Di Fulvio P, Ratti A, Pizzuti A, Stuppia L, Gambi D, Uncini A. Dysmyelinating sensory-motor neuropathy in merosin-deficient congenital muscular dystrophy. Muscle Nerve. 2003;27(4):500–6.
30. Pitt MC. Nerve conduction studies and needle EMG in very small children. Eur J Paediatr Neurol. 2012;16(3):285–91.
31. Benedetti S, Bertini E, Iannaccone S, Angelini C, Trisciani M, Toniolo D, Sferrazza B, Carrera P, Comi G, Ferrari M, Quattrini A, Previtali SC. Dominant LMNA mutations can cause combined muscular dystrophy and peripheral neuropathy. J Neurol Neurosurg Psychiatry. 2005;76(7):1019–21.
32. Mancuso M, Orsucci D, Angelini C, Bertini E, Carelli V, Comi GP, Federico A, Minetti C, Moggio M, Mongini T, Tonin P, Toscano A, Bruno C, Ienco EC, Filosto M, Lamperti C, Diodato D, Moroni I, Musumeci O, Pegoraro E, Spinazzi M, Ahmed N, Sciacco M, Vercelli L, Ardissone A, Zeviani M, Siciliano G. "Mitochondrial neuropathies": a survey from the large cohort of the Italian Network. Neuromuscul Disord. 2016;26(4–5):272–6.

33. Shah DU, Darras BT, Markowitz JA, Jones HR Jr, Kang PB. The spectrum of myotonic and myopathic disorders in a pediatric electromyography laboratory over 12 years. Pediatr Neurol. 2012;47(2):97–100.
34. Kimura J. Electrodiagnosis in diseases of nerve and muscle: principles and practice. 3rd ed. New York: Oxford University Press; 2001.
35. Batthish M, Feldman BM. Juvenile dermatomyositis. Curr Rheumatol Rep. 2011;13(3):216–24.
36. Furst DE, Amato AA, Iorga SR, Gajria K, Fernandes AW. Epidemiology of adult idiopathic inflammatory myopathies in a U.S. managed care plan. Muscle Nerve. 2012;45(5):676–83.
37. Compeyrot-Lacassagne S, Feldman BM. Inflammatory myopathies in children. Pediatr Clin N Am. 2005;52(2):493–520. vi-vii
38. Bohan A, Peter JB. Polymyositis and dermatomyositis (second of two parts). N Engl J Med. 1975;292(8):403–7.
39. Bohan A, Peter JB, Bowman RL, Pearson CM. Computer-assisted analysis of 153 patients with polymyositis and dermatomyositis. Medicine. 1977;56(4):255–86.
40. Brown VE, Pilkington CA, Feldman BM, Davidson JE, P.R.E.S. Network for Juvenile Dermatomyositis. An international consensus survey of the diagnostic criteria for juvenile dermatomyositis (JDM). Rheumatology. 2006;45(8):990–3.
41. Barsotti S, Zampa V, Talarico R, Minichilli F, Ortori S, Iacopetti V, D'Ascanio A, Tavoni AG, Bombardieri S, Mosca M, Neri R. Thigh magnetic resonance imaging for the evaluation of disease activity in patients with idiopathic inflammatory myopathies followed in a single center. Muscle Nerve. 2016;54(4):666–72.
42. Buchthal F. Electrophysiological abnormalities in metabolic myopathies and neuropathies. Acta Neurol Scand. 1970;46(Suppl 43):129+.
43. Karpati G. Disorders of Voluntary Muscle. Cambridge: Cambridge University Press; 2010.
44. Papa R, Madia F, Bartolomeo D, Trucco F, Pedemonte M, Traverso M, Broda P, Bruno C, Zara F, Minetti C, Fiorillo C. Genetic and Early Clinical Manifestations of Females Heterozygous for Duchenne/Becker Muscular Dystrophy. Pediatr Neurol. 2016;55:58–63.
45. Bushby K, Finkel R, Birnkrant DJ, Case LE, Clemens PR, Cripe L, Kaul A, Kinnett K, McDonald C, Pandya S, Poysky J, Shapiro F, Tomezsko J, Constantin C, D.M.D.C.C.W. Group. Diagnosis and management of Duchenne muscular dystrophy, part 1: diagnosis, and pharmacological and psychosocial management. Lancet Neurol. 2010;9(1):77–93.
46. Gonorazky H, Liang M, Cummings B, Lek M, Micallef J, Hawkins C, Basran R, Cohn R, Wilson MD, MacArthur D, Marshall CR, Ray PN, Dowling JJ. RNAseq analysis for the diagnosis of muscular dystrophy. Ann Clin Transl Neurol. 2016;3(1):55–60.
47. Mah JK. Current and emerging treatment strategies for Duchenne muscular dystrophy. Neuropsychiatr Dis Treat. 2016;12:1795–807.
48. Voit T, Topaloglu H, Straub V, Muntoni F, Deconinck N, Campion G, De Kimpe SJ, Eagle M, Guglieri M, Hood S, Liefaard L, Lourbakos A, Morgan A, Nakielny J, Quarcoo N, Ricotti V, Rolfe K, Servais L, Wardell C, Wilson R, Wright P, Kraus JE. Safety and efficacy of drisapersen for the treatment of Duchenne muscular dystrophy (DEMAND II): an exploratory, randomised, placebo-controlled phase 2 study. Lancet Neurol. 2014;13(10):987–96.
49. Haas M, Vlcek V, Balabanov P, Salmonson T, Bakchine S, Markey G, Weise M, Schlosser-Weber G, Brohmann H, Yerro CP, Mendizabal MR, Stoyanova-Beninska V, Hillege HL. European Medicines Agency review of ataluren for the treatment of ambulant patients aged 5 years and older with Duchenne muscular dystrophy resulting from a nonsense mutation in the dystrophin gene. Neuromuscul Disord. 2015;25(1):5–13.
50. Mendell JR, Goemans N, Lowes LP, Alfano LN, Berry K, Shao J, Kaye EM, Mercuri E, Eteplirsen Study G, D.M.D.I.N. Telethon Foundation. Longitudinal effect of eteplirsen versus historical control on ambulation in Duchenne muscular dystrophy. Ann Neurol. 2016;79(2):257–71.

51. Kishnani PS, Beckemeyer AA, Mendelsohn NJ. The new era of Pompe disease: advances in the detection, understanding of the phenotypic spectrum, pathophysiology, and management. Am J Med Genet C: Semin Med Genet. 2012;160C(1):1–7.
52. American Association of Neuromuscular & Electrodiagnostic Medicine. Diagnostic criteria for late-onset (childhood and adult) Pompe disease. Muscle Nerve. 2009;40(1):149–60.
53. van der Beek NA, de Vries JM, Hagemans ML, Hop WC, Kroos MA, Wokke JH, de Visser M, van Engelen BG, Kuks JB, van der Kooi AJ, Notermans NC, Faber KG, Verschuuren JJ, Reuser AJ, van der Ploeg AT, van Doorn PA. Clinical features and predictors for disease natural progression in adults with Pompe disease: a nationwide prospective observational study. Orphanet J Rare Dis. 2012;7:88.
54. Werneck LC, Lorenzoni PJ, Kay CSK, Scola RH. Muscle biopsy in Pompe disease. Arq Neuropsiquiatr. 2013;71(5):284–9.
55. Winkel LP, Hagemans ML, van Doorn PA, Loonen MC, Hop WJ, Reuser AJ, van der Ploeg AT. The natural course of non-classic Pompe's disease; a review of 225 published cases. J Neurol. 2005;252(8):875–84.
56. Hobson-Webb LD, Dearmey S, Kishnani PS. The clinical and electrodiagnostic characteristics of Pompe disease with post-enzyme replacement therapy findings. Clin Neurophysiol. 2011;122(11):2312–7.
57. Schoser B, Stewart A, Kanters S, Hamed A, Jansen J, Chan K, Karamouzian M, Toscano A. Survival and long-term outcomes in late-onset Pompe disease following alglucosidase alfa treatment: a systematic review and meta-analysis. J Neurol. 2017;264(4):621–30.
58. Floriach-Robert M, Cabello A, Simon De Las Heras R, Mateos Beato F. Neonatal hypotonia of muscular origin: analysis of 50 cases. Neurologia. 2001;16(6):245–53.
59. Graziano A, Bianco F, D'Amico A, Moroni I, Messina S, Bruno C, Pegoraro E, Mora M, Astrea G, Magri F, Comi GP, Berardinelli A, Moggio M, Morandi L, Pini A, Petillo R, Tasca G, Monforte M, Minetti C, Mongini T, Ricci E, Gorni K, Battini R, Villanova M, Politano L, Gualandi F, Ferlini A, Muntoni F, Santorelli FM, Bertini E, Pane M, Mercuri E. Prevalence of congenital muscular dystrophy in Italy: a population study. Neurology. 2015;84(9):904–11.
60. Falsaperla R, Pratico AD, Ruggieri M, Parano E, Rizzo R, Corsello G, Vitaliti G, Pavone P. Congenital muscular dystrophy: from muscle to brain. Ital J Pediatr. 2016;42(1):78.
61. Bonnemann CG. The collagen VI-related myopathies Ullrich congenital muscular dystrophy and Bethlem myopathy. Handb Clin Neurol. 2011;101:81–96.
62. Shorer Z, Philpot J, Muntoni F, Sewry C, Dubowitz V. Demyelinating peripheral neuropathy in merosin-deficient congenital muscular dystrophy. J Child Neurol. 1995;10(6):472–5.
63. Quijano-Roy S, Renault F, Romero N, Guicheney P, Fardeau M, Estournet B. EMG and nerve conduction studies in children with congenital muscular dystrophy. Muscle Nerve. 2004;29(2):292–9.
64. Swaiman KF. Swaiman's pediatric neurology principles and practice. Edinburgh: Elsevier Saunders; 2006.
65. Wallgren-Pettersson C, Sainio K, Salmi T. Electromyography in congenital nemaline myopathy. Muscle Nerve. 1989;12(7):587–93.
66. Lacomis D. Electrodiagnostic approach to the patient with suspected myopathy. Neurol Clin. 2012;30(2):641–60.
67. Dowling JJ, Joubert R, Low SE, Durban AN, Messaddeq N, Li X, Dulin-Smith AN, Snyder AD, Marshall ML, Marshall JT, Beggs AH, Buj-Bello A, Pierson CR. Myotubular myopathy and the neuromuscular junction: a novel therapeutic approach from mouse models. Dis Model Mech. 2012;5(6):852–9.
68. Gibbs EM, Clarke NF, Rose K, Oates EC, Webster R, Feldman EL, Dowling JJ. Neuromuscular junction abnormalities in DNM2-related centronuclear myopathy. J Mol Med. 2013;91(6):727–37.
69. Rodriguez Cruz PM, Sewry C, Beeson D, Jayawant S, Squier W, McWilliam R, Palace J. Congenital myopathies with secondary neuromuscular transmission defects; a case report and review of the literature. Neuromuscul Disord. 2014;24(12):1103–10.

70. Munot P, Lashley D, Jungbluth H, Feng L, Pitt M, Robb SA, Palace J, Jayawant S, Kennet R, Beeson D, Cullup T, Abbs S, Laing N, Sewry C, Muntoni F. Congenital fibre type disproportion associated with mutations in the tropomyosin 3 (TPM3) gene mimicking congenital myasthenia. Neuromuscul Disord. 2010;20(12):796–800.
71. Illingworth MA, Main M, Pitt M, Feng L, Sewry CA, Gunny R, Vorstman E, Beeson D, Manzur A, Muntoni F, Robb SA. RYR1-related congenital myopathy with fatigable weakness, responding to pyridostigimine. Neuromuscul Disord. 2014;24(8):707–12.
72. Natera-de Benito D, Nascimento A, Abicht A, Ortez C, Jou C, Muller JS, Evangelista T, Topf A, Thompson R, Jimenez-Mallebrera C, Colomer J, Lochmuller H. KLHL40-related nemaline myopathy with a sustained, positive response to treatment with acetylcholinesterase inhibitors. J Neurol. 2016;263(3):517–23.
73. Preston DC, Shapiro BE. Electromyography and neuromuscular disorders. Boston: Butterworth-Heinemann; 1998. p. 541–59.
74. Kimura J. Electrodiagnosis in diseases of muscle and nerve. Philadelphia: F.A. Davis; 1989. p. 252–4.
75. Fu YH, Pizzuti A, Fenwick RG Jr, King J, Rajnarayan S, Dunne PW, Dubel J, Nasser GA, Ashizawa T, de Jong P, et al. An unstable triplet repeat in a gene related to myotonic muscular dystrophy. Science. 1992;255(5049):1256–8.
76. Mahadevan M, Tsilfidis C, Sabourin L, Shutler G, Amemiya C, Jansen G, Neville C, Narang M, Barcelo J, O'Hoy K, et al. Myotonic dystrophy mutation: an unstable CTG repeat in the 3′ untranslated region of the gene. Science. 1992;255(5049):1253–5.
77. Brook JD, McCurrach ME, Harley HG, Buckler AJ, Church D, Aburatani H, Hunter K, Stanton VP, Thirion JP, Hudson T, et al. Molecular basis of myotonic dystrophy: expansion of a trinucleotide (CTG) repeat at the 3′ end of a transcript encoding a protein kinase family member. Cell. 1992;69(2):385.
78. Harper PS. Myotonic Dystrophy. Philadelphia: Saunders; 2001.
79. Gadalla SM, Lund M, Pfeiffer RM, Gortz S, Mueller CM, Moxley RT 3rd, Kristinsson SY, Bjorkholm M, Shebl FM, Hilbert JE, Landgren O, Wohlfahrt J, Melbye M, Greene MH. Cancer risk among patients with myotonic muscular dystrophy. JAMA. 2011;306(22):2480–6.
80. Logigian EL, Martens WB, Moxley RT 4th, McDermott MP, Dilek N, Wiegner AW, Pearson AT, Barbieri CA, Annis CL, Thornton CA, Moxley RT 3rd. Mexiletine is an effective antimyotonia treatment in myotonic dystrophy type 1. Neurology. 2010;74(18):1441–8.
81. Bachinski LL, Udd B, Meola G, Sansone V, Bassez G, Eymard B, Thornton CA, Moxley RT, Harper PS, Rogers MT, Jurkat-Rott K, Lehmann-Horn F, Wieser T, Gamez J, Navarro C, Bottani A, Kohler A, Shriver MD, Sallinen R, Wessman M, Zhang S, Wright FA, Krahe R. Confirmation of the type 2 myotonic dystrophy (CCTG)n expansion mutation in patients with proximal myotonic myopathy/proximal myotonic dystrophy of different European origins: a single shared haplotype indicates an ancestral founder effect. Am J Hum Genet. 2003;73(4):835–48.
82. Liquori CL, Ricker K, Moseley ML, Jacobsen JF, Kress W, Naylor SL, Day JW, Ranum LP. Myotonic dystrophy type 2 caused by a CCTG expansion in intron 1 of ZNF9. Science. 2001;293(5531):864–7.
83. Ranum LP, Rasmussen PF, Benzow KA, Koob MD, Day JW. Genetic mapping of a second myotonic dystrophy locus. Nat Genet. 1998;19(2):196–8.
84. Day JW, Ricker K, Jacobsen JF, Rasmussen LJ, Dick KA, Kress W, Schneider C, Koch MC, Beilman GJ, Harrison AR, Dalton JC, Ranum LP. Myotonic dystrophy type 2: molecular, diagnostic and clinical spectrum. Neurology. 2003;60(4):657–64.
85. Moxley RT 3rd, Meola G, Udd B, Ricker K. Report of the 84th ENMC workshop: PROMM (proximal myotonic myopathy) and other myotonic dystrophy-like syndromes: 2nd workshop. 13–15th October, 2000, Loosdrecht, The Netherlands. Neuromuscul Disord. 2002;12(3):306–17.
86. Ricker K, Koch MC, Lehmann-Horn F, Pongratz D, Speich N, Reiners K, Schneider C, Moxley RT 3rd. Proximal myotonic myopathy. Clinical features of a multisystem disorder similar to myotonic dystrophy. Arch Neurol. 1995;52(1):25–31.

87. Meola G, Moxley RT 3rd. Myotonic dystrophy type 2 and related myotonic disorders. J Neurol. 2004;251(10):1173–82.
88. Shapiro BE, Ruff R. Disorders of skeletal muscle membrane excitablity myotonia congenita, paramyotonia congenita, periodic paralysis, and related disorders. In: Katirji B, Kaminski H, Preston DC, Ruff R, Shapiro BE, editors. Neuromuscular disorders in clinical practice. Boston: Butterworth-Heinemann; 2002. p. 987–1020.
89. Becker P, Knussmann R, Kuhn E. Myotonia congenita and syndromes associated with myotonia, Topics of Human Genetics, vol. Vol. III. Stuttgart: Thieme; 1977. p. 1–178.
90. Gutmann L, Phillips LH 2nd. Myotonia congenita. Semin Neurol. 1991;11(3):244–8.
91. Stum M, Davoine CS, Vicart S, Guillot-Noel L, Topaloglu H, Carod-Artal FJ, Kayserili H, Hentati F, Merlini L, Urtizberea JA, Hammouda el H, Quan PC, Fontaine B, Nicole S. Spectrum of HSPG2 (Perlecan) mutations in patients with Schwartz-Jampel syndrome. Hum Mutat. 2006;27(11):1082–91.
92. Nicole S, Topaloglu H, Fontaine B. 102nd ENMC International Workshop on Schwartz-Jampel syndrome, 14–16 December, 2001, Naarden, The Netherlands. Neuromuscul Disord. 2003;13(4):347–51.
93. Nicole S, Davoine CS, Topaloglu H, Cattolico L, Barral D, Beighton P, Hamida CB, Hammouda H, Cruaud C, White PS, Samson D, Urtizberea JA, Lehmann-Horn F, Weissenbach J, Hentati F, Fontaine B. Perlecan, the major proteoglycan of basement membranes, is altered in patients with Schwartz-Jampel syndrome (chondrodystrophic myotonia). Nat Genet. 2000;26(4):480–3.
94. Ptacek LJ, Trimmer JS, Agnew WS, Roberts JW, Petajan JH, Leppert M. Paramyotonia congenita and hyperkalemic periodic paralysis map to the same sodium-channel gene locus. Am J Hum Genet. 1991;49(4):851–4.
95. Ptacek LJ, Gouw L, Kwiecinski H, McManis P, Mendell JR, Barohn RJ, George AL Jr, Barchi RL, Robertson M, Leppert MF. Sodium channel mutations in paramyotonia congenita and hyperkalemic periodic paralysis. Ann Neurol. 1993;33(3):300–7.
96. McClatchey AI, Trofatter J, McKenna-Yasek D, Raskind W, Bird T, Pericak-Vance M, Gilchrist J, Arahata K, Radosavljevic D, Worthen HG, et al. Dinucleotide repeat polymorphisms at the SCN4A locus suggest allelic heterogeneity of hyperkalemic periodic paralysis and paramyotonia congenita. Am J Hum Genet. 1992;50(5):896–901.
97. Brooke M. Disorders of skeletal muscle. In: Bradley WG, Daroff RB, Fenichel GM, Marsden CD, editors. Neurology in clinical practice. Boston: Butterworth-Heinemann; 2000. p. 2187–235.
98. Moxley RT III. Channelopathies. Curr Treat Options Neurol. 2000;2:31–47.
99. Amato A, Dumitru D. Hereditary myopathies. In: Dumitru D, Amato A, Zwarts M, editors. Electrodiagnostic Medicine. Philadelphia: Hanley and Belfus; 2002. p. 1265–370.
100. Fournier E, Viala K, Gervais H, Sternberg D, Arzel-Hezode M, Laforet P, Eymard B, Tabti N, Willer JC, Vial C, Fontaine B. Cold extends electromyography distinction between ion channel mutations causing myotonia. Ann Neurol. 2006;60(3):356–65.
101. Weckbecker K, Wurz A, Mohammadi B, Mansuroglu T, George AL Jr, Lerche H, Dengler R, Lehmann-Horn F, Mitrovic N. Different effects of mexiletine on two mutant sodium channels causing paramyotonia congenita and hyperkalemic periodic paralysis. Neuromuscul Disord. 2000;10(1):31–9.
102. Trudell RG, Kaiser KK, Griggs RC. Acetazolamide-responsive myotonia congenita. Neurology. 1987;37(3):488–91.
103. Buchthal F, Engbaek L, Gamstorp I. Paresis and hyperexcitability in adynamia episodica hereditaria. Neurology. 1958;8(5):347–51.
104. McManis PG, Lambert EH, Daube JR. The exercise test in periodic paralysis. Muscle Nerve. 1986;9(8):704–10.
105. Heatwole CR, Moxley RT. Channelopathies: myotonic disorders and periodic paralysis. In: Swaiman KF, editor. Pediatric neurology: principles and practice. Philadelphia: Elsevier Saunders; 2012. p. 1667–89.

106. Sansone V, Links TP, Meola G, Rose MR. Treatment for periodic paralysis. Cochrane Database Syst Rev. 2006;2
107. Sansone V, Meola G, Links TP, Panzeri M, Rose MR. Treatment for periodic paralysis. Cochrane Database Syst Rev. 2008;1:CD005045.
108. Milone M, McEvoy KM, Sorenson EJ, Daube JR. Myotonia associated with caveolin-3 mutation. Muscle Nerve. 2012;45(6):897–900.
109. Heatwole CR, Moxley RT. The non-dysmorphic myotonias. Neurotherapeutics. 2007;4:238–51.
110. Logigian EL, Ciafaloni E, Quinn LC, Dilek N, Pandya S, Moxley RT 3rd, Thornton CA. Severity, type, and distribution of myotonic discharges are different in type 1 and type 2 myotonic dystrophy. Muscle Nerve. 2007;35(4):479–85.
111. Heatwole CR, Statland JM, Logigian EL. The diagnosis and treatment of myotonic disorders. Muscle Nerve. 2013;47(5):632–48.
112. Sander HW, Scelsa SN, Conigliari MF, Chokroverty S. The short exercise test is normal in proximal myotonic myopathy. Clin Neurophysiol. 2000;111(2):362–6.
113. Nielsen VK, Friis ML, Johnsen T. Electromyographic distinction between paramyotonia congenita and myotonia congenita: effect of cold. Neurology. 1982;32(8):827–32.
114. Ricker K, Hertel G, Langscheid K, Stodieck G. Myotonia not aggravated by cooling. Force and relaxation of the adductor pollicis in normal subjects and in myotonia as compared to paramyotonia. J Neurol. 1977;216(1):9–20.
115. Kwiecinski H, Ryniewicz B, Ostrzycki A. Treatment of myotonia with antiarrhythmic drugs. Acta Neurol Scand. 1992;86(4):371–5.
116. Jurkat-Rott K, Lehmann-Horn F. Human muscle voltage-gated ion channels and hereditary disease. Curr Opin Pharmacol. 2001;1(3):280–7.
117. Lehmann-Horn F, Jurkat-Rott K. Voltage-gated ion channels and hereditary disease. Physiol Rev. 1999;79(4):1317–72.
118. Barohn RJ, Wang Y, Herbelin L, Bundy BN, Trivedi JR, Hanna MG, Rayan DR. Phase II therapeutic trial of mexiletine in non-dysmorphic myotonia. Neurology. 2011:A645.
119. Statland JM, Bundy BN, Wang Y, Rayan DR, Trivedi JR, Sansone VA, Salajegheh MK, Venance SL, Ciafaloni E, Matthews E, Meola G, Herbelin L, Griggs RC, Barohn RJ, Hanna MG, C. Consortium for Clinical Investigation of Neurologic. Mexiletine for symptoms and signs of myotonia in nondystrophic myotonia: a randomized controlled trial. JAMA. 2012;308(13):1357–65.
120. Pouget J, Serratrice G. Myotonia with muscular weakness corrected by exercise. The therapeutic effect of mexiletine. Rev Neurol. 1983;139(11):665–72.
121. Leheup B, Himon F, Morali A, Brichet F, Vidailhet M. Value of mexiletine in the treatment of Thomsen-Becker myotonia. Arch Fr Pediatr. 1986;43(1):49–50.
122. Lion-Francois L, Mignot C, Vicart S, Manel V, Sternberg D, Landrieu P, Lesca G, Broussolle E, Billette de Villemeur T, Napuri S, Portes V d, Fontaine B. Severe neonatal episodic laryngospasm due to de novo SCN4A mutations: a new treatable disorder. Neurology. 2010;75(7):641–5.
123. Campbell RW. Mexiletine. N Engl J Med. 1987;316(1):29–34.
124. Feinberg L, Travis WD, Ferrans V, Sato N, Bernton HF. Pulmonary fibrosis associated with tocainide: report of a case with literature review. Am Rev Respir Dis. 1990;141(2): 505–8.
125. Aoike F, Takahashi MP, Sakoda S. Class Ic antiarrhythmics block human skeletal muscle Na channel during myotonia-like stimulation. Eur J Pharmacol. 2006;532(1–2):24–31.
126. Finkel MJ. Phenytoin revisited. Clin Ther. 1984;6(5):577–91.
127. Lyons MJ, Duron R, Molinero I, Sangiuolo F, Holden KR. Novel CLCN1 mutation in carbamazepine-responsive myotonia congenita. Pediatr Neurol. 2010;42(5):365–8.
128. Gascon GG, Staton RD, Patterson BD, Konewko PJ, Wilson H, Carlson KM, Brumback RA. A pilot controlled study of the use of imipramine to reduce myotonia. Am J Phys Med Rehabil. 1989;68(5):215–20.

129. Antonini G, Vichi R, Leardi MG, Pennisi E, Monza GC, Millefiorini M. Effect of clomipramine on myotonia: a placebo-controlled, double-blind, crossover trial. Neurology. 1990;40(9):1473–4.
130. Milner-Brown HS, Miller RG. Myotonic dystrophy: quantification of muscle weakness and myotonia and the effect of amitriptyline and exercise. Arch Phys Med Rehabil. 1990;71(12):983–7.
131. Cleland JC, Griggs RC. Treatment of neuromuscular channelopathies: current concepts and future prospects, Neurotherapeutics: the journal of the American Society for Experimental. Neurotherapeutics. 2008;5(4):607–12.
132. Eguchi H, Tsujino A, Kaibara M, Hayashi H, Shirabe S, Taniyama K, Eguchi K. Acetazolamide acts directly on the human skeletal muscle chloride channel. Muscle Nerve. 2006;34(3):292–7.
133. Griggs RC, Moxley RT 3rd, Riggs JE, Engel WK. Effects of acetazolamide on myotonia. Ann Neurol. 1978;3(6):531–7.
134. Ohtaki E, Komori H, Yamaguchi Y, Matsuishi T. Successful dantrolene sodium treatment of a patient with myotonia congenita (Thomsen's disease). Acta Paediatr Jpn. 1991;33(5):668–71.
135. Grant R, Sutton DL, Behan PO, Ballantyne JP. Nifedipine in the treatment of myotonia in myotonic dystrophy. J Neurol Neurosurg Psychiatry. 1987;50(2):199–206.

Chapter 23
Neuromuscular Complications in the Critically Ill Child

Hugh J. McMillan and Jahannaz Dastgir

Neurophysiologists may be asked to evaluate a child in the pediatric intensive care unit (PICU) with muscle weakness, hypotonia, or inability to recover from an underlying disease at the expected rate. Some children may be difficult to wean from mechanical ventilation or fail multiple attempts at extubation.

Children in the intensive care unit can be very difficult to exam electrophysiologically due to the frequent use of sedative or paralytic medications as well as the placement of intravenous lines and endotracheal intubation. Children may demonstrate difficulty cooperating with aspects of the physical examination due to an associated encephalopathy or due to anxiety, discomfort and/or side effects of medication. Neurophysiological testing can be particularly helpful in cases where a lower motor neuron disorder is suspected. It can provide important localizing information, thereby narrowing the list of potential diagnoses and justifying appropriate genetic testing, magnetic resonance imaging and/or biopsy to be pursued as indicated [1]. Moreover, electromyography (EMG) can typically be obtained quickly at most pediatric tertiary care hospitals, which can be important for some acquired conditions such as infantile botulism where early treatment is preferred.

H.J. McMillan, MD, MSc, FRCPC, FAAN
Division of Neurology, Children's Hospital of Eastern Ontario, University of Ottawa, Ottawa, ON, Canada

J. Dastgir, DO (✉)
Atlantic Health System, Goryeb Children's Hospital, Morristown, NJ, USA
e-mail: jz.dastgir@gmail.com; jahannaz.dastgir@atlantichealth.org

© Springer International Publishing AG 2017

H.J. McMillan, P.B. Kang (eds.), *Pediatric Electromyography*,
DOI 10.1007/978-3-319-61361-1_23

Weakness in Children Admitted to the PICU

Children admitted to the pediatric intensive care unit (PICU) can demonstrate clinical weakness for a variety of reasons. Symptoms could be attributable to the acute presentation of a neuromuscular disorder such as Guillain-Barré syndrome or botulism, or an exacerbation of a chronic neuromuscular disease where clinical decompensation has been triggered by an intercurrent illness. Medications can adversely affect the function of muscles, nerves, and the neuromuscular junction, particularly in children with an underlying neuromuscular disease. Acquired diseases such as critical illness polyneuropathy (CIP) or critical illness myopathy (CIM) can also develop during hospitalization. Lastly, central nervous system disease can also produce weakness which is often but not always associated with a decreased level of consciousness, seizures and/or problems with higher order function such as language. This latter category is beyond the scope of this chapter which will focus upon neuromuscular complications in the critically ill child.

This chapter will provide a brief summary of the common and/or treatable causes of neuromuscular disease in the critically ill child; review critical illness polyneuropathy and myopathy and discuss the complications of medications in children with neuromuscular disease in the critical care setting.

Clinical Symptoms of Neuromuscular Disease in Early Childhood

Weakness that begins *in utero* can result in arthrogryposis multiplex congenita, defined as the presence of two or more congenital joint contractures. Fetal limb movements are necessary to avoid contracture formation, thus reduced mobility due to neuromuscular weakness as well as brain lesions or uterine/environmental factors can give rise to contractures. Polyhydramnios can be an indicator of impaired fetal swallowing due to bulbar weakness.

Infants may present with clinically evident weakness immediately after birth or within the first few months of life after an apparent period of normalcy. Symptoms can include feeding difficulty with ensuing failure to thrive, failure to attain expected gross motor milestones including development of head control or bringing hands to the mouth as well as symptoms of respiratory distress or respiratory failure such as that seen with a "brief resolved unexplained event (BRUE)", previously known as an "acute life threating event" (ALTE) [2].

Older children and adolescents may also be evaluated in the PICU with key diseases covered below.

Anterior Horn Cell

Children with disorders affecting the anterior horn cell or motor neurons will present with progressive muscle weakness due to the loss of motor neurons. The presence or absence of contractures as well as the involvement of other cranial nerves can provide important diagnostic clues. Electrodiagnostic test results will classically reveal robust sensory nerve action potential (SNAP) amplitudes with variable reductions in compound motor action potential (CMAP) amplitudes. Electromyography will also show classic neurogenic changes with reduced numbers of high amplitude rapidly firing motor units visible.

Spinal muscular atrophy (SMA) type I is a common cause of infantile hypotonia [3], occurring in about 1 in 11,000 individuals [4]. It is common for infants with SMA type I to show symptoms of gross motor delay and hypotonia in the first few months of life. The clinical phenotype is quite characteristic and early recognition of this disease is imperative in light of a new disease-modifying therapy [5]. Joint contractures are uncommon in SMA type I. Respiratory symptoms are common with infants demonstrating a characteristic 'bell-shaped' chest and paradoxical abdominal breathing. Most pediatric centers will have ready access to genetic testing for SMA. Nevertheless, EMG can also provide supportive evidence given the pattern of abnormalities that indicate anterior horn cell or motor neuron involvement (Table 23.1). SMA type I has been reported to mimic critical illness neuropathy, illustrating the importance of complete neurophysiological testing whenever possible [6].

Other diagnostic considerations in this age group could include riboflavin transporter deficiency or Brown-Vialetto-Van Laere syndrome or Fazio Londe Syndrome. Although children typically present in the toddler-years, onset is well documented in the first few months of life [7]. SMA with respiratory distress (SMARD) can also show phenotypic overlap with SMA, although less severe phenotypes without respiratory involvement have been increasingly reported in the literature. Congenital amyoplasia is another example of an early-onset disease affecting motor neurons [8]. Given that this disease is highly discordant among monozygotic twins [9, 10] it is generally thought to be an acquired disruption of fetal blood vessels and subsequent motor neuron development. Limb contractures are symmetric and typically involve all four limbs [11]. Shoulders are adducted and internally rotated, with elbows extended and wrists flexed, a characteristic arm position that bears some clinical resemblance to the arm position in Erb palsy except that in amyoplasia this arm position is maintained by joint contractures [12]. Needle EMG in affected children has identified symmetric, segmental anterior horn cell disease with an apparent predilection for the upper cervical myotomes (C5–6). Unlike other anterior horn cell disorders causing arthrogryposis, amyoplasia is associated with a relatively good long term outcome. Children demonstrate normal language development and normal or above-average intelligence [11]. With proper physiotherapy and orthopedic interventions approximately 60–80% of children will eventually acquire independent ambulation [11, 13]. Associated non-neurologic features include mid-facial capillary hemangioma, micrognathia, and genital, bowel and spine anomalies [9].

Older children and adolescents can also become critically unwell with motor neuronopathies. Acquired conditions are an important consideration, particularly in children who have travelled and/or have been previously well. Wildtype poliovirus infection has been largely eradicated but does remain endemic in three countries: Nigeria, Afghanistan and Pakistan with documented transmission to neighboring nations [14]. Given the ease of international air travel, polio must remain a diagnostic consideration, particularly in regions where vaccination rates may be suboptimal. Patients with acute poliovirus infection are typically asymptomatic or exhibit mild fever and gastrointestinal symptoms. Very few patients (<1%) develop central nervous system involvement (aseptic meningitis and/or paralytic disease). Other "polio-like" viruses share a similar affinity for anterior horn cell and brainstem motor nuclei. Presentations resembling that of poliomyelitis have been reported for enteroviruses [15], echoviruses [16], herpes simplex virus 1 [17], West Nile virus [18], Epstein–Barr virus [19] and human immunodeficiency virus [20]. Anterior horn cell disorders are covered in detail in Chap. 16.

Peripheral Nerve

Children with peripheral nerve disorders will most commonly demonstrate clinical signs of both sensory and motor involvement. Electrodiagnostic testing may reveal either demyelinating changes (prolonged latencies, slowed conduction velocities, temporal dispersion and conduction block) or axonal loss (low or absent SNAP and CMAP amplitudes). The documentation of sensory involvement is important to differentiate diseases of peripheral nerve from other lower motor neuron lesions. Since young children and critically ill patients may have difficulty cooperating with sensory testing, electrodiagnostic testing is particularly important in this regard.

Neonatal polyneuropathies are relatively rare, comprising only about 5% of all cases of neonatal hypotonia [21]. Many genes showing both dominant and recessive inheritance patterns have been linked to congenital or early-onset Charcot-Marie-Tooth (CMT) disease [22]. As such, many of the congenital hypomyelinating neuropathies that had previously been classified as CMT type 3 or Dejerine-Sottas disease are now known to be caused by some of the same genes that cause CMT type 1 (autosomal dominant, demyelinating), CMT type 2 (autosomal dominant axonal form) and type 4 (autosomal recessive). Nerve conduction studies can be particularly helpful at directing the choice of genetic testing since neuropathy genes are not consistently included on genetic test panels for suspected primary muscle disease. Mitochondrial and other metabolic diseases can also present with infant-onset polyneuropathies. Acquired disorders can cause peripheral nerve dysfunction at birth. Guillain-Barré syndrome also known as acute inflammatory demyelinating polyneuropathy has been diagnosed at birth due to the passive transfer of maternal auto-antibodies [23–25]. However, these inflammatory disorders are much more common in older children and adults. Among adult ICU patients with EMG confirmation of neuromuscular disorders, 13% were diagnosed with acute or chronic inflammatory demyelinating polyradiculoneuropathy [26]. While EMG is an important diagnostic criterion for GBS, abnormalities may take time to become apparent on neurophysiological testing [27]. Adult patients with clinical symptoms of GBS who undergo neurophysiological testing 1 week after symptom-onset will show: prolonged or absent H-reflexes (100% patients) and F-responses (84%), prolonged motor distal latencies (61%), temporal dispersion (58%) and conduction velocity slowing (52%) [27]. Prolonged F-wave latencies are also one of the earliest abnormalities detected in children with GBS [28]. As such, obtaining late responses should be considered in all patients with suspected GBS. One cautionary note for the critically ill patient is the observation that anesthetic agents do have the potential to attenuate or abort late responses [29, 30]. As such that this is a reminder that neurophysiological finding should not be interpreted in isolation.

Many patients will require admission to ICU since respiratory failure occurs in 16–17% of affected children [28, 31] compared to 25–30% of affected adults [32]. Autonomic symptoms, including variability in heart rate, blood pressure and thermoregulation can also be seen in 20–40% of affected children and in rare situations can be the cause of death [33]. Peripheral neuropathies are covered in detail in Chap. 18.

Neuromuscular Junction

Transient neonatal myasthenia gravis can be seen in approximately 10% of infants born to mothers with autoimmune myasthenia gravis [34]. Infants will typically demonstrate sucking, swallowing and respiratory difficulties within the first 24 hours of life. Management is typically supportive as most infants will fully recover within weeks. Rarely, infants can present with more severe clinical symptoms including congenital contractures [35, 36]. Repetitive nerve stimulation (RNS), discussed in Chap. 6, can be particularly helpful at diagnosing this acquired condition (Table 23.1).

Infantile botulism does not present at birth, but has been diagnosed in infants as young as a few days old [37, 38]. More commonly, infants will present between 1–6 months old. This age group is particularly vulnerable since the immature gut lacks the protective bacterial flora and bile acids which inhibit *Clostridum* growth [39]. Infants will typically present with constipation followed by progressive feeding difficulty (due to bulbar weakness), ophthalmoplegia including sluggish pupillary responses, descending paralysis, and apnea. RNS is also helpful at diagnosing this condition particularly higher frequency (20–50 Hz) RNS which can demonstrate an incremental CMAP due to the presynaptic nature of this problem. Early diagnosis is important since treatment with human botulism immune globulin can hasten recovery and reduce the overall duration of hospitalization [40].

Table 23.1 Neuromuscular conditions in the critical ill infant (<4 months old)

	Clinical				Electrodiagnostic		
	Facial bulbar weak	Respiratory distress	Other	Contractures	NCS	Rep stim/ SFEMG	EMG
Anterior horn cell							
Spinal muscular atrophy	Common	Possible	Bell shaped chest	Uncommon	Low CMAP	Normal	Neurogenic
Riboflavin transporter deficiency	Common (later)	Late finding	SNH loss early sign	No	May be normal	Normal	Neurogenic
SMARD	Common	Typical		No	May be normal	Normal	Neurogenic
Amyoplasia congenita	No	No	Facial hemangioma	Yes	Low CMAP	Normal	Neurogenic
Peripheral nerve							
Charcot-Marie-Tooth	No	No	Areflexic	Possible	Low SNAP CMAP	N/a	Neurogenic
Guillain-Barré syndrome	Possible	Possible	Areflexic	Uncommon	Low SNAP CMAP	N/a	Normal or neurogenic
Neuromuscular junction							
Congenital myasthenia	Common	May have apneas	Ptosis	Possible	May be normal	Abnormal	Normal
Transient myasthenia gravis	Common	May have apneas	Ptosis	Uncommon	May be normal	Abnormal	Normal
Infantile botulism	Typical	Typical	Constipation, ptosis	No	Low CMAP possible	Abnormal	Normal

	Clinical				Electrodiagnostic		
	Facial bulbar weak	Respiratory distress	Other	Contractures	NCS	Rep stim/ SFEMG	EMG
Muscle							
Congenital myopathies	Common	Possible	CK normal	Possible	Normal	Normal	Myopathic
Congenital muscular dystrophies							
Dystroglycanopathy	Common	Possible	CK elevated, brain, eye findings	Possible	Normal	Normal	Myopathic
Infantile FSH	Typical	Uncommon	CK normal or elevated	Possible	Normal	Normal	Myopathic
Congenital myotonic dystrophy	Common	Possible	CK normal	Possible	Normal	Normal	Myopathic
Mitochondrial disease	Possible	Possible	Lactate, alanine high	Possible	Normal	Normal	Myopathic
Peroxisomal disease	Possible	Uncommon	Possible seizures, renal or hepatic cysts	Uncommon	Normal	Normal	Myopathic
Pompe disease	Common	Possible	Cardiomegaly, CK elevated	Uncommon	Normal	Normal	Myopathic

Congenital myasthenic syndrome typically presents at or shortly after birth, though there are rare reports of patients presenting in adolescence [41, 42]. Typical clinical features include onset at birth or early childhood and fatigable weakness particularly affecting oculobulbar musculature. Classic electrophysiologic findings include abnormal decrement on RNS and/or increased jitter on stimulated single fiber EMG testing (SFEMG) [43]; the latter is covered in Chap. 10. Some infants with congenital myasthenic syndrome due to choline acetyltransferase (*CHAT*) mutations can present with sudden episodes of apnea that can be triggered by infection [44]. Care must be taken to differentiate congenital myasthenic syndrome from autoimmune myasthenia gravis in young children so as to avoid the inappropriate use of immunosuppressant therapies and the withholding of medications such as 3,4 di-aminopyridine, salbutamol and/or fluoxetine that may show benefit in some cases [45]. Gene panels are becoming more widely available for patients who demonstrate clinical and electrophysiological evidence for CMS.

Autoimmune juvenile myasthenia gravis (JMG) can also present with fatigable ptosis, ophthalmoplegia, dysarthria, dysphagia and generalized skeletal muscle weakness. Unlike CMS, this condition is due to an acquired autoimmune cause. RNS and/or SFEMG are important for helping establishing a diagnosis. Whereas antibodies to the nicotinic AChR are found in 80% of adults with myasthenia gravis [46], only 50% of prepubertal and 70% of peripubertal JMG patients have anti-AChR antibodies [47], most likely due to the more frequent occurrence of ocular myasthenia in prepubertal children and generalized myasthenia in peripubertal adolescents. Anti-MuSK antibodies also do not appear to be as common in JMG [48]. Intravenous immunoglobulin (IVIG) or plasma exchange (PLEX) can be used in the acute management of myasthenia gravis. Caution must be taken when initiating corticosteroid therapy in weak patients who are not yet intubated since increased weakness may occur within the first 1–2 weeks of corticosteroid treatment, potentially precipitating a myasthenic crisis [49]. Disorders of neuromuscular transmission are covered in detail in Chap. 21.

Muscle

Primary disorders of muscle are a more common cause of neonatal hypotonia. One series reported that myopathies comprised 20% of all causes of neonatal hypotonia as well as 75% of causes of 'peripheral' hypotonia [21]. Muscle disorders can include the following groups of disorders which can be grouped into the following large categories: congenital myopathies, congenital muscular dystrophies, congenital myotonic disorders, and metabolic myopathies. Electrophysiological testing will reveal normal sensory responses as well as normal or reduced CMAP amplitudes and EMG evidence of myopathic units. Muscle disorders are covered in detail in Chap. 22.

Critical Illness Polyneuropathy and Myopathy

Critical illness polyneuropathy (CIP) and critical illness myopathy (CIM) are neuromuscular disorders that develop during the course of a critical illness. This is one of the key features that allow patients with CIP to be differentiated from patients presenting with an acute motor sensory axonal neuropathy (AMSAN), namely the axonal variant of Guillain-Barré syndrome [50]. In CIP, patients do not show a preceding history of sensory or motor deficits. Moreover, they must have an associated critical illness that seems to trigger the underlying neuromuscular disease [51] with onset of weakness in the 1–2 weeks following the critical illness [52].

Critical illness polyneuropathy (CIP) and CIM can be difficult to differentiate on clinical and electrophysiological testing [26]. However there are some distinguishing features (Table 23.2). Since CIP and CIM can co-exist in the same patient, some authors have grouped them together as critical illness polyneuromyopathy (CIPNM) or critical illness myopathy and neuropathy (CRIMYNE) [53].

In adults, CIP and CIM are the most common neuromuscular conditions that develop during an ICU admission and diagnostic criteria have been created to permit them to be distinguished from other diseases as well as, whenever possible,

Table 23.2 Key features differentiating critical illness myopathy and critical illness polyneuropathy

	Critical illness myopathy	Critical illness polyneuropathy
Clinical	Triggered by critical illness	Triggered by critical illness
	Limb weakness	Limb weakness (distal)
	Onset after PICU admission	Onset 1–2 weeks after PICU admission
Serum CK	Normal or elevated	Normal
NCS	Decreased CMAP amplitudes	Decreased CMAP amplitudes
	Preserved SNAP amplitudes	Decreased SNAP amplitudes
EMG	Myogenic changes (low amplitude motor units with or without fibrillation potentials)	Neurogenic changes (large amplitude motor units with abundant fibrillation potentials)
	Decreased excitability on direct stimulation	
Muscle biopsy Histology	Loss of ATPase reaction in type I fibers	Acute & chronic denervation changes (i.e. angular fibers, fiber-type grouping)
	Type II fiber atrophy common	
	Necrotizing myopathy with vacuolization	
	Destruction of thick myosin filaments	
Ultrastructure	Selective loss of thick (myosin) filaments	
	Disorganization of myofibrils	
Nerve biopsy		Fiber loss and primary axonal degeneration

CK creatine kinase, *CMAP* compound motor action potential, *SNAP* sensory nerve action potential

from each other [51]. One center reviewed all patients admitted to ICU over 15 years who had neuromuscular disease confirmed by neurophysiological testing. Of this group, 13% patients had CIP and 41% had CIM [26]. The incidence of CIP/CIM in children is less clear. A prospective study of all children (3 months to 17 years old) admitted to the PICU of a pediatric tertiary care hospital identified generalized muscle weakness in 1.7% (14/830) patients [54]. Children with pre-existing neuromuscular diseases and Guillain-Barré syndrome were excluded from this cohort. Of the remaining children showing weakness who underwent electrophysiological testing, about half (4 out of 7) showed low CMAP amplitudes and most (4 out of 5) had myopathic units evident upon EMG analysis. When one considers the difference in study design of the adult [26] and pediatric [54] studies (including versus excluding patients GBS) the overall incidence of CIPM appears similar in the two groups, accounting for about half of all patients with confirmed neuromuscular disease in this setting.

Many adult and pediatric patients who develop CIPM have undergone a solid organ or bone marrow transplant, suffered a traumatic injury (e.g., head injury, burns) and/or have had one or more episodes of bacterial sepsis [26, 54]. The use of corticosteroids and neuromuscular blocking agents is also common. Although the precise mechanism of CIPM is not known, it is believed to result from a systemic inflammatory response syndrome (SIRS) provoked by a severe systemic infection or trauma [51]. Patients exhibit profound changes in cellular and humoral immune responses altering the microcirculation throughout the body. At the microscopic level, mitochondrial dysfunction occurs with the loss of normal ATPase staining in type 1 fibers of a muscle biopsy [51, 54]. Endothelial damage may result in the disruption of the vasa nervorum with resulting ischemia of axons. In muscles this can cause disruption of the function and structure of the basic contractile unit and, in more severe cases, areas of necrosis and vacuolar changes [51]. This evidence of microstructural damage and mitochondrial dysfunction seen on biopsy is congruent with the high rate of long-term morbidity seen in adult patients who have suffered CIM [55, 56]. Prospective studies of adult ICU patients indicate that CIPM occurs in about 50-70% of patients suffering from systemic inflammatory response syndrome [57, 58]. As such, milder cases of CIPM may even be more prevalent than that reported by Lacomis [26] and Banwell [54]. Phrenic nerve conduction studies and needle EMG of the diaphragm and chest wall muscles have been recommended in adult patients with suspected CIPM [51]; however, these particular studies are not commonly performed in pediatric EMG.

Drugs Exacerbating Underlying Neuromuscular Diseases

Medications or toxins can exacerbate underlying disorders of nerve, muscle and neuromuscular transmission.

Chemotherapy Induced Peripheral Neuropathy

Chemotherapeutic agents such as vincristine have been reported to cause significant toxicity in patients with Charcot-Marie-Tooth disease.

Most individuals will not report symptoms of a vincristine-induced sensorimotor neuropathy until after a minimum cumulative dose of vincristine 5–8 mg has been administered [59]. However patients with Charcot-Marie-Tooth disease will show marked sensitivity to this chemotherapeutic agent with dramatic sensory symptoms or even a Guillain-Barré-like phenotype apparent after a cumulative dose of only 2 mg [59, 60]. On rare occasions CMT has presented in previously asymptomatic patients after receiving vincristine to treat lymphoma [61, 62]. Reports exist of adults with no prior neurological symptoms progressing to quadriplegia and bulbar palsy after vincristine therapy [62]. As such, hereditary neuropathies must be considered among individuals showing extreme sensitivity to this drug.

The chronic use of other medications that pose a potential risk for exacerbating CMT including metronidazole, nitrous oxide, HMG co-reductase inhibitors ('statins'), nitrofurantoin and phenytoin [59].

Neuromuscular Blockade

Neuromuscular blocking agents bind to acetylcholine receptors post-synaptically, thereby inhibiting the action of the neurotransmitter acetylcholine. This blocks neuromuscular transmission, resulting in paralysis of the muscle. These medications are aimed at preventing movement in an intubated patient to avoid self-extubation and/or self-injury. Since they do not possess any sedative or amnestic properties, they are routinely used with other medications.

Children with underlying renal or hepatic dysfunction may take longer to clear these medications during which time they may appear clinically weak and show electrophysiological evidence of reduced or absent CMAP amplitudes.

Patients with disorders of neuromuscular transmission such as myasthenia gravis have a reduction in the total number of acetylcholine receptors. As such, they show increased sensitivity to non-depolarizing neuromuscular blockers [63]. For surgeries requiring muscle relaxation, it if often necessary to adjust the dosing of these medications in such patients [64].

Malignant Hyperthermia

Malignant hyperthermia (MH) is a pharmacogenetic syndrome of skeletal muscle associated with a hypermetabolic response to volatile anesthetic gas (e.g., halothane, sevoflurane) and the depolarizing muscle relaxant succinylcholine. Rarely, MH can also be triggered by heat or vigorous exercise.

An episode of MH is characterized by muscle rigidity, rhabdomyolysis, hyperthermia, tachycardia, hyperpnea, metabolic acidosis and hyperkalemia. Uncontrolled MH can lead to severe hyperthermia and rhabdomyolysis. Progressive muscle breakdown results in hyperkalemia and myoglobinuria which can cause acute renal failure and life-threatening electrolyte abnormalities and cardiac arrhythmia.

Most patients with MH susceptibility show no evidence of muscle dysfunction prior to their exposure to anesthetic. There is a smaller subset of MH susceptible patients who show clinical signs of a congenital myopathy associated with mutations in *RYR1* or *CACNA1S*. Most patients with King-Denborough syndrome, central core disease and/or multiminicore disease show MH susceptibility. As such, it is paramount that neuromuscular clinicians and anesthesiologists be aware of this risk and follow MH precautions for any child with suspected congenital myopathy that includes avoidance of potential anesthetic triggers. MH is a medical emergency that necessitates immediate action to prevent progressive tissue destruction and risk of death. When MH is suspected, inhaled anesthetics must be stopped and succinylcholine must not be re-administered. Dantrolene, the only known antidote, should be administered and active cooling initiated. Careful monitoring of blood electrolytes, gas and creatinine kinase as well as monitoring urine output and cardiac rhythm is required. Critical care monitoring is required for at least 24 hours due to risk of morbidity [65].

Muscular dystrophies including Duchenne muscular dystrophy (DMD) and Becker muscular dystrophy (BMD) have been associated with an MH-like reaction triggered by volatile anesthetic agents with or without succinylcholine. Patients exhibited hyperthermia, hyperkalemia and hyperCKemia (>40,000 U/L) that responded to dantrolene [66, 67]. Genetic testing for *RYR1*, *CACNA1S* and *STAC3* were negative in each case [66]. Some patients with DMD have also tested positive to the caffeine-halothane contracture test [68]. Although this may not fall within the strict definition of malignant hyperthermia, MH precautions should nevertheless be applied to all patients with muscular dystrophies and other inherited myopathies.

Technical Considerations in the Pediatric Intensive Care Unit

Neurophysiologists are commonly faced with several challenges in the ICU that can include limited access to typical stimulation and recording sites due to the need for intravenous access, peripheral edema, and difficulty maintaining limb temperatures in the desired range. This can result in artifacts, which are discussed in detail in Chap. 11. In order to minimize the influence of 60 Hz interference from other electrical sources it is important to disconnect as many electronic devices as possible, in consultation with the primary team and nursing staff. In the sedated patient it can be difficult to recruit motor units, which can make distinguishing a myopathic from neuropathic process more difficult. It is important to document at what time boluses of paralytic medications were given since the neuromuscular blockade can artificially depress CMAP amplitudes. Caution should be exercised when applying electrical stimulus near an intravascular line that could lie in close proximity to the heart.

References

1. Lisi EC, Cohn RD. Genetic evaluation of the pediatric patient with hypotonia: perspective from a hypotonia specialty clinic and review of the literature. Dev Med Child Neurol. 2011;53:586–99.
2. Byring RF, Pihko H, Tsujino A, Shen XM, Gustafsson B, Hackman P, et al. Congenital myasthenic syndrome associated with episodic apnea and sudden infant death. Neuromuscul Disord. 2002;12:548–53.
3. Darras BT, Jones HR Jr. Neuromuscular problems of the critically ill neonate and child. Semin Pediatr Neurol. 2004;11:147–68.
4. D'Amico A, Mercuri E, Tiziano FD, Bertini E. Spinal muscular atrophy. Orphanet J Rare Dis. 2011;6:71.
5. Finkel RS, Chiriboga CA, Vajsar J, Day JW, Montes J, De Vivo DC, et al. Treatment of infantile-onset spinal muscular atrophy with nusinersen: a phase 2, open-label, dose-escalation study. Lancet. 2016;388:3017–26.
6. Fernandez-Torre JL, Teja JL, Castellanos A, Figols J, Obeso T, Arteaga R. Spinal muscular atrophy type I mimicking critical illness neuropathy in a paediatric intensive care neonate: electrophysiological features. Brain Dev. 2008;30:599–602.
7. Jaeger B, Bosch AM. Clinical presentation and outcome of riboflavin transporter deficiency: mini review after five years of experience. J Inherit Metab Dis. 2016;39:559–64.
8. Gaitanis JN, McMillan HJ, Wu A, Darras BT. Electrophysiologic evidence for anterior horn cell disease in amyoplasia. Pediatr Neurol. 2010;43:142–7.
9. Hall JG, Reed SD, Driscoll EP. Part I. Amyoplasia: a common, sporadic condition with congenital contractures. Am J Med Genet. 1983;15:571–90.
10. Hall JG, Reed SD, McGillivray BC, Herrmann J, Partington MW, Schinzel A, et al. Part II. Amyoplasia: twinning in amyoplasia--a specific type of arthrogryposis with an apparent excess of discordantly affected identical twins. Am J Med Genet. 1983;15:591–9.
11. Sells JM, Jaffe KM, Hall JG. Amyoplasia, the most common type of arthrogryposis: the potential for good outcome. Pediatrics. 1996;97:225–31.
12. Sheldon W. Amyoplasia congenita: (multiple congenital articular rigidity: arthrogryposis multiplex congenita). Arch Dis Child. 1932;7:117–36.
13. Kroksmark AK, Kimber E, Jerre R, Beckung E, Tulinius M. Muscle involvement and motor function in amyoplasia. Am J Med Genet A. 2006;140:1757–67.
14. Nnadi C, Damisa E, Esapa L, Braka F, Waziri N, Siddique A, et al. Continued endemic wild poliovirus transmission in security-compromised areas-Nigeria. MMWR Morb Mortal Wkly Rep 2017. 2016;66:190–3.
15. Huang CC, Liu CC, Chang YC, Chen CY, Wang ST, Yeh TF. Neurologic complications in children with enterovirus 71 infection. N Engl J Med. 1999;341:936–42.
16. Kopel FB, Shore B, Hodes HL. Nonfatal bulbospinal paralysis due to ECHO 4 virus. J Pediatr. 1965;67:588–94.
17. Kyllerman MG, Herner S, Bergstrom TB, Ekholm SE. PCR diagnosis of primary herpesvirus type I in poliomyelitis-like paralysis and respiratory tract disease. Pediatr Neurol. 1993;9:227–9.
18. Heresi GP, Mancias P, Mazur LJ, Butler IJ, Murphy JR, Cleary TG. Poliomyelitis-like syndrome in a child with West Nile virus infection. Pediatr Infect Dis J. 2004;23:788–9.
19. Wong M, Connolly AM, Noetzel MJ. Poliomyelitis-like syndrome associated with Epstein-Barr virus infection. Pediatr Neurol. 1999;20:235–7.
20. Chitsike I, van FR. Paralytic poliomyelitis associated with live oral poliomyelitis vaccine in child with HIV infection in Zimbabwe: case report. BMJ. 1999;318:841–3.
21. Richer LP, Shevell MI, Miller SP. Diagnostic profile of neonatal hypotonia: an 11-year study. Pediatr Neurol. 2001;25:32–7.
22. Baets J, Deconinck T, De VE, Zimon M, Yperzeele L, Van HK, et al. Genetic spectrum of hereditary neuropathies with onset in the first year of life. Brain. 2011;134:2664–76.

23. al-Qudah AA, Shahar E, Logan WJ, Murphy EG. Neonatal Guillain-Barre syndrome. Pediatr Neurol. 1988;4:255–6.
24. Luijckx GJ, Vles J, de BM, Buchwald B, Troost J. Guillain-Barre syndrome in mother and newborn child. Lancet. 1997;349:27.
25. Buchwald B, de BM, Luijckx GJ, Toyka KV. Neonatal Guillain-Barre syndrome: blocking antibodies transmitted from mother to child. Neurology. 1999;53:1246–53.
26. Lacomis D, Petrella JT, Giuliani MJ. Causes of neuromuscular weakness in the intensive care unit: a study of ninety-two patients. Muscle Nerve. 1998;21:610–7.
27. Gordon PH, Wilbourn AJ. Early electrodiagnostic findings in Guillain-Barre syndrome. Arch Neurol. 2001;58:913–7.
28. Bradshaw DY, Jones HR Jr. Guillain-Barre syndrome in children: clinical course, electrodiagnosis, and prognosis. Muscle Nerve. 1992;15:500–6.
29. De Jong RH, Hershey WN, Wagman IH. Measurement of a spinal reflex response (H-reflex) during general anesthesia in man. Association between reflex depression and muscular relaxation. Anesthesiology. 1967;28:382–9.
30. Kerz T, Hennes HJ, Feve A, Decq P, Filipetti P, Duvaldestin P. Effects of propofol on H-reflex in humans. Anesthesiology. 2001;94:32–7.
31. Vajsar J, Fehlings D, Stephens D. Long-term outcome in children with Guillain-Barre syndrome. J Pediatr. 2003;142:305–9.
32. Hahn AF. The challenge of respiratory dysfunction in Guillain-Barre syndrome. Arch Neurol. 2001;58:871–2.
33. Jones HR Jr. Guillain-Barre syndrome: perspectives with infants and children. Semin Pediatr Neurol. 2000;7:91–102.
34. Jovandaric MZ, Despotovic DJ, Jesic MM, Jesic MD. Neonatal outcome in pregnancies with autoimmune Myasthenia Gravis. Fetal Pediatr Pathol. 2016;35:167–72.
35. Midelfart HJ, Midelfart A. Maternal myasthenia gravis: a cause for arthrogryposis multiplex congenita. J Child Orthop. 2015;9:433–5.
36. Behin A, Mayer M, Kassis-Makhoul B, Jugie M, Espil-Taris C, Ferrer X, et al. Severe neonatal myasthenia due to maternal anti-MuSK antibodies. Neuromuscul Disord. 2008;18:443–6.
37. Keet CA, Fox CK, Margeta M, Marco E, Shane AL, Dearmond SJ, et al. Infant botulism, type F, presenting at 54 hours of life. Pediatr Neurol. 2005;32:193–6.
38. Thilo EH, Townsend SF, Deacon J. Infant botulism at 1 week of age: report of two cases. Pediatrics. 1993;92:151–3.
39. Tseng-Ong L, Mitchell WG. Infant botulism: 20 years' experience at a single institution. J Child Neurol. 2007;22:1333–7.
40. Arnon SS, Schechter R, Maslanka SE, Jewell NP, Hatheway CL. Human botulism immune globulin for the treatment of infant botulism. N Engl J Med. 2006;354:462–71.
41. Chaouch A, Beeson D, Hantai D, Lochmuller H. 186th ENMC international workshop: congenital myasthenic syndromes 24-26 June 2011, Naarden, The Netherlands. Neuromuscul Disord. 2012;22:566–76.
42. Nogajski JH, Kiernan MC, Ouvrier RA, Andrews PI. Congenital myasthenic syndromes. J Clin Neurosci. 2009;16:1–11.
43. Engel AG, Shen XM, Selcen D, Sine SM. Congenital myasthenic syndromes: pathogenesis, diagnosis, and treatment. Lancet Neurol. 2015;14:420–34.
44. Ohno K, Tsujino A, Brengman JM, Harper CM, Bajzer Z, Udd B, et al. Choline acetyltransferase mutations cause myasthenic syndrome associated with episodic apnea in humans. Proc Natl Acad Sci U S A. 2001;98:2017–22.
45. Lorenzoni PJ, Scola RH, Kay CS, Werneck LC. Congenital myasthenic syndrome: a brief review. Pediatr Neurol. 2012;46:141–8.
46. Drachman DB. Myasthenia gravis. N Engl J Med. 1994;330:1797–810.
47. Andrews PI, Massey JM, Sanders DB. Acetylcholine receptor antibodies in juvenile myasthenia gravis. Neurology. 1993;43:977–82.
48. Chiang LM, Darras BT, Kang PB. Juvenile myasthenia gravis. Muscle Nerve. 2009;39:423–31.

49. Pascuzzi RM, Coslett HB, Johns TR. Long-term corticosteroid treatment of myasthenia gravis: report of 116 patients. Ann Neurol. 1984;15:291–8.
50. Bolton CF, Laverty DA, Brown JD, Witt NJ, Hahn AF, Sibbald WJ. Critically ill polyneuropathy: electrophysiological studies and differentiation from Guillain-Barre syndrome. J Neurol Neurosurg Psychiatry. 1986;49:563–73.
51. Bolton CF. Neuromuscular manifestations of critical illness. Muscle Nerve. 2005;32:140–63.
52. Tabarki B, Coffinieres A, Van Den Bergh P, Huault G, Landrieu P, Sebire G. Critical illness neuromuscular disease: clinical, electrophysiological, and prognostic aspects. Arch Dis Child. 2002;86:103–7.
53. Mohamed A, Ryan MM. Neuromuscular complications of intensive care. Handb Clin Neurol. 2013;113:1481–3.
54. Banwell BL, Mildner RJ, Hassall AC, Becker LE, Vajsar J, Shemie SD. Muscle weakness in critically ill children. Neurology. 2003;61:1779–82.
55. Guarneri B, Bertolini G, Latronico N. Long-term outcome in patients with critical illness myopathy or neuropathy: the Italian multicentre CRIMYNE study. J Neurol Neurosurg Psychiatry. 2008;79:838–41.
56. Latronico N, Shehu I, Seghelini E. Neuromuscular sequelae of critical illness. Curr Opin Crit Care. 2005;11:381–90.
57. Leijten FS, De Weerd AW, Poortvliet DC, De Ridder VA, Ulrich C, Harink-De Weerd JE. Critical illness polyneuropathy in multiple organ dysfunction syndrome and weaning from the ventilator. Intensive Care Med. 1996;22:856–61.
58. Witt NJ, Zochodne DW, Bolton CF, Grand'Maison F, Wells G, Young GB, et al. Peripheral nerve function in sepsis and multiple organ failure. Chest. 1991;99:176–84.
59. Weimer LH, Podwall D. Medication-induced exacerbation of neuropathy in Charcot Marie Tooth disease. J Neurol Sci. 2006;242:47–54.
60. Igarashi M, Thompson EI, Rivera GK. Vincristine neuropathy in type I and type II Charcot-Marie-Tooth disease (hereditary motor sensory neuropathy). Med Pediatr Oncol. 1995;25:113–6.
61. Geny C, Gaio JM, Mallaret M, Goy A, Reymond F, Pegourie B, et al. Charcot-Marie-Tooth disease disclosed by a treatment with vincristine in familial Hodgkin's disease. Ann Med Int (Paris). 1990;141:709–10.
62. Uno S, Katayama K, Dobashi N, Hirano A, Ogihara A, Yamazaki H, et al. Acute vincristine neurotoxicity in a non-Hodgkin's lymphoma patient with Charcot-Marie-Tooth disease. Rinsho Ketsueki. 1999;40:414–9.
63. Buzello W, Noeldge G, Krieg N, Brobmann GF. Vecuronium for muscle relaxation in patients with myasthenia gravis. Anesthesiology. 1986;64:507–9.
64. Itoh H, Shibata K. Comparison between sevoflurane and propofol neuromuscular effects in a patient with myasthenia gravis: effective doses of vecuronium. Anesthesiology. 2001;95:803–5.
65. Rosenberg H, Pollock N, Schiemann A, Bulger T, Stowell K. Malignant hyperthermia: a review. Orphanet J Rare Dis. 2015;10:93.
66. Bamaga AK, Riazi S, Amburgey K, Ong S, Halliday W, Diamandis P, et al. Neuromuscular conditions associated with malignant hyperthermia in paediatric patients: a 25-year retrospective study. Neuromuscul Disord. 2016;26:201–6.
67. Brownell AK, Paasuke RT, Elash A, Fowlow SB, Seagram CG, Diewold RJ, et al. Malignant hyperthermia in Duchenne muscular dystrophy. Anesthesiology. 1983;58:180–2.
68. Takagi A. Malignant hyperthermia of Duchenne muscular dystrophy: application of clinical grading scale and caffeine contracture of skinned muscle fibers. Rinsho Shinkeigaku. 2000;40:423–7.

Part VI
Appendices

Chapter 24
Normal Values Tables

Peter B. Kang

There is a long history and a significant corpus of published literature on normal values for nerve conduction studies in adults [1–3]. The earliest attempts to codify normal values for nerve conduction studies in the pediatric population date to the 1960s [4, 5]. Since then, a number of other studies have been published, as cited in Tables 24.1, 24.2, and 24.3.

Reference values for nerve conduction studies and needle electromyography in children have historically been difficult to determine in a true healthy cohort, as the discomfort of the test, albeit mild, introduces ethical issues that limit the ability to collect such data on a large scale in a prospective manner. However, data on ranges of normal values have been published, and those data have been collected, compared, and distilled to yield the following tables for sensory responses (Table 24.1), motor responses (Table 24.2) and F-responses (Table 24.3). Much of the data in the source literature are presented as means with standard deviations; in those cases, two standard deviations from the mean were used to determine the upper limit of normal in the case of latencies and lower limits of normal in the case of amplitude or conduction velocity. For focal neuropathies, consideration can also be given to comparing the response in the affected limb to that of the contralateral, unaffected side.

Children over the age of five years old have generally been found to have normal values in the adult range, thus these tables range from birth to 5 years, with standard adult values also listed to provide perspective. As a general rule of thumb for conduction velocities, a full term neonate has normal values about half those of an adult, and these gradually increase with age until 3–5 years, when adult values are reached. F response latencies do not mature until later, as they are heavily dependent upon a patient's height. When the data show normal values that may go beyond adult values, the adult values are presented.

P.B. Kang, M.D., F.A.A.N., F.A.A.P.
Division of Pediatric Neurology, Shands Children's Hospital, University of Florida College of Medicine, Gainesville, FL, USA
e-mail: pbkang@ufl.edu

© Springer International Publishing AG 2017

H.J. McMillan, P.B. Kang (eds.), *Pediatric Electromyography*,
DOI 10.1007/978-3-319-61361-1_24

Table 24.1 Suggested normal values for sensory nerve conduction studies

Age	Amplitude (μV)	Conduction velocity (m/s)
Median nerve		
Term newborn	≥3.5	≥22
0–1 month	≥3.5	≥24
1–3 months	≥5	≥25
3–6 months	≥5	≥32
6–12 months	≥5	≥33
1–2 years	≥9	≥41
2–4 years	≥13	≥45
4–6 years	≥14	≥48
Ulnar nerve		
34–36 weeks gestation	–	≥10
Term neonate	≥4	≥13
2–4 weeks	≥6	≥17
1–3 months	≥6	≥20
3–6 months	≥6	≥26
6–12 months	≥6	≥28
1–3 years	≥6	≥29
4–6 years	≥6	≥33
Sural nerve		
Term neonate	Any response	≥18
0–1 month	Any response	≥21
1–3 months	Any response	≥23
3–6 months	Any response	≥26
6–12 months	Any response	≥30
1–2 years	≥6	≥34
2–4 years	≥6	≥38
4–6 years	≥6	≥41
Medial plantar nerve		
Term neonate	≥10	–
1–6 months	≥15	≥35
6–12 months	≥15	≥40
1–2 years	≥15	≥40

Note: Data are derived from material in [6–13]. Nearly all the source articles used the orthodromic approach [6–13], but data from an antidromic study [8] was also determined to be valuable to include both due to the frequent use of that approach and also in light of the paucity of published data. Some values are marked "any response" due to large standard deviations in the source data. Of note, sural nerve responses are often difficult to elicit in infants

Table 24.2 Suggested normal values for motor nerve conduction studies

Age	Distal latency (ms)	Amplitude (mV)	Conduction velocity (m/s)
Median nerve			
23–29 weeks gestation		Any response	≥7
29–33 weeks gestation		Any response	≥16
33–38 weeks gestation	≤3.8	Any response	≥19
Term neonate (38–42)	≤3.5	≥2.5	≥20
2–4 weeks	≤3.0	≥2.5	≥23
1–6 months	≤3.0	≥3.5	≥30
6–12 months	≤3.0	≥2.3	≥35
12–18 months	≤3.0	≥3.7	≥40
18–24 months	≤3.0	≥3.7	≥45
2–3 years	≤3.1	≥2.0	≥47
3–4 years	≤3.1	≥2.0	≥48
4–5 years	≤3.2	≥3.0	≥49
Adult	≤4.5	≥4.1	≥49
Ulnar nerve			
34–37 week gestation	≤3.0	–	≥15
Term neonate	≤3.5	≥1.0	≥20
0–1 months	≤3.5	≥2.0	≥20
1–6 months	≤3.0	≥2.5	≥30
6–12 months	≤2.5	≥3.0	≥35
1–2 years	≤2.5	≥3.0	≥40
2–3 years	≤2.5	≥3.0	≥45
3–4 years	≤2.5	≥3.0	≥50
4–5 years	≤2.7	≥3.0	≥50
Adult	≤3.7	≥6.0	≥50
Peroneal (fibular) nerve			
Term neonate	≤4.5	≥0.5	≥20
0–1 months	≤4.5	≥0.5	≥20
1–6 months	≤3.2	≥0.5	≥27
6–12 months	≤3.2	≥0.7	≥36
1–2 years	≤3.2	≥0.7	≥38
2–3 years	≤4.1	≥0.9	≥39
3–4 years	≤4.1	≥1.0	≥40
4–6 years	≤4.1	≥1.3	≥40
Adult	≤6.5	≥2.0	≥40
Tibial nerve			
23–29 weeks	–	–	≥6
29–33 weeks	–	–	≥9
33–38 weeks	≤4.7	–	≥13
Term (38–42 weeks)	≤4.1	≥0.9	≥17
1–3 months	≤4.0	≥1.2	≥20

(continued)

Table 24.2 (continued)

Age	Distal latency (ms)	Amplitude (mV)	Conduction velocity (m/s)
3–6 months	≤3.5	≥1.2	≥25
6–9 months	≤3.5	≥3.4	≥30
9–12 months	≤3.5	≥3.4	≥32
1–3 years	≤4.0	≥4.8	≥33
3–6 years	≤4.7	≥4.8	≥40
Adult	≤6.1	≥4.4	≥40

Note: data are derived from material in [8–17]. Note that distal latencies tend to follow a "U-shaped" curve during infancy, most likely due to the competing influences of myelination and lengthening of distances between landmarks. Based on the published literature [9, 12, 13], mean median motor amplitudes rise steadily through childhood, but the standard variation peaks during the toddler years, leading to a dip in expected minimum amplitudes during that period. One can speculate that the excessive movement of the toddlers led to the higher standard deviations, but that is not certain. Adult values are adapted from [2]. Expected young adult values are often higher than the standard adult values listed above [2], but for simplicity adult values are not divided by age categories as the focus is on pediatric values in this table

Table 24.3 Suggested normal values for F-wave response minimum latencies

Age	Minimum latency (ms)
Median nerve	
0–1 months	≤22
1–6 months	≤20
6–12 months	≤20
1–2 years	≤20
2–4 years	≤20
4–6 years	≤22
6–14 years	≤28
Adult	≤33
Ulnar nerve	
0–1 months	≤22
1–6 months	≤19
6–12 months	≤18
1–2 years	≤18
2–4 years	≤19
4–6 years	≤22
Adult	≤33
Peroneal nerve	
0–1 months	≤35
1–6 months	≤28
6–12 months	≤29
1–2 years	≤30
2–4 years	≤34

Table 24.2 (continued)

Age	Minimum latency (ms)
4–6 years	≤36
6–14 years	≤43
Adult	≤57
Tibial nerve	
0–1 months	≤28
1–6 months	≤25
6–12 months	≤26
1–2 years	≤28
2–4 years	≤31
4–6 years	≤35
Adult	≤57

Note: data are derived from material in [9, 11–13]. Note that the F response latencies tend to follow a "U-shaped" curve during childhood due to the competing influences of myelination and lengthening of the extremities with age. Adult values are adapted from [18]

References

1. Benatar M, Wuu J, Peng L. Reference data for commonly used sensory and motor nerve conduction studies. Muscle Nerve. 2009;40:772–94.
2. Chen S, Andary M, Buschbacher R, Del Toro D, Smith B, So Y, Zimmermann K, Dillingham TR. Electrodiagnostic reference values for upper and lower limb nerve conduction studies in adult populations. Muscle Nerve. 2016;54:371–7.
3. Hodes R, Larrabee MG, German W. The human electromyogram in response to nerve stimulation and the conduction velocity of motor axons; studies on normal and on injured peripheral nerves. Arch Neurol Psychiatr. 1948;60:340–65.
4. Baer RD, Johnson EW. Motor nerve conduction velocities in normal children. Arch Phys Med Rehabil. 1965;46:698–704.
5. Gamstorp I. Normal Conduction Velocity of Ulnar, Median and Peroneal Nerves in Infancy, Childhood and Adolescence. Acta Paediatr. 1963;52(146):68–76.
6. Bye A, Fagan E. Nerve conduction studies of the sural nerve in childhood. J Child Neurol. 1988;3:94–9.
7. Martinez AC, Ferrer MT, Conde MC, Bernacer M. Motor conduction velocity and H-reflex in infancy and childhood. II. -Intra and extrauterine maturation of the nerve fibres. Development of the peripheral nerve from 1 month to 11 years of age. Electromyogr Clin Neurophysiol. 1978;18:11–27.
8. Sladky JT. Neuropathy in childhood. Semin Neurol. 1987;7:67–75.
9. Parano E, Uncini A, De Vivo DC, Lovelace RE. Electrophysiologic correlates of peripheral nervous system maturation in infancy and childhood. J Child Neurol. 1993;8:336–8.
10. Wagner AL, Buchthal F. Motor and sensory conduction in infancy and childhood: reappraisal. Dev Med Child Neurol. 1972;14:189–216.
11. Miller RG, Kuntz NL. Nerve conduction studies in infants and children. J Child Neurol. 1986;1:19–26.
12. Garcia A, Calleja J, Antolin FM, Berciano J. Peripheral motor and sensory nerve conduction studies in normal infants and children. Clin Neurophysiol. 2000;111:513–20.
13. Cai F, Zhang J. Study of nerve conduction and late responses in normal Chinese infants, children, and adults. J Child Neurol. 1997;12:13–8.

14. Dunn HG, Buckler J, Morrison GC, Emery AW. Conduction velocity of motor nerves in infants and children. Pediatrics. 1964;34:708–27.
15. Cruz Martinez A, Ferrer MT, Martin MJ. Motor conduction velocity and H-reflex in prematures with very short gestational age. Electromyogr Clin Neurophysiol. 1983;23:13–9.
16. Cruz Martinez A, Perez Conde MC, Ferrer MT. Motor conduction velocity and H-reflex in infancy and childhood: 1—study in newborns, twins and small-for-dates. Electromyogr Clin Neurophysiol. 1977;17:493–505.
17. Thomas JE, Lambert EH. Ulnar nerve conduction velocity and H-reflex in infants and children. J Appl Physiol. 1960;15:1–9.
18. Preston DC, Shapiro BE, editors. Electromyography and neuromuscular disorders: clinical-electrophysiologic correlations. London: Elsevier; 2013.

Chapter 25
Case Presentations

Hugh J. McMillan

Case 1

Clinical Summary

A 16-year-old, right-handed young man presented with left hand weakness. He was an accomplished musician who would spend long hours playing piano, cello and guitar. He first noted mild left hand weakness 12 months prior to presentation. His symptoms worsened and he stopped playing piano and cello about 6 months prior to presentation. He continued to play guitar, but noticed increased difficulty holding more complicated chords with his left hand. He could still fasten small buttons and tie his shoe laces. He has not experienced any sensory symptoms or neck pain. His right arm and both legs were asymptomatic. He was not taking any medications. His past medical history was unremarkable, with no prior trauma, no fever or other infectious symptoms, no bowel or bladder symptoms, and no dysphagia. Family history was unremarkable. He did well academically.

On physical examination, he was an alert and well-appearing young man. Height was 50th percentile and weight was 75th percentile. General medical examination was normal. Cranial nerve examination was unremarkable. Motor exam revealed moderate muscle wasting of his left hypothenar and thenar eminences as well as his left first dorsal interosseous (FDI). No fasciculations were noted. Muscle bulk was otherwise intact. Muscle strength testing revealed the following in his left upper extremity, using the Medical Research Council (MRC) scale: deltoids 5, supraspinatus 5, infraspinatus 5, biceps 5, triceps 5, pronator teres 5, supinator 5,

H.J. McMillan, MD, MSc, FRCPC, FAAN
Division of Neurology, Children's Hospital of Eastern Ontario, University of Ottawa, Ottawa, ON, Canada
e-mail: hmcmillan@cheo.on.ca

© Springer International Publishing AG 2017

H.J. McMillan, P.B. Kang (eds.), *Pediatric Electromyography*,
DOI 10.1007/978-3-319-61361-1_25

Table 25.1

Nerve conduction studies

	Normal	Right	Left		Normal	Right	Left
Sensory				Motor			
Median				Median (at wrist to APB)			
PL (ms)	<3.2	2.6	2.1	DML (ms)	<4.2	3.7	3.9
SNAP (mV)	>14.0	29.0	35.8	CMAP (mV)	>3.9	12.4	7.9
Ulnar				CV (m/s)	>50	56	55
PL (ms)	<3.3		2.0	Ulnar (at wrist to ADM)			
SNAP (mV)	>9.0		25.1	DML (ms)	<3.4	2.5	3.0
Dors Ulnar Cut				CMAP (mV)	>5.9	11.5	**5.4**
PL (ms)	<3.3		1.3	CV (m/s)	>50	61	59
SNAP (mV)	>4.0		16.1	Radial (proximal forearm to EIP)			
Radial				DML (ms)		4.4	4.3
PL (ms)	<2.9		2.2	CMAP (mV)		5.4	3.2
SNAP (mV)	>11.0		38.7	CV (m/s)		63	50
MAC							
PL (ms)	<3.3	1.3	1.7				
SNAP (mV)	>4.0	13.1	8.5				

Concentric needle EMG

Side	Muscle	Root	Insert	Fib	PSW	Amp	Dur	Poly	Recruit
Left	First dorsal interosseous	C8–T1	**Incr**	**2+**	Nml	**Incr**	**Incr**	Nml	**2- to 3-**
Left	Flexi carpi radialis	C6–C7	**Incr**	Nml	**1+**	**Incr**	**Incr**	**1+**	**1-**
Left	Flex pollicus longus	C7–C8	**Incr**	Nml	**3+**	**Incr**	Nml	Nml	**1-**
Left	Extensor digit comm	C7–C8	**Incr**	**1+**	**1+**	**Incr**	Nml	Nml	**2- to 3-**
Left	Biceps	C5–C6	Nml	Nml	Nml	Nml	Nml	Nml	Nml
Left	Triceps	C6–C8	Nml	Nml	Nml	**Incr**	**Incr**	**1+**	**1-**
Right	First dorsal interosseous	C8–T1	Nml	**1+**	Nml	**Incr**	**Incr**	Nml	**1-**
Right	Abductor pollicus brev	C8–T1	Nml	Nml	Nml	**Incr**	**Incr**	**1+**	**1-**
Right	Extensor digit comm.	C7–C8	Nml	Nml	Nml	**Incr**	**Incr**	**1+**	**1-**
Left	Vastus lateralis	L2–L4	Nml	Nml	Nml	Nml	Nml	Nml	Nml
Left	Tibialis anterior	L4–L5	Nml	Nml	Nml	Nml	Nml	Nml	Nml

Bold = abnormal. Abbreviations: *PL* peak onset latency, *SNAP* sensory nerve action potential, *DML* distal motor onset latency, *CMAP* compound motor action potential, *EDB* extensor digitorum brevis, *AH* abductor hallucis, *Fib* fibrillation potential, *PSW* positive sharp wave, *Amp* amplitude, *Dur* duration, *Poly* polyphasic, *Recruit* recruitment pattern

EDC 4-, EIP 4-, EPB 3, FPL 4+, APB 4, FDI 4-, ADM 4-, FDP (2nd digit) 4, FDP (5th digit) 4-. Right upper extremity strength was normal. Lower extremity strength testing was normal. Deep tendon reflexes were intact (2+) throughout. Plantar responses were flexor, bilaterally. Sensory testing (pin-prick, cold, vibration and propriocepton) was normal. A mild intention tremor was noted in his left upper extremity. Routine MRI of the cervical-spine and brachial plexus revealed no abnormalities.

Neurophysiological testing revealed the following (Table 25.1).

Nerve conduction studies provided electrophysiological evidence for a disorder affecting motor nerves, motor neurons or ventral roots at the C7/8/T1 level (left > right). Given the patient's age and clinical progression (over many months), Hirayama syndrome was considered. There was no prior illness to point to an infectious myelitis. There was no family history and no clinical evidence of upper motor neuron involvement to suggest juvenile amyotrophic lateral sclerosis.

One additional study was performed to confirm the diagnosis.

Hirayama disease is characterized by insidious onset of distal weakness and atrophy of hand muscles. Symptoms typically progress for several years before stabilizing. Onset is typically in the late teenage years or early 20's, similar to this patient. Findings are most often unilateral but can appear bilateral in a smaller proportion of patients. The mechanism of injury is thought to be focal trauma and ischemia of the anterior horn cells at the level(s) where the spinal cord is compressed against the vertebrae (Fig. 25.1c). Nerve conduction studies may show low ulnar and/or median CMAP amplitudes. Since this affects only motor neurons, sensory responses remain unaffected. Differential diagnosis includes: poliomyelitis, juvenile amyotrophic lateral sclerosis (ALS), spinal muscular atrophy (SMA) or spinal cord lesions (syrinx, tumor).

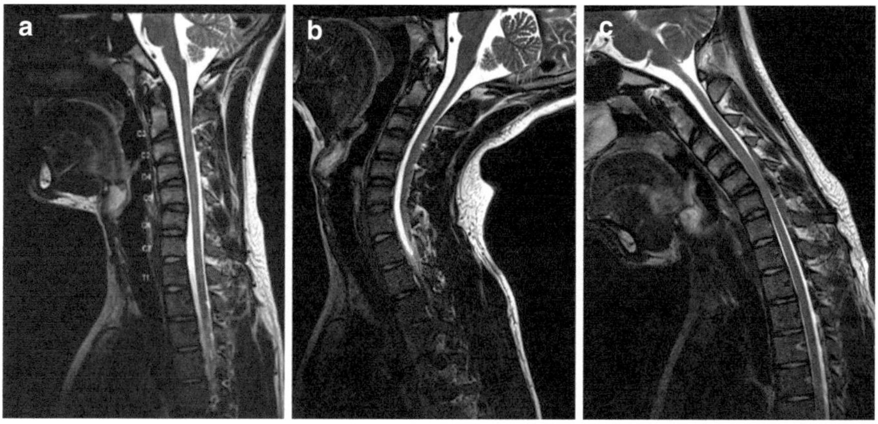

Fig. 25.1 MRI of the cervical spine, T2-weighted sagittal sequences (Fig 25.1) with flexion-extension views confirmed Hirayama disease. (**a**) revealed a mild loss of normal cervical spine lordosis. Extension view (**b**) revealed CSF anterior to the spinal cord. Upon neck flexion (**c**), MRI demonstrates loss of CSF spaces and compression of the cord at C5–6

Case 2

Clinical Summary

A 3 year old girl presented with a 4 week history of foot pain. The pain was initially thought to be intermittent and was particularly bothersome at bedtime. She became increasingly irritable. Her gait became abnormal 1–2 weeks prior to presentation, as she began to walk with both feet inverted which had been attributed to increasing foot pain. She also began falling more frequently. On the day of presentation and hospitalization, she refused to walk and appeared unable to bear weight on her legs. No bowel or bladder incontinence was noted. Her medical history was otherwise unremarkable. Birth history and neurodevelopmental history had been unremarkable.

Physical examination noted an alert but irritable girl. Height was 50th percentile and weight was 50th percentile. General medical examination was unremarkable. Cranial nerve examination was unremarkable. Muscle bulk was intact. Muscle strength testing revealed proximal and distal weakness of her upper and lower extremities. When placed in a standing position she could bear weight on her legs (with knees locked) but was unable to take any steps. She complained of back pain when standing. Deep tendon reflexes were reduced to absent in the upper and lower extremities. Plantar responses were flexor, bilaterally. Sensory testing showed decreased response to tickle and pin-prick. No sensory level was noted.

Serum CK was 48 U/L (normal <175 U/L).

Nerve conduction studies provided electrophysiological evidence for a sensorimotor polyneuropathy with demyelinating features (Table 25.2). The waveforms for the left median nerve and tibial nerve motor conduction studies revealed delayed distal onset latencies as well as temporal dispersion (Fig. 25.2). Late responses (F-responses, H-reflex) were not performed given low CMAP amplitudes observed. Left median and tibial motor CMAPs showed temporal dispersion (Fig. 25.2 above).

Additional testing included the following:

Lumbar puncture revealed CSF leukocytes 1/hpf (normal <5), CSF erythrocytes 0/hpf, CSF protein 1.07 g/L (normal 0.15–0.6 g/L) and CSF glucose 3.7 mmol/L (normal 2.0–4.4 mmol/L).

MRI of the spine revealed nerve root enhancement.

Given the clinical, electrophysiological and biochemical evidence she was diagnosed with Guillain-Barré syndrome (see Chap. 18). She was treated with intravenous immunoglobulin (IVIG) 1 g/kg for each of two consecutive days. She demonstrated signs of clinical recovery within days and was able to walk cautiously 7 days later. Her physical examination was entirely normal when re-examined 4 months later.

Table 25.2

Nerve conduction studies					
	Normal	Left		Normal	Left
Sensory			Motor		
Median			Median (at wrist to APB)		
SNAP (μV)	>13.0	**NR**	DML (ms)	<3.1	**22.8**
CV (m/s)	>45		CMAP (mV)	>3.9	**0.1**
Ulnar			CV (m/s)	>48	**14**
SNAP (μV)	>6.0	**NR**	Ulnar (at wrist to ADM)		
CV (m/s)	>29		DML (ms)	<2.5	**23.3**
Superficial peroneal			CMAP (mV)	>3.0	**0.3**
SNAP (μV)	>6.0	**NR**	CV (m/s)	>50	**27**
CV (m/s)	>38		Tibial (ankle to AH)		
Sural			DML (ms)	<4.7	**18.1**
SNAP (μV)	>6.0	**NR**	CMAP (mV)	>4.8	**0.2**
CV (m/s)	>38		CV (m/s)	>40	**26**

Concentric needle EMG

Side	Muscle	Root	Insert	Fib	PSW	Amp	Dur	Poly	Recruit
Left	Tibialis anterior	L4–L5	Nml	Nml	Nml	Nml	**1+**	**1+**	**1-**

Bold = abnormal. Abbreviations: *PL* peak onset latency, *SNAP* sensory nerve action potential, *DML* distal motor onset latency, *CMAP* compound motor action potential, *EDB* extensor digitorum brevis, *AH* abductor hallucis, *Fib* fibrillation potential, *PSW* positive sharp wave, *Amp* amplitude, *Dur* duration, *Poly* polyphasic, *Recruit* recruitment pattern

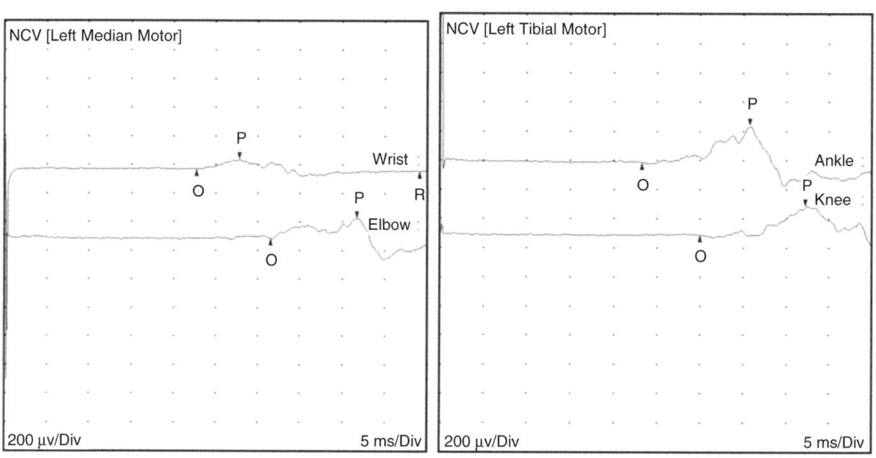

Fig. 25.2 The waveforms for the left median nerve and tibial nerve motor conduction studies (above) revealed evidence for delayed distal motor onset latency and temporal dispersion

Case 3

Clinical Summary

After undergoing cardiac surgery, a 10-year-old boy awoke complaining of numbness of the plantar and dorsal surfaces of his left foot. He also had weakness of his left lower extremity.
Physical exam of his left leg on post-operative day #1 noted: gluteus maximus 5, gluteus medius 5, hamstrings 5, tibialis anterior 1, peroneus longus 1, gastrocnemius 1, tibialis posterior 1, extensor halluces longus 1. Left patellar reflex 2+, left ankle reflex was absent. Sensation was reduced over the left tibial and peroneal distributions; however, sensation was intact over the left saphenous distribution. MRI brain was performed due to post-operative concern of potential ischemic brain injury. However, brain imaging was entirely normal.

He showed improvement in his symptoms during the 4 weeks between his cardiac surgery and his presentation for electrophysiological testing. He was now able to walk and bear weight on his left leg; however, he noted persistent weakness. He states that when he touches his left foot this sensation has improved. He notes markedly decreased sensation to the left plantar surface of the foot; however, he states that sensation over the left dorsal surface of the foot has improved.

On physical examination 1 month after the surgery, he was noted to be an alert and well-appearing boy. Height was 90%ile and weight 70%ile. Cranial nerves were intact. Muscle strength of his left leg was as follows (according to the Medical Research Council scale): gluteus maximus 5, gluteus medius 5, hip flexors 5, adductors 5, hamstrings 4, tibialis anterior 4+, tibialis posterior 4, peroneus longus 4+, gastrocnemius 3, EHL 4, toe flexors 4-. Mild atrophy was noted to his left EDB and left gastrocnemius. Strength testing of right leg was normal. Deep tendon reflexes were graded as 2+ at the patellae bilaterally, 2+ at the right ankle, and 0 at the left ankle. Sensation was decreased over the sole of the left foot in the tibial nerve distribution. However, sensation appeared intact over the saphenous and common peroneal distributions. He was able to walk with no discernable foot drop. He could not rise up on his heels on the left side. He also was unable to do a toe raise when standing on his left foot alone. Neurophysiological testing 1 month after surgery revealed the following (Table 25.3).

Neurophysiological testing, specifically the pattern of abnormality on needle EMG, provided evidence for a left sciatic neuropathy. Given his clinical improvement, a large proportion of the injury was attributed to neurapraxia; however, his mild persistent weakness and evidence of denervation in sciatic-innervated muscles also indicated some degree of axontnesis. The intact superficial

Table 25.3

Nerve conduction studies

	Normal	Left		Normal	Left
Sensory			Motor		
Median			Median (at wrist to APB)		
PL (ms)	<3.2		DML (ms)	<4.2	3.0
SNAP (μV)	>14.0		CMAP (mV)	>3.9	7.9
Ulnar			CV (m/s)	>50	58
PL (ms)	<3.3	2.3	Common peroneal (ankle to EDB)		
SNAP (μV)	>9.0	27.3	DML (ms)	<6.0	3.4
Superficial peroneal			CMAP (mV)	>2.4	6.3
PL (ms)	<3.8	2.4	CV (m/s)	>40	48
SNAP (μV)	>5.0	15.0	Tibial (ankle to AH)		
Sural			DML (ms)	<6.0	4.5
PL (ms)	<4.2	2.3	CMAP (mV)	>3.9	10.8
SNAP (μV)	>5.0	12.0	CV (m/s)	>40	44

Concentric needle EMG

Side	Muscle	Root	Insert	Fib	PSW	Amp	Dur	Poly	Recruit
Left	Medial gastrocnemius	S1–S2	**Incr**	**1+**	**2+**	Nml	**Incr**	**Incr**	**1-**
Left	Tibialis anterior	L4–L5	**Incr**	**1+**	**1+**	Nml	**Incr**	**Incr**	**1-**
Left	Biceps femoris (short)	L5–S1	**Incr**	**1+**	**1+**	Nml	**Incr**	**Incr**	**1-**
Left	Biceps femoris (long)	L5–S2	**Incr**	**1+**	**2+**	Nml	**Incr**	**Incr**	**1-**
Left	Gluteus medius	L4–S1	Nml	Nml	Nml	Nml	Nml	Nml	Nml
Left	Paraspinal muscle (L5)	L4–S1	Nml	Nml	Nml	Nml	Nml	Nml	Nml

Bold = abnormal. Abbreviations: *PL* peak onset latency, *SNAP* sensory nerve action potential, *DML* distal motor onset latency, *CMAP* compound motor action potential, *EDB* extensor digitorum brevis, *AH* abductor hallucis, *Fib* fibrillation potential, *PSW* positive sharp wave, *Amp* amplitude, *Dur* duration, *Poly* polyphasic, *Recruit* recruitment pattern

peroneal and sural SNAP amplitudes as well as the intact common peroneal nerve (EDB) and tibial (AH) CMAP amplitudes also suggest that axontmesis was a relatively minor component of the overall injury.

The lack of clinical or electrographic changes in the left gluteus medius (L5-root, superior gluteal nerve innervated muscles) or left paraspinal muscles (L5-root) were helpful for excluding the possibility of a left lumbosacral or nerve root injury.

Clinical re-examination 6 months post-operatively demonstrated full recovery.

Case 4

Clinical Summary

A 9-year-old boy was evaluated for coordination problems and frequent falling. His parent noted him to have 'always been clumsy'. However, over the past 1–2 years it has become more evident. Over the past few months he had fallen three times in the shower, bringing the curtain down with him when he fell. He has done well academically. He has had increasing problems keeping up with his peers in sports, particularly skating. He reports no paresthesiae or pain. No weakness was reported; he can run up a set of stairs or climb up one foot per step. His parents had noted subtle voice changes; he has been noted to speak more slowly and hesitantly. Past medical history was otherwise unremarkable. His neurodevelopment was appropriate. He was on no regular medication. Family history was unremarkable.

Physical examination noted a boy with height at 25th percentile and weight at 50th percentile. General medical exam was notable for slight pes cavus and early hammertoeing. Cranial nerve examination was notable only for mild dysarthria. Muscle strength testing was entirely normal. Complete areflexia was evident. Plantar responses were extensor, bilaterally. Heel contractures were noted; with his knees straight his ankles could be passively dorsiflexed to neutral position only. Sensory testing confirmed decreased vibration sense at both toes. Proprioception was diminished. Cold and fine touch was intact. He demonstrated sensory ataxia, with difficulty touching his nose with his eyes closed. The Romberg test was positive; he swayed considerably. He could not perform a tandem gait. He could not stand on one leg (either side).

Nerve conduction studies demonstrated electrophysiological evidence for a severe sensory neuropathy or ganglionopathy (Table 25.4).

This pattern of selective sensory loss without pain can be due to many conditions including vitamin or other micronutrient deficiencies (e.g., vitamin B12 or E, copper) as well as vitamin toxicity (vitamin B6) or drug toxicity (tamoxifen, cisplatin). Genetic conditions including Friedrich ataxia and spinocerebellar ataxias (SCA4), as well as a-β-lipoproteinemia or mitochondrial diseases. Autoimmune and paraneoplastic causes are rare but important cases in childhood.

Genetic testing confirmed >100 GAA expansions within the *FRDA* gene, consistent with the diagnosis of Friedreich ataxia.

Echocardiogram also identified a mild cardiomyopathy.

Table 25.4

Nerve conduction studies

	Normal	Right		Normal	Right
Sensory			Motor		
Median			Median (at wrist to APB)		
PL (ms)	<3.2		DML (ms)	<4.2	3.3
SNAP (mV)	>14.0	**NR**	CMAP (mV)	>3.9	9.2
Ulnar			CV (m/s)	>50	52
PL (ms)	<3.3		Ulnar (at wrist to ADM)		
SNAP (mV)	>9.0	**NR**	DML (ms)	<3.4	2.7
Superficial peroneal			CMAP (mV)	>5.9	7.4
PL (ms)	<3.8		CV (m/s)	>50	57
SNAP (mV)	>5.0	**NR**	Common peroneal (ankle to EDB)		
Sural			DML (ms)	<6.0	4.5
PL (ms)	<4.2		CMAP (mV)	>2.4	3.5
SNAP (mV)	>5.0	**NR**	CV (m/s)	>40	43

Bold = abnormal. Abbreviations: *PL* peak onset latency, *SNAP* sensory nerve action potential, *DML* distal motor onset latency, *CMAP* compound motor action potential, *EDB* extensor digitorum brevis, *AH* abductor hallucis, *Fib* fibrillation potential, *PSW* positive sharp wave, *Amp* amplitude, *Dur* duration, *Poly* polyphasic, *Recruit* recruitment pattern.

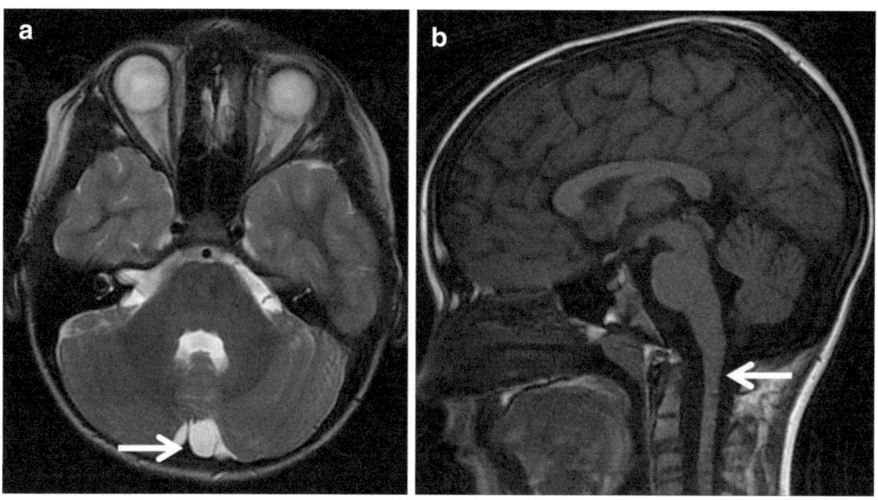

Fig. 25.3 Biochemical testing noted serum CK 344 U/L (normal <175 U/L). MRI brain (Fig. 25.3) identified a small mid-line subarachnoid cyst in the posterior fossa (**a**; *arrow*) that was determined to be an incidental finding. There was no cerebellar atrophy, although later re-examination did show mild thinning of the cervical spinal cord (**b**; *arrow*)

Case 5

Clinical Summary

A 2-year-old boy was referred for progressive muscle weakness over at least 4 months. He began sitting independently at 6–7 months of age and took his first independent steps at 14 months. He had been more hesitant with walking compared to other children and has had a definite decline in his muscle strength particularly over the past 4 months. His parents believed that his right leg was slightly weaker than the left leg. He had difficulty rising from a seated to a standing position. He was able to walk for at least 5 minutes, but fatigued afterwards and the falling became more frequent. He had a tendency to lock his knees when walking. He could not lower himself to the ground, compensating by attempting controlled falls onto his knees. He was not experiencing sensory symptoms, including pain. There were no diurnal fluctuations of his symptoms. He was not experiencing dysphagia, ptosis, dysarthria, dysconjugate gaze, back pain, or bowel or bladder symptoms. Medical history was otherwise unremarkable. He was born at term after an uneventful pregnancy.

Physical exam noted his height to be 90th percentile and weight 85th percentile. He was well-appearing, and general medical examination was unremarkable. Cranial nerve exam was unremarkable. His palate was not high arched. His tongue bulk and power were normal with no fasciculations seen. Muscle strength testing noted definite weakness in the lower extremities. His quadriceps were most affected with quadriceps strength 3 bilaterally on the Medical Research Council scale. Hip flexors also seemed weak at 4-. He demonstrated ankle dorsiflexion and plantar flexion. He had good grip strength. He was able to reach with both arms in the air. Deep tendon reflexes were 2+ at the biceps, 0 at the patellae, and 1+ at the ankles. Abdominal reflexes were absent. Plantar responses were flexor, bilaterally. Sensory testing appeared intact (he withdrew to tickling on his feet).

MRI brain and spine was unremarkable. Serum CK was 122 U/L (normal <175 U/L).

Neurophysiologic testing provided evidence for a diffuse disorder affecting motor nerves or motor neurons (Table 25.5).

Motor neuropathies or neuronopathies in childhood are most commonly attributable to spinal muscular atrophy. Other diagnostic considerations (covered in Chap. 16) could include other genetic causes (e.g., spinal muscular atrophy with respiratory distress or SMARD) and non-5q SMA. Acquired conditions could include poliomyelitis or a polio-like infection as well as toxins (e.g., dapsone).

Table 25.5

Nerve conduction studies

	Normal	Right	Left		Normal	Right	Left
Sensory				Motor			
Median				Median (at wrist to APB)			
PL (ms)	<3.2		1.8	DML (ms)	<4.2		2.5
SNAP (μV)	>14.0		27.0	CMAP (mV)	>3.9		4.1
Ulnar				CV (m/s)	>50		53
PL (ms)	<3.3			Common peroneal (ankle to EDB)			
SNAP (μV)	>9.0			DML (ms)	<6.0	3.8	3.4
Superficial peroneal				CMAP (mV)	>2.4	2.4	**2.1**
PL (ms)	<3.8			CV (m/s)	>40	45	45
SNAP (μV)	>5.0			Tibial (ankle to AH)			
Sural				DML (ms)	<6.0	3.3	4.1
PL (ms)	<4.2	1.8	1.7	CMAP (mV)	>3.9	**2.5**	**2.3**
SNAP (μV)	>5.0	14.6	14.9	CV (m/s)	>40	42	48

Concentric needle EMG

Side	Muscle	Root	Insert	Fib	PSW	Amp	Dur	Poly	Recruit
Right	Tibialis anterior	L4–L5	**Incr**	**1+**	**1+**	**Incr**	**Incr**	**1+**	**1-**
Right	Vastus lateralis	L2–L4	**Incr**	**3+**	**2+**	**Incr**	**Incr**	**1+**	**2-**
Right	Vastus medialis	L2–L4	**Incr**	**3+**	**2+**	**Incr**	**Incr**	**3+**	**2-**
Right	Iliopsoas	L2–L3	**Incr**	**1+**	**1+**	**Incr**	**Incr**	**1+**	**1-**
Right	Adductor longus	L2–L4	**Incr**	**2+**	**2+**	**Incr**	**Incr**	**1+**	**1-**
Left	Vastus lateralis	L2–L4	**Incr**	**3+**	**3+**	**Incr**	**Incr**	**1+**	**2-**
Right	Biceps	C5–6	Nml	**1+**	Nml	Nml	**Incr**	**1+**	**1-**

Bold = abnormal. Abbreviations: *PL* peak onset latency, *SNAP* sensory nerve action potential, *DML* distal motor onset latency, *CMAP* compound motor action potential, *EDB* extensor digitorum brevis, *AH* abductor hallucis, *Fib* fibrillation potential, *PSW* positive sharp wave, *Amp* amplitude, *Dur* duration, *Poly* polyphasic, *Recruit* recruitment pattern

Diagnostic considerations in older children could also include Hirayama syndrome or juvenile amyotrophic lateral sclerosis (ALS).

Genetic testing in this patient revealed 0 copies of *SMN1* and 4 copies of *SMN2*, confirming the diagnosis of spinal muscular atrophy (SMA). Given that he was ambulatory and had 4 copies of *SMN2*, his phenotype was deemed most consistent with SMA type III.

Case 6

Clinical Summary

A 12-year boy was referred for progressive weakness over at least 6 months. He had a known history of autistic spectrum disorder but was able to communicate verbally. He initially developed problems eating. He was taking longer to finish his dinner, demonstrated decreased appetite with progressive weight loss. He had occasional episodes of choking when eating solid foods. Over the next 2–3 months his mother noted that he appeared to be moving his eyes less, turning his head to look at objects. In the month prior to hospital admission he developed generalized fatigue and muscle weakness. Pregnancy and birth histories were unremarkable. Neurodevelopment was significant for language delays but his gross motor and fine motor milestones progressed appropriately. Family history was unremarkable.

Physical exam on admission noted a thin, underweight boy. His height was 15th percentile and weight just below 3rd percentile. Vital signs were stable. He had a marked hypophonia and had an inaudible laugh. On cranial nerve exam, his pupils were equal and reactive to light. Fundi were normal with no papilledema. He had markedly decreased extraocular eye movements with mild ptosis and no nystagmus. He demonstrated ocular apraxia—needing to turn his head to fixate on an object as he was unable to generate normal saccadic pursuits. Facial movements were decreased. The orbicularis oculi were weak (forced eye closure could be broken) and his orbicularis oris were also weak (he could not whistle or puff out his cheeks). He was able to smile but it was less expressive than normal. Corneal reflexes were intact. Palate, uvula and tongue movements were normal. Muscle strength testing revealed the following, according to the Medical Research Council scale: neck flexors 4-, deltoids 4-, biceps 4, triceps 4, gluteus medius 4-, and distal muscles were intact. Deep tendon reflexes were reduced at 1+. Sensation was intact. Coordination testing was normal.

Serum CK was 38 U/L (normal <175 U/L). MRI brain was negative.

Neurophysiological testing provided evidence for a disorder affecting neuromuscular transmission (Table 25.6). Repetitive nerve stimulation (3 Hz) of the left ulnar nerve (at ADM), left median nerve (at APB) and left spinal accessory nerve (at trapezius) all showed an abnormal decrement, defined as a >10 % decrease in CMAP amplitude between the first and the fifth (or fourth) stimulation (Fig. 25.4). His serum anti-AChR antibody titre was negative at <0.20 nmol/L (normal <0.40 nmol/L); however his serum anti-MuSK antibody titre was markedly elevated at 1:5120 (normal <1:10) consistent with the diagnosis of juvenile myasthenia gravis (see Chap. 21). His CT chest was negative with no evidence for thymoma or thymic hyperplasia. He was treated with IVIG 1 g/kg (x2 doses), and began pyridostigmine and prednisone therapies. Doses were gradually increased to pyridostigmine 7 mg/kg/day and prednisone 20 mg/daily. Mycophenolate mofetil was started. He remained on IVIG 1 g/kg (q4-weeks), pyridostigmine, prednisone 20 mg/day and mycophe-

Table 25.6

Nerve conduction studies					
	Normal	Left		Normal	Left
SensorySensory			Motor		
Median			Median (at wrist to APB)		
PL (ms)	<3.2	1.7	DML (ms)	<4.2	3.1
SNAP (μV)	>14.0	69.5	CMAP (mV)	>3.9	5.1
Ulnar			CV (m/s)	>50	56
PL (ms)	<3.3	1.3	Ulnar (wrist to ADM)		
SNAP (μV)	>9.0	43.9	DML (ms)	<3.4	2.5
Radial			CMAP (mV)	>5.9	**2.2**
PL (ms)	<2.9	1.8	CV (m/s)	>50	52
SNAP (μV)	>11.0	19.6	Common peroneal (ankle to EDB)		
Superficial peroneal			DML (ms)	<6.0	4.0
PL (ms)	<3.8	1.8	CMAP (mV)	>2.4	**1.1**
SNAP (μV)	>5.0	19.6	CV (m/s)	>40	52
Sural			Tibial (ankle to AH)		
PL (ms)	<4.2	2.1	DML (ms)	<6.0	3.0
SNAP (μV)	>5.0	35.9	CMAP (mV)	>3.9	11.1
			CV (m/s)	>40	48

Repetitive nerve stimulation (3 Hz)			
Trial #	Amplitude 1 (mV)	Amplitude 5 (mV)	Difference (%)
Left ulnar nerve (to abductor digiti minimi)			
Baseline	3.65	2.67	**–27.0**
Post-exercise (immediate)	3.57	2.56	**–28.3**
Post-exercise (1-min)	3.53	2.69	**–23.7**
Left median nerve (to abductor pollicis brevis)			
Baseline	4.75	3.43	**–27.7**
Post-exercise (immediate)	4.04	3.18	**–21.4**
Post-exercise (1-min)	3.99	3.26	**–18.4**
Left spinal accessory nerve (to trapezius)			
Baseline	2.13	1.60	**–24.9**
Post-exercise (immediate)	2.25	1.75	**–22.2**
Post-exercise (1-min)	2.29	1.79	**–22.1**

Concentric needle EMG

Side	**Muscle**	**Root**	**Insert**	**Fib**	**PSW**	**Amp**	**Dur**	**Poly**	**Recruit**
Left	Deltoid	C5–C6	Nml	Nml	Nml	Nml	Nml	Nml	Nml
Left	Tibialis anterior	L4–L5	Nml	Nml	Nml	Nml	Nml	Nml	Nml
Left	Ext digitorum brev	L5–S1	Nml	Nml	Nml	Nml	Nml	Nml	Nml
Left	Abd Hallucis	S1–S2	Nml	Nml	Nml	Nml	Nml	Nml	Nml

Bold = abnormal. Abbreviations: *PL* peak onset latency, *SNAP* sensory nerve action potential, *DML* distal motor onset latency, *CMAP* compound motor action potential, *EDB* extensor digitorum brevis, *AH* abductor hallucis, *Fib* fibrillation potential, *PSW* positive sharp wave, *Amp* amplitude, *Dur* duration, *Poly* polyphasic, *Recruit* recruitment pattern.

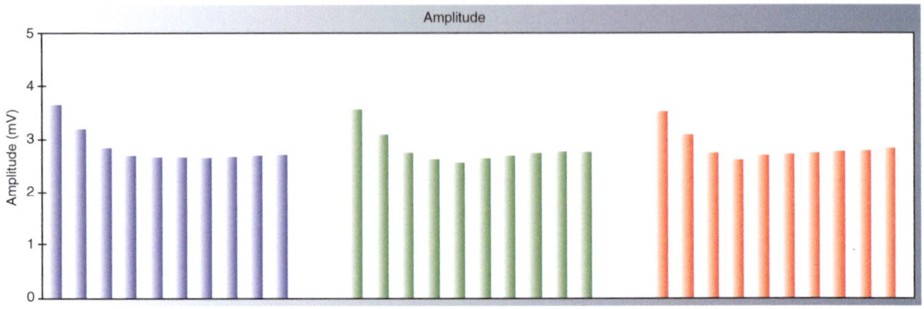

Fig. 25.4 Repetitive nerve stimulation (RNS) at 3 Hz of the left ulnar nerve (to abductor digiti minimi) shows a significant decrement (>10%) when the compound motor action potential (CMAP) of wave #1 and wave #5 are compared at baseline (*blue*); immediately after exercise (*green*) and 1-min after exercise (*red*). RNS is discussed in Chap. 6

nolate mofetil 750 mg 2x/day. He demonstrated slow but constant improvement of symptoms over the following months. His swallowing improved and his weight increased to 10th percentile. By 6 months after initiation of immunomodulation therapy, he was able to run without fatigue; at this time he began slowly weaning-off predisone. His neurological exam was entirely normal 9-months later. He remains in remission 18-months later on mycophenolate mofetil monotherapy. His symptoms of marked oculobulbar weakness for many months prior to the onset of more generalized weakness is typical of juvenile myasthenia gravis associated with anti-MuSK antibodies.

Case 7

Clinical Summary

A 12-year-old right-handed young woman was referred for possible myopathy. She had bilateral calf pain for about the past 3–4 years. Her pain was exacerbated by exercise and it was commonly experienced during gym class. She reported that if she ran or sprinted, her muscles became tight with spasms or cramps. She also noted similar symptoms with her hands. Her symptoms worsened with initial activity or with short bursts of exercise. Low intensity, cardiopulmonary exercise such as walking was less troublesome. Her handwriting was okay and she did not have problems with her hands "freezing up" while writing. Cold worsened her symptoms slightly. She reported no muscle weakness, diplopia, dysphagia, dysarthria, pigmenturia or hematuria. Medical history was otherwise unremarkable. Neurodevelopmental milestones were appropriate. She did well academically. Her mother recalled that she walked and reached developmental milestones at similar ages as her peers. Her younger sibling had similar symptoms.

On physical examination, her height was 50–75th percentile and weight 90th percentile. General medical examination was unremarkable. Cranial nerve exam was unremarkable. There was no evidence of eyelid paramyotonia with repeated forceful contraction of orbicularis oculi. Muscle strength testing revealed the following according to the Medical Research Council scale: neck flexors 4, deltoids 5, biceps 5, triceps 5, flexor pollicus longus 5, first dorsal interosseous 5, iliopsoas 4, quadriceps 4+, tibialis anterior 5, gastrocnemius 5. Hypertrophy of the biceps and gastrocnemius muscles was appreciated. Deep tendon reflexes were normal. Plantar responses were flexor, bilaterally. Ankle flexion was full with no contractures. Grip myotonia was present, along with percussion myotonia at both thenar eminences. Sensory testing (fine touch, cold, and vibration) was intact. There was no dysmetria.

Serum CK was 435 U/L (normal <175 U/L).

Her neurophysiologic studies demonstrated electrophysiological evidence for a primary disorder of muscle given the abundant myotonic discharges noted on concentric needle EMG (Table 25.7). Although nerve conduction studies were unrevealing, the short exercise test (see Chap. 6) showed a >20% drop in CMAP amplitude that rapidly recovered. This pattern of abnormality supported a chloride channelopathy (given the rapid recovery of CMAP amplitude) rather than a sodium channelopathy (which typically shows a more prolonged drop in CMAP amplitude).

Table 25.7

Nerve conduction studies

	Normal	Right		Normal	Right
Sensory			Motor		
Median			Median (at wrist to APB)		
PL (ms)	<3.2	1.8	DML (ms)	<4.2	3.1
SNAP (μV)	>14.0	73.5	CMAP (mV)	>3.9	14.8
Superficial peroneal			CV (m/s)	>50	54
PL (ms)	<3.8	2.9	Tibial (ankle to AH)		
SNAP (μV)	>5.0	14.9	DML (ms)	<6.0	5.1
Sural			CMAP (mV)	>3.9	14.8
PL (ms)	<4.2	3.7	CV (m/s)	>40	43
SNAP (μV)	>5.0	22.0			

Repetitive nerve stimulation

Trial #	Amplitude 1 (mV)	Amplitude 5 (mV)	Difference (%)	Comment (Hz)
Right ulnar nerve (to abductor digiti minimi)				
Baseline	10.5	10.7	+2.7	3
Post-exercise (immediate)	10.3	10.5	+1.9	3
Post-exercise (1-min)	10.7	10.9	+1.8	3

Short exercise test

Trial #	Onset (ms)	Amplitude (mV)	CMAP (%)[a]
Right median nerve (to abductor pollicus brevis)			
Baseline	3.2	17.6 mV	100
Exercise x10-s			
Post-exercise (immediate)	3.6	**14.0**	**79.5**
Post-exercise (10-s)	3.2	17.3	98.3
Post-exercise (20-s)	3.2	17.1	97.2
Post-exercise (30-s)	3.2	16.8	95.5
Post-exercise (40-s)	3.1	17.0	96.5

[a]Relative to baseline

Concentric needle EMG

Side	Muscle	Root	Ins	Fib	PSW	Amp	Dur	Poly	Recr	Comment
Right	Biceps	C5–C6	**Incr**	Nml	Nml	Nml	Nml	Nml	Nml	**Myotonia+**
Right	Vastuslat	L2–L4	**Incr**	Nml	Nml	Nml	Nml	Nml	Nml	**Myotonia+**

BoldBold = abnormal. Abbreviations: *PL* peak onset latency, *SNAP* sensory nerve action potential, *DML* distal motor onset latency, *CMAP* compound motor action potential, *EDB* extensor digitorum brevis, *AH* abductor hallucis, *Fib* fibrillation potential, *PSW* positive sharp wave, *Amp* amplitude, *Dur* duration, *Poly* polyphasic, *Recruit* recruitment pattern

Genetic testing confirmed mutations in both *CLCN1* genes consistent with the diagnosis of myotonia congenita.

Case 8

Clinical Summary

An 11-year-old right-handed boy presented with right arm weakness following a traumatic injury. He was active in competitive dirt biking. On the day of the accident, he had lost control of his bike and crashed into a jump landing on his right side. He may have briefly lost consciousness for about 30 seconds but when he began moving he had excruciating pain in his right arm. His parents stated that when his jersey was being taken off the pain suddenly subsided, which may have represented reduction of a right shoulder dislocation. X-rays of his right clavicle and upper arm revealed no fractures. CT head and cervical spine revealed no abnormalities. He had bothersome pain during the two months following the injury. He reported pain in the region of his right levator scapula region that extended to his right glenohumeral joint. He also noticed severe proximal right arm weakness. He also noted persistent numbness in the right upper and lateral arm. No hand weakness was noted. Past medical and family histories were unremarkable.

Physical exam revealed an alert and cooperative boy. General medical examination was unremarkable. His cranial nerves were intact. His right deltoid had a strength of 3 on the Medical Research Council scale, with marked wasting of that muscle. His strength was otherwise normal at the right trapezius, supraspinatus, infraspinatus, rhomboids, biceps, triceps, brachioradialis, wrist extensors, wrist flexors, extensor digitorum communis, flexor pollicis longus, first dorsal interosseous, abductor digiti minimi, and abductor pollicis brevis. Left arm strength was intact. No wasting was noted over his scapula, and there was no scapular winging. Reflexes were normal at the brachioradialis, biceps, and triceps, bilaterally. Sensory testing revealed absent fine touch and absent cold sensation in a 5 × 5 cm (2″ × 2″) patch over the right proximal arm.

Neurophysiological testing performed 2 months after the injury revealed the following (Table 25.8).

The nerve conduction studies and EMG revealed electrophysiological evidence for a severe right axillary neuropathy. Given the intact right median sensory response (C5/6; upper trunk) and right lateral antebrachial cutaneous nerve (upper trunk, lateral cord) as well as the absence of any denervation in right biceps and infraspinatus (upper trunk) and triceps (posterior cord) there was no evidence for a brachial plexopathy.

Although he had marked reduction in recruitment, there was evidence for axonal continuity pointing to axontmesis. His symptoms gradually improved over the ensuing 9 months with normal strength noted at that time.

Table 25.8

Nerve conduction studies							
	Normal	Right	Left		Normal	Right	Left
Sensory				Motor			
Median				Median (at wrist to APB)			
PL (ms)	<3.2	2.4		DML (ms)	<4.2	3.1	3.0
SNAP (mV)	>14.0	14.4		CMAP (mV)	>3.9	11.2	9.7
Ulnar				CV (m/s)	>50	57	56
PL (ms)	<3.3	2.1					
SNAP (mV)	>9.0	10.2					
Lateral antebrachial cutaneous							
PL (ms)	<3.3	1.4	1.4				
SNAP (mV)	>5.0	8.3	4.6				
Medial antebrachial cutaneous							
PL (ms)	<3.3	1.3					
SNAP (mV)	>4.0	9.8					

Concentric needle EMG									
Side	Muscle	Root	Insert	Fib	PSW	Amp	Dur	Poly	Recruit
Right	Biceps	C5–C6	Nml	Nml	Nml	Nml	Nml	Nml	Nml
Right	Deltoid	C5–C6	**Incr**	**2+**	**2+**	Nml	**Incr**	**Incr**	**3-**
Right	Infraspinatus	C5–C6	Nml	Nml	Nml	Nml	Nml	Nml	Nml
Right	Triceps	C6–C8	Nml	Nml	Nml	Nml	Nml	Nml	Nml

Bold = abnormal. Abbreviations: *PL* peak onset latency, *SNAP* sensory nerve action potential, *DML* distal motor onset latency, *CMAP* compound motor action potential, *Fib* fibrillation potential, *PSW* positive sharp wave, *Amp* amplitude, *Dur* duration, *Poly* polyphasic, *Recruit* = recruitment pattern

Case 9

Clinical Summary

A 15-year-old right-handed young woman was referred for a history of bilateral hand numbness for about 12 months. She initially had intermittent numbness of the fourth and fifth digits of both hands (left hand greater than right). However, her symptoms worsened such that for the past 3 months, she now experiences constant numbness of the left fourth and fifth digits. Symptoms at the right fourth and fifth digits remained intermittent. She awoke about every 2 hours at night as a result of numbness and pain in the forearm. She had a tendency to sleep with her elbows flexed. She also enjoyed playing the piano but was only able to play for about 15–20 minutes at a time before the pain became bothersome and forced her to stop. Her lower extremities were not involved. Past medical history was otherwise unremarkable. General medical health is otherwise unremarkable. Neurodevelopmentally she has progressed well and she does extremely well academically. Family history was significant for her father experiencing bilateral carpal tunnel in his early 20s that was treated with decompressive surgery in his late 20s. He has not had any other problems, though he was noted to have high arched feet.

On physical examination, she was an alert and well appearing young woman. Height was 75th percentile and weight 75th percentile. General medical examination was unremarkable. Cranial nerve examination was unremarkable. Muscle strength according to the Medical Research Council scale was 4/5 at the first dorsal interosseous and abductor digiti minimi bilaterally, while the left abductor pollicis brevis was 4+. Muscle strength was otherwise normal in the upper and lower extremities, including the following muscles: deltoid, biceps, triceps, wrist extensors, wrist flexors, flexor pollicis longus, iliopsoas, quadriceps, hamstrings, tibialis anterior, gastrocnemius, extensor hallucis longus, and extensor digitorum brevis. No wasting was observed at the intrinsic foot muscles. There was no pes cavus, but mild hammertoeing was evident. Deep tendon reflexes were normal at the biceps, triceps, patella, and ankle jerk. Plantar responses were flexor, bilaterally. Sensory testing revealed decreased fine touch sensation in the ulnar distribution bilaterally with both the dorsal and palmar surfaces of her hands affected. Splitting of the ring finger was noted in the right hand. No definite splitting of the ring finger was noted in the left hand. There was normal cold sensation, and normal proprioception in the upper and lower extremities.

Neurophysiological testing revealed the following (Table 25.9):

Nerve conduction studies and EMG revealed electrophysiological evidence for the following: 1) bilateral ulnar neuropathies that appeared to localize to the elbow; 2) left median neuropathy that localized to the wrist. Mild demyelinating changes were also noted in the leg.

Nerve conduction studies showed findings that supported the diagnosis of hereditary neuropathy with liability to pressure palsy (HNPP). The studies confirmed

Table 25.9

Nerve conduction studies

	Normal	Right	Left		Normal	Right	Left
Sensory				Motor			
Median				Median (at wrist to APB)			
PL (ms)	<3.2	3.0	**3.3**	DML (ms)	<4.2	3.8	**4.4**
SNAP (mV)	>14.0	**13.1**	**12.7**	CMAP (mV)	>3.9	10.3	**4.5**
Ulnar				CV (m/s)	>50	56	55
PL (ms)	<3.3			Ulnar (at wrist to ADM)			
SNAP (mV)	>9.0	**NR**	**NR**	DML (ms)	<3.4	3.0	3.3
Sural				CMAP (mV)	>5.9	6.3	**4.9**
PL (ms)	<4.2	**5.1**		CV (m/s)	>50	55/**34**[a]	54/**27**[a]
SNAP (mV)	>5.0	**3.9**		Peroneal (at ankle to EDB)			
				DML (ms)	<6.0	**6.7**	**6.8**
				CMAP (mV)	>2.4	3.7	7.1
				CV (m/s)	>40	42	**38**

[a]Indicates velocity in forearm (from below elbow to wrist)/across elbow (from above to below elbow)

Concentric needle EMG

Side	Muscle	Root	Insert	Fib	PSW	Amp	Dur	Poly	Recruit
Left	Abd Pollicus Brev	C8–T1	Nml	Nml	Nml	Nml	Nml	**1+**	Nml
Left	Pronator Teres	C6–C7	Nml	Nml	Nml	Nml	Nml	Nml	Nml
Left	First Dors Inteross	C8–T1	**Incr**	**Nml**	**1+**	**Incr**	**Incr**	**Incr**	**1-**
Left	Ext Digit Brev	L5–S1	Nml	Nml	Nml	Nml	**Incr**	**2+**	Nml

Bold = abnormal. Abbreviations: *PL* peak onset latency, *SNAP* sensory nerve action potential, *DML* distal motor onset latency, *CMAP* compound motor action potential, *Fib* fibrillation potential, *PSW* positive sharp wave, *Amp* amplitude, *Dur* duration, *Poly* polyphasic, *Recruit* = recruitment pattern

conduction slowing across multiple compression sites (carpal tunnel, cubital tunnel as well as across the fibular head). As is typical of adolescents and young adults with HNPP, electrophysiological findings were noted at some compression sites (across the fibular head) that were not associated with any clinical changes.

Genetic testing confirmed a *PMP22* deletion consistent with HNPP.

Case 10

Clinical Summary

A 15-year-old right-handed young woman was referred for a 2-month history of right-sided foot-drop. Her symptoms progressed over 3–4 weeks before reaching a nadir. She thinks there may have been slight improvement over the past couple weeks with regards to her ankle strength. She has not experienced tripping, stumbling, back pain, or knee pain. She reported some paresthesiae on the dorsal aspect of the right foot. There was no trauma around the time of onset. She had a tendency to sit crosslegged a great deal of the time. She has not had any transient weakness or sensory loss involving any other limbs. Past medical history is unremarkable. Family history is non-contributory.

On physical examination, she was an alert, well-appearing young woman. Cranial nerve examination was unremarkable. Muscle strength testing of the right lower extremity showed the following, according to the Medical Research Council scale: iliopsoas 5, gluteus medius 5, hip abductors 5, quadriceps 5, hamstrings 5, tibialis anteior 4- peroneal longus 4, tibialis posterior 5, gastrocnemius 5, extensor hallucis longus 3, extensor digitorum brevis 3. Muscle wasting was noted at the right extensor digitorum brevis. Left lower extremity strength was normal. Deep tendon reflexes were normal at the biceps, brachioradialis, triceps, patellae, and ankles. She had a positive Tinel sign at the right fibular head. She had decreased light touch sensation over the dorsal aspect of her right foot, which she estimated was about 60% of the sensation on the other side. Neurophysiological testing revealed the following (Table 25.10).

Nerve conduction studies showed electrophysiological evidence for a right peroneal neuropathy that appeared to localize around the fibular head region. Given the intact strength and the absence of EMG abnormalities when studying other L5-root innervated muscles (i.e., L5-paraspinals, gluteus medius, tibialis posterior) there was no evidence for a right L5 radiculopathy. The absent superficial peroneal nerve sensory response as well as the focal slowing and amplitude drop across the fibular head also pointed to the fibular head region as the site of compression.

MRI knee was obtained. There was no evidence for an extrinsic nerve compression (e.g., ganglionic cyst) and no evidence for an intrinsic nerve tumor. The etiology was deemed to be right peroneal neuropathy resulting from chronic leg-crossing. The patient made a concerted effort to avoid this and her symptoms resolved.

Table 25.10

Nerve conduction studies					
	Normal	Right		Normal	Right
Sensory			Motor		
Superficial peroneal			Common peroneal (ankle to EDB)		
PL (ms)	<3.8		DML (ms)	<6.0	5.7
SNAP (μV)	>5.0	**NR**	CMAP (mV)	>2.4	**2.0/1.8/0.6**[a]
Sural			CV (m/s)	>40	55/**32**[b]
PL (ms)	<4.2	3.5	Tibial (ankle to AH)		
SNAP (μV)	>5.0	12.1	DML (ms)	<6.0	4.3
			CMAP (mV)	>3.9	12.0
			CV (m/s)	>40	43

[a]Indicates CMAP amplitude in leg when stimulated at the ankle/below knee/above knee revealing an >50% amplitude drop across the fibular head consistent with conduction block
[b]Indicates conduction velocity in the leg when measured: between below knee and ankle/above knee and below knee indicating conduction slowing across the knee

Concentric needle EMG									
Side	Muscle	Root	Insert	Fib	PSW	Amp	Dur	Poly	Recruit
Right	Tibialis anterior	L4–L5	**Incr**	**1+**	**3+**	Nml	**1+**	**1+**	**2-**
Right	Peroneus longus	L5–S1	**Incr**	**1+**	Nml	Nml	**1+**	**1+**	**1-**
Right	Tibialis posterior	L5–S1	Nml	Nml	Nml	Nml	Nml	Nml	Nml
Right	Medial gastrocnemius	S1–S2	Nml	Nml	Nml	Nml	Nml	Nml	Nml
Right	Extensor Dig Brevis	L5–S1	**Incr**	**1+**	**1+**	Nml	**1+**	**1+**	**2-**
Right	Biceps femoris (short)	L5–S2	Nml	Nml	Nml	Nml	**1+**	**1+**	Nml
Right	Gluteus medius	L5–S1	Nml	Nml	Nml	Nml	Nml	Nml	Nml
Right	Paraspinal (L5)	L4–S1	Nml	Nml	Nml	Nml	Nml	Nml	Nml

Bold = abnormal. Abbreviations: *PL* peak onset latency, *SNAP* sensory nerve action potential, *DML* distal motor onset latency, *CMAP* compound motor action potential, *Fib* fibrillation potential, *PSW* positive sharp wave, *Amp* amplitude, *Dur* duration, *Poly* polyphasic, *Recruit* = recruitment pattern.

Chapter 26
Epilogue

Peter B. Kang and Hugh J. McMillan

When we completed our training in clinical neurophysiology, many textbooks still referred to nerve conduction studies and electromyography (EMG) as relatively novel diagnostic tests. Indeed, despite the important foundations laid by giants in the history of medicine such as Duchenne in the nineteenth century, EMG only came into widespread clinical use in the latter half of the twentieth century, in part due to the advances in computer technology that occurred during that time. Pediatric EMG remained a small niche for much of that period. However, an increasing number of child neurologists have embarked upon fellowship training in this field, and it is now expected that all major pediatric hospitals will have access to this diagnostic test. EMG will remain an important tool in modern medicine for the foreseeable future. For many children, neurophysiological testing provides a rapid means of confirming if weakness or gait difficulty is indeed attributable to a disorder affecting motor neurons, peripheral nerves, neuromuscular junction, or muscle.

Since the turn of the century, we have witnessed tremendous advances in genetic testing including: increased availability of testing and increased speed of obtaining test results, as well as improved access to comprehensive gene panels and whole exome sequencing (WES). For example, in cases of suspected spinal muscular atrophy it is now common to proceed directly to genetic testing. However, in critically ill infants and children with atypical presentations of spinal muscular atrophy or many other suspected neuromuscular diseases, neurophysiological testing remains an extremely valuable test. In other cases, the identification of a sensorimotor

P.B. Kang, MD, FAAN, FAAP (✉)
Division of Pediatric Neurology, Shands Children's Hospital, University of Florida College of Medicine, Gainesville, FL, USA
e-mail: pbkang@ufl.edu

H.J. McMillan, MD, MSc, FRCPC, FAAN (✉)
Division of Neurology, Children's Hospital of Eastern Ontario, University of Ottawa, Ottawa, ON, Canada
e-mail: hmcmillan@cheo.on.ca

© Springer International Publishing AG 2017

H.J. McMillan, P.B. Kang (eds.), *Pediatric Electromyography*,
DOI 10.1007/978-3-319-61361-1_26

polyneuropathy versus a myopathy or disorder of neuromuscular transmission may direct the clinician to consider specific gene panels. With the advent of enormous neuromuscular panels that cover all these categories, EMG can help with the interpretation of these comprehensive genetic test reports, especially as the oftentimes baffling variants of unknown significance (VUS) that appear will persist for the foreseeable future.

Moreover, neurophysiological testing continues to play a key role in the correct diagnosis and management of numerous acquired neuromuscular disorders. Nerve conduction studies help fulfill important diagnostic criteria for the evaluation of suspected acute or chronic inflammatory demyelinating polyradiculoneuropathies. Similarly, EMG can provide evidence of muscle inflammation in children with dermatomyositis, and repetitive nerve stimulation or single fiber EMG can assist with the diagnosis of autoimmune juvenile myasthenia gravis.

Neurophysiological testing provides invaluable information in acquired focal neuropathies. The localization provided by this test modality allows imaging studies to be focused on smaller areas of potential injury. This has important implications both from a patient safety perspective by reducing anesthetic time for young children undergoing MRI but also economic implications by reducing unnecessary sequence acquisition and imaging time. Intraoperative monitoring has provided a dynamic way of monitoring the integrity of the peripheral and central nervous systems during surgery which allows for the early detection of nerve or root injury and affords an opportunity to reduce patient morbidity associated with increasingly sophisticated and delicate surgical procedures. In traumatic neuropathies, EMG provides important information regarding the presence or absence of axonal continuity which can help differentiate axonotmesis from neurotmesis. Since axonotmesis shows a greater potential for spontaneous peripheral nerve regeneration and reinnervation this may provide support for watchful waiting as opposed to earlier surgical exploration and nerve grafting.

Specialized tests such as motor unit number estimation (MUNE) have been developed for specific applications. MUNE has become an important outcome measure in clinical trials of patients with spinal muscular atrophy (SMA), helping provide another objective means of documenting response to treatment.

EMG is now an established and maturing field, with an extensive body of literature that supports the performance and interpretation of this test throughout the world. Pediatric EMG is increasingly acquiring the same stature, with a rapidly growing supply of both pediatric neurophysiologists and peer-reviewed research articles that enable this diagnostic test modality to be applied rigorously and gently to children of all ages, usually without sedation or general anesthesia. Despite the stunning recent advances in genetic testing and imaging technologies, EMG yields a unique diagnostic dataset that will remain relevant and useful in the care of children for many decades to come.

Index

© Springer International Publishing AG 2017
H.J. McMillan, P.B. Kang (eds.), *Pediatric Electromyography*,
DOI 10.1007/978-3-319-61361-1

MIX
Papier aus verantwortungsvollen Quellen
Paper from responsible sources
FSC® C105338

If you have any concerns about our products,
you can contact us on
ProductSafety@springernature.com

In case Publisher is established outside the EU,
the EU authorized representative is:
Springer Nature Customer Service Center GmbH
Europaplatz 3, 69115 Heidelberg, Germany

Printed by Libri Plureos GmbH
in Hamburg, Germany